CAFFEINE AND ACTIVATION THEORY

Effects on Health

and Behavior

CAFFEINE AND ACTIVATION THEORY

Effects on Health

and Behavior

Edited by
Barry D. Smith
University of Maryland, College Park, Maryland
Uma Gupta
Institute of Medical Sciences, Banaras Hindu University, Varanasi, India

B.S. Gupta
Banaras Hindu University, Varanasi, India

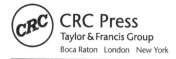

CRC Press
Taylor & Francis Group
Boca Raton London New York

CRC Press is an imprint of the
Taylor & Francis Group, an informa business

CRC Press
Taylor & Francis Group
6000 Broken Sound Parkway NW, Suite 300
Boca Raton, FL 33487-2742

First issued in paperback 2019

No claim to original U.S. Government works

ISBN 13: 978-0-367-45341-1 (pbk)
ISBN 13: 978-0-8493-7102-8 (hbk)

Visit the Taylor & Francis Web site at
http://www.taylorandfrancis.com

and the CRC Press Web site at
http://www.crcpress.com

Library of Congress Cataloging-in-Publication Data

Caffeine and activation theory : effects on health and behavior / edited by Barry
   D. Smith, Uma Gupta, B.S. Gupta.
      p. cm.
      Includes bibliographical references (p.).
      ISBN 0-8493-7102-3
      1. Caffeine--Physiological effect. 2. Caffeine--Health aspects. I. Smith, Barry D.
II. Gupta, Uma. III. Gupta, B.S.

QP801.C24C332 2006
613.8'4--dc22   2006045651

Dedication

For my wife, Liz, dedicated companion, mother, and teacher.
A pillar of strength and model of courage, her passing in
2003 left a chasm in the lives of all those she touched.

Barry Smith

For my parents, Mr. Jai Prakash and Mrs. Subhashini,
who left for their heavenly abodes on May 15, 2000 and
January 10, 2003, respectively.

Uma Gupta

For my granddaughter, Harshita, a promising small bud,
who left for her heavenly abode on February 24, 2004
(1996-2004).

B. S. Gupta

Preface

Arousal theories have long sought to explain how cortical arousal and its downstream effects on a wide range of body systems function to affect personality, behavior, and health. In that effort, we must first distinguish between trait arousal and state arousal. The former refers to the individual's typical or average level of arousal, and the latter indicates current arousal at a given moment. Both are influenced by a complex set of genetic factors that affect, among other things, structure of the reticular activating system and the limbic system, together with their neurotransmitter substrates. The phenotype for trait arousal then results when these genetic predispositions interact with specific aspects of early life experience.

State arousal at any time is a product of a three-way interaction that involves trait arousal, the presence of substances that can increase or decrease arousal, and cognitions that represent, in part, the individual's perceptual interpretation of current environmental stimulus situations. The focus of this book is on caffeine, one of the major substances known to increase arousal. The genetic factors, trait arousal, and cognitions that contribute to arousal level are taken into account by the chapter authors as appropriate.

The virtually universal popularity of caffeine, together with concerns about its potential pathogenic effects, has made it one of the most extensively studied drugs in history. Research has addressed the sources of caffeine, its pharmacokinetics and pharmacodynamics, its effects on neural substrates, and its impact on a variety of aspects of health and behavior. One reason why caffeine is so widely consumed is that it is found in many foods and drinks, such as coffee, tea, soft drinks, medicines, and chocolate. Indeed, it is difficult to avoid consuming at least some of this potent drug.

The other major reason for its widespread consumption is that caffeine quite consistently has an arousing, alerting effect. It is a morning eye-opener for millions of people worldwide, can provide increased attentional focus at almost any time, helps drivers and workers to stay awake and alert, and enhances athletic performance. *Caffeine and Activation Theory: Effects on Health and Behavior* brings together the scientific work of major theorists and researchers, who review the entire literature in their respective areas of endeavor. From these in-depth reviews, we hope to provide an integrated body of knowledge that represents much of what is currently known about the effects of caffeine on arousal and behavior, as well as on physical and emotional health.

Barry D. Smith

Uma Gupta

B. S. Gupta

Acknowledgments

In an edited book, one of the most difficult and time-consuming tasks is going through every chapter before the book goes to the publisher to make certain that the references are all listed in the proper format and that each manuscript is correctly formatted consistent with the guidelines for the book. The person primarily responsible for this entire process has been Administrative Assistant Julia Coldren, and we would like to give her very special recognition for all her efforts. She has done an outstanding job of finalizing all aspects of the chapters and has made numerous helpful, creative suggestions that have improved the entire book. Thank you, Julia!

Publishing a book is a lengthy and often difficult process for the authors and editors, but it also requires great effort on the parts of many other people, particularly those at the publishing house. They can make the work of the authors more or less difficult, and we sincerely thank everyone at Taylor & Francis/CRC Press involved with this book for making our work far less difficult than it might have been. We first thank Barbara Norwitz, our Taylor & Francis publisher, who fully supported our work throughout the entire publishing process. Kari Budyk, our editor, could not have been better. She has worked with us every step of the way, providing guidance, answering our incessant questions, and moving the manuscript through the entire publishing process. In addition, Editorial Assistant Randy Brehm was very helpful in getting the publishing process underway. Finally, we would like to thank our project editor at Taylor & Francis, Judith Simon.

The Editors

Barry Smith is professor of psychology and director of the Laboratory of Human Psychophysiology at the University of Maryland, College Park, Maryland, where he has also served as acting chair of the department, associate chair, and director of graduate studies. He received his B.S. degree at Pennsylvania State University and his Ph.D. at the University of Massachusetts at Amherst. He has authored or edited nine books and numerous journal articles and book chapters and served on review panels and study sections at the National Science Foundation, the Office of Naval Research, and the National Aeronautics and Space Administration. Dr. Smith has been a consulting or associate editor for a number of journals. His interests are centered in the field of arousal, where he has developed and tested his own theory. This work has included numerous studies of the effects of caffeine on neurophysiological and cardiovascular functioning, as well as cognition, emotion, personality, and behavior.

Uma Gupta is a research scientist in the Department of Basic Principles, Institute of Medical Sciences, Banaras Hindu University, Varanasi, India. She received her M.A., M.Phil., and Ph.D. degrees in psychology from Meerut University, Meerut, India. She has completed a number of research projects sponsored by the Indian Council of Social Science Research and the University Grants Commission, New Delhi. She has coedited three books: *Advances in Psychopharmacology, Neuropsychology & Psychiatry*, *Readings in Environmental Toxicology and Social Ecology*, and *Caffeine and Behavior: Current Views and Research Trends*. Dr. Gupta has coauthored one book, *Psycho-educative Dynamics of Indian Classical Music*, and published numerous research articles and book chapters. She is the coeditor of *Pharmachopsychoecologia*. Her research currently focuses on behavioral (especially in cognitive and affective domains) effects of caffeine intake, caffeinism, psychodynamics of music, music therapy, and environmental schematization.

B. S. Gupta is a retired professor of psychology from Banaras Hindu University, Varanasi, India. He received his M.A. and Ph.D. degrees from the Department of Psychology at Panjab University, Chandigarh, India. Before moving to Banaras Hindu University, he taught at Meerut University in Meerut and Guru Nanak Dev University in Amritsar, India. Dr. Gupta has published numerous research articles and book chapters. He has served as consulting or advisory editor on a number of journals, including the *International Journal of Psychology*. He is now the coeditor of *Pharmacopsychoecologia* and president of the Pharmacopsychoecological Association.

Contributors

Katherine Aldridge
Department of Psychology
University of Maryland
College Park, Maryland

Raymond Cooper
PhytoScience, Inc.
Los Altos, California

Solmaz Elmi
Department of Psychology
University of Maryland
College Park, Maryland

Radha Gholkar
Department of Psychology
University of Maryland
College Park, Maryland

Jean Golding
Department of Community
Community-Based Medicine
University of Bristol
Bristol, United Kingdom

B. S. Gupta
Department of Psychology
Banaras Hindu University
Varanasi, India

Uma Gupta
Department of Basic Principles
Institute of Medical Sciences
Banaras Hindu University
Varanasi, India

Iulian Iancu
POB 1
Beer Yaakov, Israel

Jack E. James
Department of Psychology
National University of Ireland
Galway, Ireland

Talash A. Likimani
Herbalife International
Century City, California

Mark Mann
Trauma Recovery Program
VA Medical Health Care System
Baltimore Medical Center
Baltimore, Maryland

D. James Morré
Department of Medicinal Chemistry
  and Molecular Pharmacology
Purdue University
West Lafayette, Indiana

Dorothy Morré
Department of Foods
  and Nutrition
Purdue University
West Lafayette, Indiana

Astrid Nehlig
INSERM U 666
Faculty of Medicine
Strasbourg, France

Kate Northstone
Department of Community-Based
  Medicine
University of Bristol
Bristol, United Kingdom

Ahikam Olmer
POB 1
Beer Yaakov, Israel

Peter J. Rogers
Department of Experimental
  Psychology
University of Bristol
Bristol, United Kingdom

Jennifer Rusted
Department of Psychology
University of Sussex
Brighton, United Kingdom

Harvey A. Schwertner
Wilford Hall Medical Center
Lackland Air Force Base, Texas

Rachel Shapiro
Department of Psychology
University of Maryland
College Park, Maryland

Hendrik J. Smit
Department of Experimental
  Psychology
University of Bristol
Bristol, United Kingdom

Barry D. Smith
Department of Psychology
University of Maryland
College Park, Maryland

Lorenzo D. Stafford
Department of Psychology
University of Portsmouth
Portsmouth, United Kingdom

Rael D. Strous
POB 1
Beer Yaakov, Israel

Nancy Toward
Department of Psychology
University of Maryland
College Park, Maryland

Hoa T. Vo
Department of Psychology
University of Maryland
College Park, Maryland

Ming Wei
Bureau of Epidemiology
Pennsylvania Department of Health
Harrisburg, Pennsylvania

Thom White
Department of Psychology
University of Maryland
College Park, Maryland

Martin R. Yeomans
Department of Psychology
University of Sussex
Brighton, United Kingdom

Table of Contents

SECTION III Menstrual and Reproductive Effects

SECTION IV Mood and Performance and Psychopathology

SECTION V Green and Black Teas

SECTION VI Integration and Conclusion

1 Arousal and Caffeine: Physiological, Behavioral, and Pathological Effects

Barry D. Smith, Uma Gupta, and B. S. Gupta

CONTENTS

INTRODUCTION

It has long been recognized that physiological arousal is a basic and important factor in health and behavior (Smith, Osborne, Mann, Jones, & White, 2004). So important are its effects that numerous theories have focused on the arousal concept in an ongoing series of attempts to explain its origins, substrates, and consequences. In 1951, Elizabeth Duffy published her classic *Psychological Review* article, "The Concept of Energy Mobilization," and later expanded on her ideas in *Activation and Behavior* (1962). She argued that physiological arousal, or activation, is more basic to behavior and performance than is the learning process.

Duffy was soon joined by Donald Lindsley (1957), Robert Malmo (1959), Magda Arnold (1960), and other theorists, who detailed the neurophysiological substrates of arousal and its effects on behavior and health. Another major theorist, Hans Eysenck (1967), proposed that the principal dimensions of human personality functioning—extraversion and neuroticism in his theory—are based in cortical arousal and activation. With many others, he argued that the reticular activating system and the limbic system are central to the integration of arousal functions and that arousal ultimately has an impact on and is dealt with by the cerebral cortex.

Smith has also proposed an arousal theory of personality, behavior, and health, called dual interaction theory (Smith, 1983; Smith, Davidson, & Green, 1993; Smith, Tola, & Mann, 1999; Smith et al., 2004). It differentiates between arousal traits and arousal states and between chronic and acute arousal as these affect health and behavior. The theory also proposes three basic dimensions that characterize arousal: An *intensity* dimension specifies a continuum that differentiates between very high and very low levels of arousal; a *type* dimension specifies two primary types of arousal, general and emotional, and recognizes that other types and subtypes may later be identified; and an *individual differences* dimension specifies multiple continua along which arousal can vary from one person to another. These include anxiety, extraversion, neuroticism, sensation seeking, and hostility, among others.

Dual interaction theory, in agreement with much of the theoretical and empirical literature, recognizes that multiple sources of and contributions to arousal. Stress, for example, has been extensively studied with regard to the increases in arousal that it produces and the adverse effects on health that it can have (Smith et al., 2004). Similarly, such widely varied mood states as anger, depression, and ecstasy can increase arousal, as can many cognitions. In addition, a substantial literature identifies and studies drugs that contribute to arousal. In particular, these include caffeine, which is arguably the single most common source of increments in arousal.

It is a common observation that caffeine is the most widely consumed drug in the world. Its multiple sources include coffee, tea, chocolate, soft drinks, energy drinks, and medications; the overall quantities in which these sources are produced and consumed are almost incalculable. More than 100 million bags of coffee beans, amounting to 6 million tons, are produced each year (International Coffee Organization [ICO], 2006). Add to this an annual production of over 3 million tons of tea (FAO, 2006) and 2.8 million tons of chocolate (Al-Ahram Weekly On-Line, 2005), along with the annual consumption of 53 gallons of soft drinks per person (Nestle, 2000), and it becomes clear that the average individual consumes a substantial amount of caffeine each year.

Heightened arousal has widespread physiological and behavioral consequences. For example, it can increase heart rate, blood pressure, and the output of adrenal corticosteroids, as well as shift EEG patterns to those associated with cortical activation. At the same time, increments in arousal are associated with elevations in anxiety, hostility, and irritability; chronically high arousal may contribute to anxiety, somatoform, and depressive disorders, among others. It is no wonder, then, that the scientific literature on caffeine is larger than that on any other drug. A search of Medline revealed 20,107 publications on caffeine, far more than the number for such drugs as marijuana and phencyclidine. With such a vast and growing literature, it is essential to review and evaluate theory and research periodically to achieve a more integrative understanding of its implications. This book provides this integration on a number of topics concerning the acute and chronic impact of caffeine consumption on health and behavior.

ORGANIZATION OF THE BOOK

We begin the first section of the book on caffeine basics with a chapter by Barry Smith, Thomas White, and Rachel Shapiro that provides detailed information concerning major sources of caffeine, including coffee, tea, chocolate, soft drinks, energy drinks, and medications. For the principal sources, the chapter provides brief histories and discusses production and consumption. In chapter 3, Astrid Nehlig details caffeine physiology. This chapter deals with the biochemical impact of the drug, including adenosine receptor inhibition, release of intracellular calcium, and inhibition of cyclic nucleotide phosphodiesterases. Nehlig also discusses the neurophysiological effects of caffeine and their downstream consequences in locomotor activity, sleep, behavior, and pathology.

Section II of the book deals with one of the major concerns about caffeine: its potentially adverse effects on the cardiovascular system. The four central issues in this section all revolve around the arousal effects of the drug and their possible cardiovascular consequences. One major theme in this literature is concerned with the potentially adverse effects of acute caffeine intake on heart function. Another addresses the contribution of chronic caffeine consumption to coronary heart disease (CHD) and myocardial infarction (MI). A third assesses the role of the drug in hypertension, and a final chapter examines its effects on serum lipid profile.

In chapter 4, Barry Smith and Katherine Aldridge address cardiac effects of acute caffeine intake, including its effects on heart rate and rhythm; this literature has yielded some surprising findings. Chapter 5, by Barry Smith, Radha Gholkar, Mark Mann, and Nancy Toward, provides a detailed analysis of the CHD literature. It begins with a review of the major factors known to contribute to CHD and then investigates the role of caffeine in relation to other causal factors.

In chapter 6, Jack James makes the point that chronic caffeine consumption is a risk factor for hypertension. Pointing out that numerous epidemiological studies have been conducted, he provides careful, in-depth review and analysis of this sizable scientific literature to support his conclusions regarding the caffeine–blood pressure relationship. In chapter 7, the final chapter in this section, Ming Wei and Harvey Schwertner review the numerous epidemiological studies and clinical trials that have addressed the effect of coffee and caffeine consumption on serum lipids. They consider and evaluate discrepancies among studies and also discuss the important observation that various coffee brewing methods affect serum lipids differently.

Section III deals with the effects of caffeine as they relate to the menstrual cycle and reproduction. In chapter 8, Hoa Vo, Barry Smith, and Solmaz Elmi deal with the relationship between caffeine and the menstrual cycle, as well as effects of the drug in women with premenstrual syndrome (PMS). Vo provides an overview of the physiology and psychology of the menstrual cycle and shows how caffeine pharmacokinetics are affected by changing menstrual physiology, as well as how caffeine affects menstrual function. She then reviews the scientific literature concerned with the possible role of caffeine in PMS.

In the second chapter in this section (chapter 9), Kate Northstone and Jean Golding address another important question concerning caffeine effects: Does this widely consumed drug reduce fertility? They point out that fertility levels in the population have been decreasing for a number of years and address the possible detrimental effects of caffeine on fertility. This chapter provides an in-depth scientific analysis of all prospective and retrospective studies of the caffeine–fertility relationship, taking into consideration sample sizes, power, and likely confounds.

Section IV deals with the effects of caffeine on mood state, cognition, and performance. Hendrik Smit and Peter Rogers review the literature on mood state effects in chapter 10 and discuss the impact of caffeine intake and caffeine deprivation on affect. Their review points out the potentially important effects of differing individual sensitivities to caffeine, time of day at which the drug is consumed, and age. They also provide a detailed methodological analysis of relevant studies and suggest the need to employ modified methods in the effort to understand the caffeine–mood relationship further.

In chapter 11, Lorenzo Stafford, Jennifer Rusted, and Martin Yeomans detail the literature concerned with effects of caffeine and its deprivation on cognitive functioning and performance. They review the substantial body of research on psychomotor performance involving such tasks as tapping and pursuit rotor, as well as the cognitive literature, which examines effects of caffeine on attention and memory. Finally, they point to a number of factors affecting study outcomes, including drug dosage, placebo effects, arousal threshold, and fatigue.

In chapter 12, Uma Gupta and B. S. Gupta review scientific research dealing with effects of caffeine on multicomponent task performance. They point out that human performance is affected by multiple factors, including basal arousal, caffeine dosage, and habituation, as well as task complexity and such personality traits as extraversion. The authors then report two experiments involving performance on a letter-transformation task. In the first, participants received one of four caffeine doses or placebo; the second employed the highest dose of the drug and examined its effect on three individual processing components of the task.

The remaining two brief sections deal with psychopathology (section V) and the potentially beneficial effects of green and black tea (section VI). In chapter 13, Iulian Iancu, Ahikam Olmer, and Rael Strous review literature on "caffeinism" and, more generally, the impact of caffeine on psychopathology. They detail what is known about caffeinism as a diagnostic entity and analyze the scientific literature on physiology of caffeine intoxication, its clinical features, and available treatments. They also consider the role of caffeine in other pathologies, including anxiety disorders, depression, eating disorders, restless-legs syndrome, and suicide.

Chapter 14, by Ray Cooper, Talash Likimani, Dorothy Morré, and James Morré, addresses the scientific literature on green and black teas. The authors discuss the effects of caffeine in tea and also hypothesized health benefits studied in recent years. They consider the possible role of polyphenols—particularly catechins—in preventing some cancers, such as colon and bladder, and the interaction of caffeine with the polyphenols as it may affect cancer prevention. Also considered is the literature on caffeine and polyphenols in weight loss and exercise endurance.

Section VII ends the book with a broad overview of the literature on arousal and caffeine in chapter 15 by Barry Smith, Uma Gupta, and B. S. Gupta. There, the health effects of the drug and its impact on behavior are considered.

REFERENCES

Al-Ahram Weekly On-Line. (2005). Death by chocolate. Retrieved on 2/20/2006 weekly. ahram.org.eg/2005/743/pe2.htm.

Arnold, M. B. (1960). *Emotion and personality.* New York: Columbia University Press.

Duffy, E. (1951). The concept of energy mobilization. *Psychology Review, 58,* 30–40.

Duffy, E. (1962). *Activation and behavior.* New York: John Wiley & Sons.

Eysenck, H. J. (1967). *Biological basis of personality.* Springfield, IL: Charles C Thomas.

FAO. (2006a). Retrieved February 17, 2006, from http://www.fao.org/DOCREP/003/X6939E/X6939e02.htm.

International Coffee Organization. (2006). About coffee: Caffeine contents. Retrieved on 2/17/2006, from http://www.ico.org/caffeine.asp.

Lindsley, D. B. (1957). Psychophysiology and motivation. In M. R. Jones (Ed.), *Nebraska symposium on motivation, 1957.* Lincoln: University of Nebraska Press.

Malmo, R. B. (1959). Activation: A neurophysiological dimension. *Psychological Review, 66,* 267–386.

Nestle, M. (2000). Soft drink pouring rights: Marketing empty calories. In *Public Health Reports.* Oxford University Press.

Smith, B. D. (1983). Extraversion and electrodermal activity: Arousability and the inverted-U. *Personality and Individual Differences, 4,* 437–440.

Smith, B. D., Davidson, R. R., & Green, R. L. (1993). Effects of caffeine on physiology and performance: Further tests of a biobehavioral model. *Physiological Behavior, 54,* 415–432.

Smith, B. D., Osborne, A., Mann, M., Jones, H., & White, T. (2004). Arousal and behavior: The biopsychological effects of caffeine. In A. Nehlig (Ed.), *Coffee, tea, chocolate and the brain.* Boca Raton, FL: CRC Press.

Smith, B. D., Tola, K., & Mann, M. (1999). Caffeine and arousal: A biobehavioral theory of physiological, behavioral, and emotional effects. In B. S. Gupta and U. Gupta (Eds.), *Caffeine and behavior: Current views and research trends* (pp. 87–135). Boca Raton, FL: CRC Press.

Section I

Caffeine: The Drug

2 The Arousal Drug of Choice: Sources and Consumption of Caffeine

Barry D. Smith, Thom White, and Rachel Shapiro

CONTENTS

Caffeine is the most widely consumed drug in the world and the principal pharmacological source of arousal, alertness, and wakefulness for millions of people (Smith, Osborne, Mann, Jones, & White, 2004). Although the thrust of this book is the scientific study of caffeine and its effects, this chapter provides a backdrop against which to understand the science of the drug by detailing the major sources of caffeine and their social and cultural history.

The principal forms in which caffeine is consumed are coffee and tea, and we therefore devote the most in-depth coverage to these two beverages. In each case, a brief history is followed by information concerning the major producing countries, nomenclature, and harvesting and processing involved in the product. We also consider the varieties of coffee and tea, their caffeine content, and current production trends. Briefer coverage is provided for soft drinks, energy drinks, chocolate, and medications containing the drug.

Caffeine occurs naturally in the leaves, seeds, or fruit of over 60 plants, including those that produce coffee beans, tea leaves, and cocoa beans. Coffee, tea, and chocolate are, of course, produced quite directly from these plant sources. In addition, the caffeine derived from the plants is often added to carbonated drinks and to such medications as analgesics, diet aids, and cold remedies (Smith et al., 2004).

COFFEE: A BOHEMIAN BLEND

History of Coffee

From its legendary origins to modern times, coffee has been praised and valued for its taste and, more importantly, its effects on arousal. As a result, this simple fruit of the coffee plant became the basis for an industry that has grown over the centuries to multibillion dollar proportions. World coffee exports average six million tons annually (International Coffee Organization [ICO], 2006) or over 100 million bags of coffee beans (Food and Agricultural Organization [FAO], 2006a).*

---

* Please note that a number of our citations in this chapter involve websites, rather than journals. The reason is that most of the current information on caffeine consumption and production is found only on Internet sites and is not in the professional journal literature. In some cases, this means that the information is provided by commercially oriented organizations. As a result, we have cross-checked the information we report as thoroughly as possible, but prudence in accepting and interpreting the data is certainly appropriate.

Although humans have been drinking coffee for centuries, it is not clear just where coffee originated or who first discovered it. However, the predominant legend has it that an observant goatherd named Kaldi discovered coffee in the Ethiopian highlands. Various dates for this legend include 900 B.C. (Nescafe, 2006), 800 B.C. (North Coast Coffee, 2006), 300 A.D. (Kaldi Coffee, 2006), 600 to 800 A.D. (The Roast and Post Coffee Company, 2006), and 800 A.D. (National Geographic Society, 2006). Regardless of the actual date, it is said that Kaldi noticed that his goats did not sleep at night after eating berries from what would later be known as a coffee tree. When Kaldi reported his observation to the local monastery, the abbot became the first person to brew a batch of coffee and note its alerting effect when he drank it. Word of the arousing effects and pleasant taste of this new beverage soon spread beyond the monastery, initially east to the Arabian Peninsula and eventually throughout the world (James, 1997).

The story of Kaldi might be more fable than fact, but at least some historical evidence indicates that coffee did originate in the Ethiopian highlands. Indeed, most, if not all, coffees have been traced to that part of the world, whether they are now grown in Asia, Africa, Central and South America, or the Pacific and Caribbean Islands.

The first known reference to coffee in Arabic writings came from an Islamic physician, Abu Bakr Muhammad ibn Zakariya El Razi (known as "Rhazes"), who wrote a now lost medical textbook circa 900 A.D. Rhazes made the first reference to what can be reliably identified as coffee, and archaeologists have found iron roasting pans dating to 1000 A.D. However, Rhazes' textbook has been lost to the ages, and only more recent references in other Arabian literature exist citing his book (see Dufour, 1685, for a French-language account of the secondary sources). The oldest extant accounts of coffee roasting date to the writings of the famous Islamic physician Ibn Sina, traditionally referred to in English-language texts by his Latinized name, "Avicenna." Avicenna's praises of coffee were published in Arabic circa 1000 A.D. and translated into Latin circa 1200 A.D. (Goodman, 1992).

The coffee industry began on the Arabian Peninsula, where Arabs became the first to recognize the commercial value of the lowly bean. They cultivated coffee and, by the 15th century, were growing it in quantity in the Yemeni district, from which it spread, by the next century, to Syria, Egypt, Persia, and Turkey. As the coffee industry expanded throughout the Arab countries, coffee became a highly popular drink, perhaps in part because the Koran forbids Muslims from drinking alcoholic beverages. Nonetheless, some orthodox Islamic jurists were concerned about the popularity of coffee among the masses and attempted to justify banning the drink based on interpretations of Koran verses. They did not succeed, and three types of coffee-serving establishments spread across the Islamic world: stalls, shops, and *qahveh khaneh* (coffeehouses).

Stalls were small take-out counters in business districts (foreshadowing today's drive-through coffee stands). Shops were buildings where customers could buy coffee to go, but offered a few tables (antedating such modern coffee giants as Starbucks and Peet's by a millennium). The *qahveh khaneh* were the most lavish and prestigious of the three establishments. They offered garden-like surroundings, live music, and tree-covered tables, foreshadowing the high-end establishments found in large cities today. Not surprisingly, the *qahveh khaneh* became centers of social activity, where one could engage in pleasant conversation over a cup of coffee, play games, hear music, see plays, and stay up to date on the news. This latter function earned coffee houses the title of "schools of the wise" (National Coffee Association of the U.S.A. [NCAUSA], 2006a).

It was perhaps inevitable that the popularity of coffee would spread beyond the Islamic world, and it soon did. By the early 17th century, coffee had made its way to Venice, where it was at first decried as "the bitter invention of Satan" and condemned by local clergymen (NCAUSA, 2006a). However, Pope Clement VIII soon tasted it, liked it, and gave it the official imprimatur of the Church. The pope's approval added fuel to the caffeine fire, and the popularity of coffee rapidly spread throughout Europe. Coffee houses were opened in Marseilles in 1644, Venice in 1645, Oxford in 1650, London in 1652, Paris in 1657, and Vienna in 1683 (Ukers, 1935).

By 1675, 25 years after the opening of the first English coffee house (in Oxford), the number of coffee houses in England had grown to nearly 3,000, and King Charles II announced that year that coffeehouses were "seditious" meeting places. Nonetheless, their popularity was unstoppable. Each coffee house catered to its own segment of society, and members of a profession or industry would gather to discuss news of the day and conduct business. Some of these coffee houses went on to become major companies, such as Lloyd's of London. This world-famous business originated simply as Edward Lloyd's Coffee House (James, 1997).

As profits rolled in from the European centers, Arabian countries tried hard to maintain a coffee monopoly, with harsh penalties for those caught trying to smuggle out live trees. However, industrial espionage was alive and well, and Dutch entrepreneurs were successfully growing coffee in Ceylon and Java following their 1690 smuggling of a coffee plant out of Arabia. In 1714, the mayor of Amsterdam gave a young coffee plant to King Louis XIV of France for the Royal Botanical Garden in Paris, and this plant is said to be the origin of the coffee trees now found throughout the Caribbean and South and Central America (NCAUSA, 2006a).

CURRENT COUNTRIES OF ORIGIN

Today, coffee plants are cultivated in more than 50 countries, resulting in a wide variety of coffees, each with its own combination of flavor, body, and aroma. Depending on the type of coffee bean, where it is grown, the conditions under which it thrives, and how it is harvested and processed, coffee can have a wide variety of flavors and textures. For example, Kona coffee from Hawaii is always in high demand as a result of its rich taste and aroma and its medium body. Mexican coffee, on the other hand, has a pronounced sharpness that makes it desirable for dark roasts and blends. Puerto Rico produces coffee known for its balanced body and acidity with a fruity aroma. Guatemalan coffee has a complex taste that is almost chocolaty. Brazilian coffee is known worldwide for its mild taste.

Nomenclature

Linnaeus was first to describe and classify the coffee plant in his book *Species Plantarum*, published in 1753. The plants that yield coffee beans as their fruit are

TABLE 2.1
Botanical Classification of Coffee

Kingdom	Vegetable
Subkingdom	Angiospermae
Class	Dicotyledoneae
Subclass	Sympetalae
Order	Rubiales
Family	Rubiaceae
Genus	Coffea
Subgenus	Eucoffea
Species	C. arabica
	C. canephora

Source: Adapted from the National Coffee Association website. Retrieved on March 13, 2006, from http://www.ncausa.org/.

members of the genus *Coffea*, which is in the Rubiaceae family, a part of the subkingdom Angiospermae (Table 2.1) (NCAUSA, 2006b). Other members of that family include the gardenia and plants from which quinine is derived. Coffee plants are quite varied. They can range in size from small shrubs to 30-foot trees, and their leaves vary in color from purple to yellow. Because of this variability, botanists have failed to agree on a precise classification system, but there appear to be at least 25— perhaps as many as 100—species (NCAUSA, 2006; ICO, 2006b). However, the two varieties of coffee that its drinkers are most familiar with are *Arabica* and *Canephora* (commonly called *Robusta*).

The Arabica plant is a descendent of the original Ethiopian coffee trees and is typically a large bush that can reach a height of 14 to 20 feet. Its fruit, which has a fine, mild, aromatic taste, represents about 70% of world coffee production (ICO, 2006), and Arabica coffees typically command the highest market prices. The Arabica plant reaches maturity in 3 to 4 years and then continues to bear fruit for 20 to 30 years. It requires a mild climate, ideally with temperatures between 59 and 75° and rainfall of about 60 inches per year. The best Arabica coffees come from plants grown at altitudes between 2,000 and 6,000 feet. The ideal altitude within this range varies with distance from the equator (NCAUSA, 2006b).

The Robusta plant is similar to Arabica in size, shape, and time to maturity, but produces smaller and rounder beans that contain nearly twice the amount of caffeine found in Arabica. Robusta plants are cheaper to cultivate because they are heartier, more disease resistant, and can withstand warmer climates (preferring temperatures between 75 and 85°). Nonetheless, Arabica is widely preferred over Robusta because its taste is considered superior (James, 1997).

When they reach maturity, coffee trees of either variety bear fruits commonly referred to as "cherries" that turn red when they are ready for harvesting. The Arabica bean usually ripens in about 9 months, and the Robusta needs 10 or 11 months (ICO, 2006). Coffee beans are the seeds of these cherries.

Harvesting and Processing Coffee

Harvesting of the cherry typically occurs once a year, though the time varies by region, and equatorial countries can harvest all year round. The cherries can be harvested by strip picking, in which the entire crop is picked at one time, or by selective picking, when only the ripest cherries are harvested, leaving others to ripen and be harvested later. The latter method is very expensive and is used primarily for the Arabica cherries, where it is more cost effective. Once picked, the cherries are processed using one of two methods.

The older, simpler, and cheaper method is the more widely used "dry" or "natural" approach: the cherries are sorted and cleaned, spread out in the sun to dry, and raked frequently to ensure even drying and to prevent fermentation. When they are nearly dry, the outer shells turn brown and brittle and the beans are loosely contained inside. At this point, the cherries are stored in silos, where they continue to lose moisture. They are then hulled, sorted, graded, and bagged (ICO, 2006).

The wet method of processing coffee is more expensive than the dry method because it uses specialized equipment and large amounts of water. It is better suited for climates that are very rainy or where the humidity is high, preventing successful use of the dry method. It also protects the integrity of the bean and hence produces fewer defective beans (ICO, 2006). The main difference from the dry method is that the pulp is removed from the bean within 24 hours of harvesting instead of allowing the cherries to dry. The pulping is done by a machine that squeezes the cherries between fixed and moving surfaces. The beans are then vibrated to separate them and are washed. Next, they are stored in fermentation tanks and monitored carefully to prevent them from souring. Finally, the beans are dried in a manner similar to that used in the dry method.

Regardless of the initial processing method, beans, once dry, must be hulled. Hulling the wet processed beans means removing a final parchment-like covering around the bean. For the dry processed beans, the husks, which contain the whole of the dried coverings, are removed. All the beans are then sorted by density and size and are graded. The details of the grading system vary from one country to another. However, most employ variants of a five-grade system. The green-coffee grading categories of the Specialty Coffee Association of America (SCAA) appear in Table 2.2. The top grade beans are often designated "strictly hard bean" or "strictly high grown," which means the coffee was grown at least 4,000 feet above sea level.

After grading, the beans are exported, still in their green state, and sent directly to roasters or initially to warehouses, from which they later go to roasters. Roasting houses have experts who initially roast a small amount of the coffee, taste samples of the beans, and rate them for body, acidity, age, defects, aroma, and fullness. The remaining coffee beans are then roasted, typically at an air temperature that gradually reaches 550°F. When a bean reaches about 400°, its oil starts to emerge; this process, called pyrolosis, produces the flavor and aroma of the coffee we drink. Beans can be roasted anywhere in a range from very light to very dark. A light roast results in no oil reaching the surface of the bean, yielding a milder coffee, whereas a

TABLE 2.2
SCAA Green-Coffee Grading Schedules

Grade	Description of grade including defects per 300 g of green coffee beans
Grade 1	Specialty grade: No primary defects are allowed and a maximum of three full defects is allowed. Only 5% of beans may be above or below the specified screen size.
Grade 2	Premium grade: Primary defects are allowed and a maximum of eight full defects is allowed. Only 5% of beans may be above or below the specified screen size.
Grade 3	Exchange grade: Beans must be free from faults and a maximum of 23 full defects is allowed. Fifty percent of beans may be above the specified screen size, but only 5% may be below the specified screen size.
Grade 4	Below standard grade: 24 to 86 full defects.
Grade 5	Off grade: More than 86 full defects.

Source: Adapted from Coffee Research. Retrieved on March 13, 2006, from http://www.coffeeresearch. org/.

dark-roasted bean will be shiny with oil and very bitter, but less acidic than the lighter roasts. Regardless of the level of roasting, the end products are the familiar aromatic brown nuggets sold in coffee shops.

DECAFFEINATION

Contemporary concerns about possible adverse effects of caffeine are by no means unique to this century. Consumers long ago realized that the widely desired and sought after alerting effects of the brown bean could get out of hand and cause uncomfortably high levels of arousal in some instances. It became clear that some individuals reacted with hyperarousal and anxiety even to fairly small amounts of caffeine. Moreover, most who consumed very large quantities of the drug experienced these same adverse effects. As a result, early 19th-century scientists searched for methods of removing the caffeine from coffee. In 1820, Friedrich Ferdinand Runge, a German chemist, was asked by the poet Goethe to determine why he was unable to sleep after drinking coffee. Runge soon identified caffeine as the culprit and developed a crude method of decaffeination. However, this early approach weakened the structure of the coffee bean and substantially modified the taste and aroma of the resulting brew, rendering it virtually undrinkable.

Significant advances in decaffeination awaited the 20th century, at which time Ludwig Roselius brought about the development of a new approach. There are several versions of the Roselius story, but it appears that he was a coffee importer from Bremen, Germany, who, in 1903, enticed a team of chemists to help him develop a better method of decaffeination. Roselius and his colleagues decided to steam the beans first, causing them to swell and allowing the caffeine to be more easily removed by the solvent benzene. The benzene containing the caffeine was then removed from the beans. Roselius called his process "sans caffeine," later shortening the term to create his world-famous brand name, Sanka.

Pretreatment with steam is still used in modern decaffeination procedures, but many changes in technology and the solvents used have occurred. Currently, three major decaffeination methods are used; one uses chemical solvents, another supercritical gases, and a third the so-called Swiss water process:

In the chemical solvent process, the beans are steamed and then boiled under pressure with a solvent that extracts the caffeine without affecting the coffee in any other way. The chemicals currently deemed safe for this purpose by the FDA are methylene chloride, which has the advantage of a lower boiling point, and ethyl acetate, which is found in many fruits. Some of the solvent remains in the beans, though the amount can be reduced by using a second steaming to force it out.

The supercritical gas method requires beans be exposed to supercritical carbon dioxide (CO_2). The "critical point" of the gas under pressure is the point at which the gas behaves more like a liquid. As such, the supercritical CO_2 acts like a liquid, enters the coffee bean, extracts the caffeine, and leaves the bean intact.

The Swiss water process method was developed and so named to assuage fears of the consuming public that the chemicals used in decaffeination were dangerous, despite FDA approval. Surely, the public would agree that decaffeination using water must be harmless! In the Swiss water method, green coffee beans are immersed in hot water, allowing the caffeine to pass out of the bean and into the water. This extract is next passed through activated carbon, removing the caffeine. The caffeine-free mixture is then added back to the partially dried beans.

Any of these methods will remove at least 97% of the caffeine present in natural coffee beans, resulting in a cup of brewed coffee that contains only about 1.5 mg of caffeine.

AMOUNT OF CAFFEINE IN COFFEE

The amount of caffeine in coffee beans ranges from 1.01 to 1.42% by weight (Owen, 2006). The variability in percentage is a function of variety of coffee, blend, and how the coffee beans were roasted (i.e., light or dark roast). Table 2.3 indicates the amount of caffeine in each of a number of different types of coffee. The highest amount of caffeine by weight and variety is found in the Tanzania Peaberry bean, with 1.42 g of caffeine per kilogram of coffee. Using the SCAA recommendation of 10 g of ground coffee per 6-oz (168-ml) serving (Owen, 2006), Tanzania Peaberry would yield approximately 142 mg of caffeine per serving of coffee. Other highly caffeinated coffees include Columbia Supremo, Colombia Excelso, and Indian Mysore (each at 1.37%), Kenya AA (1.36%), and Costa Rica Tarrazu (1.35%). At the other end of the scale are the mild Mocha Mattari (1.01%) and Zimbabwe (1.10%) coffees. Because different coffee manufacturers use different blends of coffees and roast them differently, brand-to-brand and even day-to-day variability in caffeine content is the norm. Additionally, the coarseness of the grind also affects caffeine content of the finished coffee.

TABLE 2.3
Amount of Caffeine by Coffee Blend

Source of caffeine	% Caffeine	Source of caffeine	% Caffeine
Varietals and straights		**Blends and dark roasts**	
Brazil Bourbons	1.20	Colombia Supremo Dark	1.37
Celebes Kalossi	1.22	Espresso Roast	1.32
Colombua Excelso	1.37	French Roast	1.22
Colombia Supremo	1.37	Vienna Roast	1.27
Ethiopian Harrar–Moka	1.13	Mocha–Java	1.17
Guatemala Antigua	1.32	**Decaffeinated**	
Indian Mysore	1.37	All blends (Swiss process)	0.02
Jamaican Blue Mountain	1.24		
Java Estate Kuyumas	1.20		
Kenya AA	1.36		
Kona Extra Prime	1.32		
Mexico Pluma Altura	1.17		
Mocha Matari (Yemen)	1.01		
New Guinea	1.30		
Panama Organic	1.34		
Sumatra Mandheling–Lintong	1.30		
Tanzania Peaberry	1.42		
Zimbabwe	1.10		

Source: Adapted from Coffee FAQ, 2006a. Retrieved March 13, 2006, from http://coffeefaq.com/.

Brewing Method and Caffeine Yields

The amount of caffeine in a serving of coffee depends not only on variety and blend, but also on brewing method. According to Bunker and McWilliams (1979), the amount of caffeine in a 7-oz serving (196 ml) of coffee by any method ranges from 65 to 175 mg. Thus, the number of milligrams of caffeine per serving of brewed coffee is not determined entirely by the grams of caffeine per kilogram of coffee beans discussed earlier. The major brewing methods can be categorized by drip coffee (which involves water near boiling) versus a number of methods that involve fully-boiling water versus a number of methods that make use of pressurized water. The most common of the boiling water methods are press (also called French press), percolation, and instant coffee. The most common of the pressure methods are vacuum filtering, espresso, and crema. In Table 2.4, the amount of caffeine found in a 7-oz serving (196 ml) of coffee is listed by brewing method.

Drip coffee is the most common brewing method in the United States, although it is used worldwide. The drip method involves flowing water near boiling into medium-coarse ground coffee. The liquid coffee then drips through a metal, plastic, or paper filter into a carafe. Compared to paper filters, using metal or plastic filters results in a larger amount of sediment and essential oils being filtered through to

TABLE 2.4
Amount of Caffeine in 7-oz Serving
(196 ml) Coffee by Brewing Method

Source	Range (mg)
Drip	115–175
Espresso[a]	100
Brewed	80–135
Instant	65–100
Decaf, brewed	3–4
Decaf, instant	2–3

[a]One serving of espresso is 1.5 to 2 oz (42 to 56 ml).
Source: Adapted from Bunker, M. L., & McWilliams, M. (1979). *Journal of the American Dietician, 74,* 28–32.

the final product (Owen, 2006). Metal filters are usually made of stainless steel, although gold-plated mesh filters, which are said to leave less of an aftertaste in the brewed coffee, are available. Drip coffee has between 115 and 175 mg of caffeine per 7-oz serving (196 ml) (Bunker & McWilliams, 1979).

The boiling methods include the Turkish ibrik, French press, percolator, and Neapolitan coffee makers. The Turkish ibrik is a brass or copper container. The ibrik is a brass or copper container that is wide at its base but narrower toward the top. Water is brought to a boil in the ibrik and then finely ground coffee is placed in the water, which is again brought to a boil. The French press or plunger method is popular in Europe and is increasing in popularity in the United States. When coffee is brewed in a French press, boiling water is poured over coarse-ground coffee in a covered glass carafe. The grounds are brewed in the water for 2 to 3 minutes and then pressed to the bottom of the carafe by using a plunger with wire mesh attached. The resulting cup of coffee is laden with sediment and essential oils (Owen, 2006). Coffee made this way has between 80 and 135 mg of caffeine per 7-oz serving (196 ml) (Bunker & McWilliams, 1979).

Percolated coffee, popular in Europe and the United States, is made by boiling water in the base of the percolator, causing the water to rise up a central tube, spray over the coffee grounds in a basket, drip back down, without filtration, into the base, and then recirculate continuously (Owen, 2006). In the Neapolitan method, water is boiled in the base of the pot, which is flipped upside down, allowing the water to pass through the coffee grounds in a basket (Sally's Place, 2006). The average 7-oz serving (196 ml) contains about 140 mg of caffeine. A less common approach to making coffee, although popular in Japan, is the vacuum method. A buildup of steam in a lower bowl forces the water into a funnel, where it mixes with the ground coffee. This is stirred and allowed to brew for 2 minutes. A vacuum is created and the coffee mixture is drawn through a filter to get the final product (Owen).

In producing instant coffee, which has between 65 and 100 mg of caffeine per 7-oz serving (196 ml), the manufacturer first percolates, then dries the coffee.

The process of percolation dissolves the coffee extractables and causes the complex carbohydrates to become soluble and partially hydrolyzed. This yields 36% of the water-soluble extract. The sediment is then discarded and the rest is dehydrated. This dehydrated extract can be spray- or freeze dried. Spray drying the coffee involves passing 480°F air over the extract. The solids drop, and the result is coffee granules with 3% moisture. This method of drying yields a less powerful flavor and is used with Robusta beans.

In freeze drying, the coffee extract is frozen, causing the soluble coffee solids to separate out and form slabs, which are then broken for packaging. As a final step, flavor aroma is added back into the coffee. This can be done by mixing the granules with aqueous gelatin or gum Arabica, spray drying or coating the granules with oily droplets of the flavor aroma compounds, and then drying in a lattice (Spiller, 1998).

Espresso coffee, long a mainstay in Europe, has grown increasingly popular in the United States over the last decade or so. Enterprising Italian manufacturer Luigi Bezzera invented espresso between 1901 and 1903. He observed that the long coffee breaks taken by his employees were reducing their productivity and wanted a quick method of making coffee to shorten the breaks. He found that by using steam pressure, he could reduce brewing time to 20 seconds—and espresso coffee was born. Bezzera soon saw the financial potential in his espresso machine and proceeded to patent it. By 1905, he had sold the patent to Desidoro Pavoni, and the machines were soon available to the public. The only problem with the Bezzera machine was that his steam pressure method produced coffee with a slightly burnt taste. That problem was eliminated in 1938, when Cresemonesi developed a piston pump to force hot water through the coffee. A bonus feature of the Cresemonesi pump was the now much desired layer of foam or crema that tops the cup of espresso.

Espresso is made with coffee that is ground very finely, often almost to a powder. Using a short brewing cycle, very high pressure sends hot (not boiling) water through the grounds. Once the extraction begins, the entire process lasts about 25 seconds for a 2-oz serving (Arabee Coffee, 2006). One serving or "shot" of espresso (1.5 to 2 oz, or 42 to 56 ml) has about 100 mg of caffeine (Bunker & McWilliams, 1979). Espresso can be consumed as "straight" coffee or in a variety of specialty forms, such as cappuccino and latte. Table 2.5 presents definitions of the major espresso-based drinks.

One of the newest forms of coffee, increasingly popular in Europe and the United States, is crema coffee, which is essentially a weaker version of espresso. Crema is made using the same pressure method as that used in espresso, but instead of the usual 1.5- to 2.0-oz cup (42 to 56 ml), the machine produces a full-size cup of 6 to 8 oz (168 to 224 ml) containing the same amount of caffeine as in a regular espresso shot. A cup of coffee produced by the crema process has the traditional espresso crema on top—hence, its name. Some of the newer "superautomatic" espresso machines include separate settings for automatically producing crema coffee. The taste of crema coffee can be quite different from that of a cup of drip coffee made with the same beans.

As previously mentioned, the method of brewing coffee has an impact on the amount of caffeine per ounce. Although espresso has less caffeine per serving than brewed coffee, this is because the serving of espresso is much smaller (2 oz) than a serving of brewed coffee (7 oz). Using a 7-oz standard for all methods, espresso has

TABLE 2.5
Contents of Different Espresso-Based Drinks

Caffe latte	Single shot of espresso with steamed milk in a 3:1 milk-to-coffee ratio
Café au lait	Not an espresso drink, but similar to caffe latte; brewed coffee (instead of espresso) with steamed milk in a 1:1 milk-to-coffee ratio; sugar often added for flavor
Cappuccino	Equal parts espresso (usually one shot), steamed milk, and frothed milk
Americano	Single shot of espresso in a coffee cup; 6 to 8 oz of hot water then added to fill the cup
Hammerhead	Single shot of espresso in a coffee cup; 6 to 8 oz of drip coffee then added to fill the cup
Mocha	Cappuccino or caffe latte with chocolate syrup added
Espresso con panna	Single shot of espresso with whipped cream on top
Double shot	Any of the above espresso drinks with two shots of espresso instead of a single shot
Ristretto	Any of the above espresso drinks, but with restricted amount of water allowed to come through the grounds, yielding a 0.75-oz shot
Lungo	Any of the above espresso drinks, but with longer "pull" and twice as much water coming through the grounds, yielding a 2- to 3-oz shot

Source: Adapted from Coffee FAQ, 2006a. Retrieved March 13, 2006, from http://coffeefaq.com/.

by far the most caffeine. There is between 350 and 475 mg of caffeine in 7 oz of espresso, compared to 115 to 175 mg in drip coffee. The variability within each method is due to individual differences in the ratio of coffee grounds to water while brewing, the type of coffee bean used, and the roast of the bean.

Total world coffee production for 2005 and 2006 is forecast at 113.2 million bags, down 7% from the 2004–2005 growing season (USDA, 2006). The production forecast for major coffee-producing countries for the 2005–2006 coffee growing season is given in Table 2.6. Production of Arabica coffee in 2004 and 2005 amounted to 58.97 million bags, an increase of 2.34%, compared with 57.62 million bags in 2003 and 2004. Robusta production amounted to 29.98 million bags, a decrease of 3.64%, compared with 31.11 million bags recorded in 2003 and 2004 (ICO, 2006).

In terms of coffee consumption, in the United States, Germany, and Japan, the younger populations have shown an overall decrease in coffee consumption. It is possible that this decrease can be attributed to the advertising tactics of soft-drink makers, whose consumption rates increased by 13.7% in the United States in the 1990s. Conversely, among older populations, coffee consumption is stable or increasing in West Germany and the United States.

This trend is not evident in Japan, whose older population remains loyal to the Japanese habit of tea drinking. According to Garattini (1993), a Japanese survey showed that Japanese who drank more coffee were less traditional than those who drank less: those who drank less coffee were more likely to have breakfast with their families and to consume more rice; those who drank more coffee were more likely to skip breakfast, eat breakfast alone, or eat a breakfast with higher bread content (i.e., to have more Westernized "bad" habits). This survey also showed that those

TABLE 2.6
Coffee Production Forecast for the 2005–2006 Coffee-Growing Season

Country	Arabica production (millions of bags)	Robusta production (millions of bags)
Brazil	26.00	10.10
Colombia	11.55	0
Vietnam	0.33	12.00
Indonesia	0.75	6.00
Mexico	4.05	0.15
India	1.75	2.88
Cote d'Ivoire	0	2.50
Guatemala	3.65	0.03
Honduras	2.99	0
Costa Rica	2.00	0
Ecuador	0.55	0.40
Venezuela	0.82	0
United States	0.17	0

Source: Adapted from USDA Foreign Agricultural Service. Retrieved March 13, 2006, from http://www.fas.usda.gov/.

with a higher stress level, more urban lifestyle, and preference for gourmet foods consumed more coffee than those with a more traditional lifestyle. It can be concluded from these observations that those who drink more coffee in Japan are evidently marked as having been more Westernized (Garattini).

SPECIALTY COFFEES

Specialty coffees include everything from espresso-based beverages to frozen coffee mixtures. Consumers are having a field day with these specialty coffees, as reflected in the seemingly exponential increase in coffee bars across the United States and the fact that U.S. sales of regular coffees have slightly decreased over the past few years, while gourmet coffee sales have consistently increased at a rate of about 20% a year. In 1989, gourmet coffee sales were at $1.5 billion. By 2000, they reached $5 billion. It should be noted, however, that specialty coffees are not expected to replace their commercial counterparts, but rather to complement them.

TEA: A DECOROUS DRINK

The second most common worldwide source of caffeine is tea. Like coffee, it is consumed on a daily basis by millions of people. In some countries, like England, it is virtually a way of life, with "tea time" defining the day for many drinkers. In others, it is less central and symbolic, but is nevertheless consumed regularly by much of the populace. Recent evidence suggests, in fact, that tea is rapidly increasing in popularity in the United States (Lee & Levine, 2000).

The word "tea" appears to be a derivative of an early Chinese term for the drink. In most of China, where tea likely originated, and in Japan, the word for tea is "cha," but in Fujian Province it is "te," which is pronounced "tay." It was in Fujian that the Dutch—first world marketers of tea—did most of their early business. The drink later entered England pronounced as "tay," but the pronunciation was still later changed to "tee." It is still pronounced "tay" in Scotland and Ireland.

A Brief History of Tea

As with coffee, the history of tea is more a matter of legend than of fact. Although some accounts date the origin of tea to at least the 10th century, B.C., the most widely subscribed accounts place it somewhat later in time. The tea plant is native to China and India and thus there are two dominant legends concerning the discovery of this source of caffeine, both noting the arousing effects of the drug in the drink. The Chinese version attributes the discovery of tea to the Second Emperor Shen Nung, who reigned from 2737 to 2697 B.C. Apparently, for health reasons, he insisted that all water be boiled before drinking. Legend has it that on one occasion some tea leaves fell in water that the emperor was boiling. He found the aroma so pleasing that he drank the tea, experiencing its pleasant taste and the arousing effects of the caffeine (In Pursuit of Tea, 2006).

The second legend is of Buddhist origin and attributes tea to the Bodhisattva Bodhidharma, the founder of Zen Buddhism. To prove his faith, Bodhidharma swore to travel to China without sleep. However, after several days of travel, his eyelids closed and he fell into a deep sleep. When he awoke, he was so angry that his vow was broken by his disobedient eyelids that he threw them to the ground. They quickly disappeared into the soil, from which there soon arose a tea bush. Upon chewing the leaves of the bush, he felt a surge of energy (In Pursuit of Tea, 2006).

Whether tea originated in China or India, it certainly became a staple in both cultures. In China, it was soon the most popular national drink, eventually becoming a part of the economy. Its economic value was recognized in the eighth century, when a guide to producing tea, the Ch'a Ching (Classic of Tea), was published in 780 A.D. by the poet Lu Yu (In Pursuit of Tea, 2006). It detailed the process of growing, manufacturing, brewing, and consuming tea; commercial production soon led to even more widespread use. In India, tea became a central feature of the Buddhist faith. A tea master prepared the brew for the faithful, who gathered in a small, bare room and consumed it as part of the ritualistic, symbolic, Buddhist tea ceremony. The pleasant, arousing effects of the large quantities of caffeine that could be consumed in these ceremonies may well have had much to do with the popularity of tea as a part of fervent religious ceremony.

Despite its widespread popularity in Asia, it was not until the 16th century that tea reached Europe. The first European to write about his contact with tea was Father Jasper da Cruz. Da Cruz was the first Portuguese Jesuit to be a missionary in China, and he wrote about tea upon his return home to Portugal in 1560. Tea would not be mentioned in English until 1597, when the Dutch navigator Jan Hugo van Lin–Schooten's writings about the *chaa* drink were translated into English (Gepts, 2002; Stashtea, 2006). Subsequently, Portugal became the first European nation to import tea. Between 1652 and 1654, tea reached England, a country that reveres its aroma, flavor, and pleasant alerting effect to this day.

By 1664, the East India Company, founded by Queen Elizabeth to import spices, cloth, and other products from the East, was also bringing tea in quantity to British shores, and its popularity and economic success grew rapidly. Although the East India Company held exclusive trade rights with the Orient for nearly the next two centuries, so valuable was the drink that a tea "underground" provided considerable amounts illegally, frequently offering it at a lower price and contributing to its widespread consumption. By 1699, tea had spread like wildfire throughout Holland and France, and 40,000 pounds were imported each year. By 1708, that figure had grown to 240,000 pounds per year (Stashtea, 2006).

Tea would shortly come to play an important role in the newly founded United States, as well. In fact, it came to America in 1650, even before it reached England, when Peter Stuyvesant brought it to the Dutch colony known as New Amsterdam (now New York). Once tea did become popular in England, the British could hardly be expected to travel abroad without their precious drink and, as a result, tea made a second entrée to the United States with the British colonists. By the beginning of the 18th century, it was available in major American cities, but primarily through trade with England. As the British raised tariffs higher and higher, the colonists grew angrier and angrier, and action against the British became inevitable. On December 16, 1773, the infuriated colonists, dressed as Indians, went to Griffin's Wharf and dumped several hundred pounds of tea from docked British ships into Boston Harbor. This famous Boston Tea Party marked the beginning of the end for British rule in America. The Declaration of Independence and the Revolutionary War soon followed and, since then, coffee has always been more popular in America than tea (Stashtea, 2006).

The late 19th and early 20th centuries saw further developments in the world of tea. Perhaps most notable were the coming of Lipton Tea, iced tea, tea bags, and herbal teas. In 1890, Sir Thomas Lipton, who had already helped to popularize tea in England, brought his business acumen to the United States. Purchasing tea estates in Ceylon (now Sri Lanka), Lipton shipped large quantities of tea to America, advertised his wares widely, and soon became the prime mover in bringing tea to the U.S. masses (Every, 2001). Iced tea was invented by tea peddler Richard Blechynden on a hot summer day at the World's Fair in St. Louis in 1904 and soon became a warm-weather staple among tea lovers.

Tea bags came a few years later, in 1908, when Thomas Sullivan developed them and tea drinkers learned that steeping them in hot water was a quick and convenient way to make tea (Every, 2001). Herbal teas came still later, with a claim to being healthier because many of them had no caffeine and, indeed, no tea leaves. In fact, "herbal tea" is a misnomer because these "teas" consist of spices, berries, seeds, flowers, and the leaves and roots of a variety of plants, but typically do not include products of the tea bush.

TEA-PRODUCING COUNTRIES

Although tea is now consumed in most parts of the world, it is still grown and processed primarily in the East. In 2003, world tea production reached 3.15 million tons, a 75,000-ton increase over 2002 (FAO, 2006b). The leading tea-producing countries include India, China, Sri Lanka, and Kenya. Tea production in these countries is summarized in Table 2.7.

TABLE 2.7
Major Tea-Producing Countries

Country	2004 Tea production	% Change from 2003	% World production
India	857,000	−3.4	27.4
China	791,000	2.4	24.6
Sri Lanka	N/A	N/A	9.75
Kenya	N/A	N/A	9.4

Note: N/A = data not available.

Source: Adapted from FAO (2006b). Retrieve0d March 13, 2006, from http://www.fao.org/ newsroom/en/ news/2004/51815/.

Nomenclature

By the time the nomenclaturist Linnaeus published his *Species Plantarum* (1753), tea had, of course, already been grown and consumed for centuries, and he was aware of the availability of green and black teas. Accordingly, he identified two separate species of plants that yield tea: *Thea viridis* (green) and *Thea bohea* (black). That inaccurate classification held until the early 19th century, when it was determined that these two plants were, in fact, one and the same. The species of the tea plant is *Camellia sinensis*. It is in the family Theaceae of order Theales (Table 2.8). Interestingly enough, over 2000 varieties of tea are derived from this one plant species. The differences are a function of the way in which the tea leaves are processed.

Processing and Varieties of Tea

Tea has more naturally occurring caffeine than does coffee. However, the brewing process typically dilutes tea more than coffee, resulting in one quarter to one third less caffeine per cup (Barone & Roberts, 1984). The processing of all teas begins with the *Camellia sinensis* plant. Only the top two leaves and the unopened leaf bud

TABLE 2.8
Botanical Classification of Tea

Kingdom	Plantae
Division	Magnoliophyta
Class	Magnoliopsida
Order	Ericales
Family	Theaceae
Genus	Camellia
Species	sinensis

Source: Adapted from Wikipedia. Retrieved March 13, 2006, from http://www.wikipedia.org/.

from the plant are used. There are four principal methods for processing the plant, and they result in the major types of tea that are the most widely consumed. These are white, green (or unfermented), oolong (or semifermented), and black (or fermented) tea.

White tea is derived by the simplest of the four processing methods and, in some classification schemes, is grouped with green tea. Only the youngest leaves are picked for white tea, and these leaves still contain short white "hair." The leaves are simply steamed and dried, and their appearance is relatively unaltered (AATea.com, 2001). Brewing then produces a pale yellow cup of tea with a fresh flavor. Examples of white teas are Imperial Silver Needles, Drum Mountain White Cloud, Pai Mu Tan, and Poobong White Tea Darjeeling. Table 2.9 lists some examples of the major types of tea along with flavor descriptions of each.

Tea leaves for the production of green tea are handled with special care because preservation of the healthy, natural, active substances in the fresh leaves is essential for the tea to be at its best (see chapter 14 in this volume for a review of the scientific literature on the potential benefits of tea). After picking, the leaves are set out in hot air to wither and then usually pan fried to prevent oxidation or fermentation. Otherwise, this chemical process produces polyphenic bodies, which lead to color and flavor changes in the tea. The more oxidation that takes place, the darker and more pungent the tea is. Once fried, the leaves are rolled, giving them a twisted, curly, or balled appearance and increasing their durability. This process also helps regulate release of natural substances during steeping.

The leaves are next dried, using a process called firing, in which the leaves are placed in a heat-controlled environment. The most common approach is to move the tea on a conveyor through a rotating drum. The drum is heated by fire to a temperature that is constantly controlled to ensure even firing of the leaves. The goal is to reduce the moisture in the leaves to about 4%. In addition, some sugars are caramelized in the process and the polyphenols undergo epimerization. Firing stabilizes the fragrance and flavor of the tea. The resulting green colored leaves yield a cup of tea high in nutrients and minerals that is the subject of many medical studies. Examples of green teas are Genmaicha, Gyokuro, and Bancha (Table 2.9).

During production of oolong tea, the leaves are allowed to mature longer before picking, which results in fuller body. Upon picking, the leaves are withered, much as they are in green tea. However, after withering, their edges are bruised by shaking. Bruising mixes the cellular constituents and starts the oxidation process. Bruising is typically repeated several times, and the leaves are then spread out to dry. The next step is oxidation, which continues until 20 to 60% of the tea leaf is fermented, depending on the variety of oolong. Although avoided in creating green teas, this process is essential in oolong and black teas because it yields the heartier, richer flavors characteristic of these varieties. Fermentation is finally stopped by pan firing and the leaves are ready for export. Oolong teas include Tie Guan Yin (Mainland China) and Formosa Oolong (Taiwan).

Unlike other teas, black tea is completely fermented, giving the leaves their characteristic color as well as a strong, rich flavor. The first treatment of the leaves for black tea is again withering, followed by rolling. Then the leaves are piled up in cool, humid rooms to ferment. After full fermentation, the leaves are fired to

TABLE 2.9
Descriptions of Varieties of Tea by Type

Variety	Origin	Description
White		
Flowery Pekoe	China	Slightly sweet, creamy
Mutan	China	Delicate, light with no astringency
White Peony	China	Delicate, sweet flavor
Silver Needles	China	Slightly sweet, nutty overtones
Yunnan Snow Tea	China	Delicate, sweet flavor
Green		
Dragon's Well	China	Subtle, chestnut flavor
Brown Rice Tea	Japan	Nutty, toasty flavor
Pearl Tea	China	Pungent, astringent, may be nutty
Jewel Dew	Japan	Mild, fresh
Mao Feng	China	Mellow, slightly sweet
Macha	Japan	Bitter
Pi Lo Chun	China	Peach, plum, apricot
Oolong		
Formosa	Taiwan	Flowery, delicate
Pu-her	China	Earthy
Tue Guan Yin	Taiwan and China	Rich, floral
Wu Lung	China	Flowery, delicate
Black		
Assam	Assam, India	Hearty, robust, malty
Ceylon	Sri Lanka	Flowery, sweet, very delicate
Darjeeling	Darjeeling, India	Pungent, astringent
Kalgar	India	Similar to Assam, but lighter
Keemun	China	Sweet, full bodied, mellow
Keemun Hao Ya	China	Fruity, sweet flavor, orchid aroma
Lapsang	Taiwan	Flavored with pine root smoke
Nilgiri	Nilgiri, India	Mild, fresh, full bodied
Sikkim	Sikkim, India	Malty but light and delicate
Yunnan	China	Strong and somewhat peppery

Source: Adapted from CNN Food. Retrieved March 13, 2006, from http://www.cnn.com/ HEALTH/ indepth.food/beverages/tea/.

stop the process, and the juices that are the product of fermentation dry on the surfaces of the leaves and remain until steeping. The processed leaves have budding tips called pekoe from the Chinese Pak-Ho, meaning hair, probably a reference to the white "down" that appears on the budding leaves. The tea is thus often referred to as orange pekoe, though the origin of the term "orange" is unclear. The black teas are exemplified by Sonarie Assam (India) and Newara Eliya Ceylon (Sri Lanka).

Tea-Leaf Grading

The grading of the tea leaf differs by country and by processing method. By way of example, black teas are usually divided into four categories: whole leaf, broken leaf, fannings, and dust. The tea is then graded within each category. For the whole-leaf category, the four grades of tea are flowery orange pekoe (FOP), derived from the very ends or tips of the young leaf buds; orange pekoe (OP), harvested when the terminal buds open into leaf; pekoe (P), which uses shorter, coarser leaves; and souchong (S), derived from large leaves often rolled lengthwise. The other types of tea are also graded, using somewhat less complex schemes.

Amount of Caffeine by Variety, Form, and Brew

The varied processing that produces the several varieties of tea also results in somewhat different levels of caffeine. In particular, different processing methods remove varied percentages of caffeine from the tea leaves. Table 2.10 indicates the differences in the amount of caffeine in a serving of tea by variety. Fermenting results in the highest final level of caffeine content; hence, black tea, which is fully

---

TABLE 2.10
Amount of Caffeine in 5-oz Serving of Tea (140 ml) by Variety and Brewing Time

Brew time	Range (mg)	Mean (mg)
Black, bagged		
Brewed 1 minute	21–33	28
Brewed 3 minutes	35–46	N/A
Brewed 5 minutes	39–50	46
Green, bagged		
Brewed 1 minute	9–19	14
Brewed 3 minutes	20–33	27
Brewed 5 minutes	26–36	31
Darjeeling, loose		
Brewed 1 minute	N/A	19
Brewed 3 minutes	N/A	25
Brewed 5 minutes	N/A	28
Japanese panfried, loose		
Brewed 1 minute	N/A	14
Brewed 3 minutes	N/A	20
Brewed 5 minutes	N/A	21
Most herbal and mint teas	N/A	0

Note: N/A = data not available.

Source: Adapted from Bunker & McWilliams (1979).

TABLE 2.11
Amount of Caffeine in a 12-oz Serving of
Tea by Brand and Variety

Brand	Caffeine (mg)
Lipton, brisk	9
Mistic	18
Nestea sweetened	26
Nestea unsweetened	26
Snapple sweet tea	12
Snapple flavored teas	31.5

Source: Adapted from NSDA. Retrieved March 13, 2006, from http://www.ameribev.org/.

fermented, has the highest caffeine content of all teas. Conversely, green and white teas are not fermented, and they contain lower levels of caffeine. The size of the tea leaves also has an effect on the amount of caffeine per cup; smaller leaves result in higher caffeine content.

Another factor is the method of brewing. Tea that is broken up and placed in tea bags has a higher caffeine yield than tea brewed directly from whole leaves through a filter (The Tea House, 2006). Finally, brewing time has a slight effect on caffeine content. In particular, when tea is brewed for over 3 minutes—some experts recommend 3 to 5 minutes for black tea—caffeine yield increases slightly (Lipton Tea Company, 2006). Table 2.11 presents caffeine data for various brands of tea.

TEA PRODUCTION TRENDS

Asia produces the most tea each year, with Indian and Chinese yields constituting over 80% of the worldwide crop (Spiller, 1998). Interestingly enough, much of the product is consumed domestically, in contrast to coffee production and consumption per country. Table 2.12 shows the tea production trends for major producing countries. The year 1971 is included to show the substantial (30%) increase in tea production over time. The increase over the first half of the 1990s, by contrast, was only 4%. The rate of increase for China and India slowed considerably (Spiller, 1998). Despite the reduced rate of increase in the aforementioned countries, world tea production is still on the rise (Table 2.12).

TEA CONSUMPTION TRENDS

After water and coffee, tea is the most widely consumed beverage in the world; approximately 1.9 trillion cups are consumed each year worldwide (Rasmussen & Rhinehart, 1998).

TABLE 2.12
Tea Production Trends

Year	World production (millions of metric tons)
1971	1.09
1994	2.49
1995	2.50
1996	N/A
1997	2.72
1998	2.19
1999	2.85
2000	2.96
2001	3.03
2002	N/A
2003	N/A
2004	3.20

Note: N/A = data not available.

Sources: Community Integrated Pest Management (http://www.communityipm. org/); European Fair Trade Association (http://www.eftafairtrade.org/); FAO (http://www. fao.org/); Hawaiian Agricultural Products (http://hawaiianagricul-turalproducts.com/); NewCROP (http://www.hort.purdue.edu/newcrop/default. html/); Tea and Coffee (http://www.teaandcoffee.net/).

CAFFEINATED HOLLY TEAS OF THE AMERICAS

Far less commonly consumed and less known to consumers than Asian tea, several holly teas indigenous to the Americas are sources of caffeine. Although these drinks are caffeinated teas, they are not nearly as popular or as widespread as Asian teas made from *Camellia sinensis*. Of the 25 identified holly plants of the *Ilex* genus, only three are known to contain caffeine: *Ilex guayasa, Ilex paraguariensis*, and *Ilex vomitoria* (Hu, 1979).

Excavation of Bolivian burial sites has found tea-producing paraphernalia alongside the leaves of *Ilex guayusa*, a caffeine-containing holly plant, suggesting that caffeinated holly teas were brewed as early as 500 A.D. in the Western hemisphere. *Ilex guayasa* is not known to be in use at the present time. However, the leaves of *Ilex paraguariensis*, a similar holly plant native to Paraguay, Uruguay, Argentina, Chile, and southern Brazil, is still consumed as *mate* (Hudson, 1979).

Cassina, also known as "black drink," is made from twigs and leaves of Yaupon holly (*Ilex vomitoria*), an ornamental shrub indigenous to the southeastern United States, from Virginia to Florida, along the Atlantic coast, and west to Texas along the Gulf coast. *Cassina* was discovered by Native Americans (perhaps the Timuacan tribe) and is produced by parching twigs and leaves of the Yaupon holly, then boiling them to produce a potent, dark drink nearly black in appearance. As its scientific name suggests, the emetic properties of the Yaupon holly were touted by Native Americans. However, to induce vomiting, the leaves must be eaten raw. Made into tea, *Cassina* does not induce vomiting and is said to taste like a bitter variant of black or oolong tea. It became briefly popular in Europe following its introduction to Europe in the 16th and 17th centuries by Spanish colonizers. However, it eventually lost out to coffee and Asian tea in Europe and America (Hu, 1979). In fact, the relative obscurity of caffeinated holly teas is reflected in the lack of extant literature on them in over two decades.

SOFT DRINKS: AN INCREASING SOURCE OF CAFFEINE

In addition to coffee and tea, caffeine is found in many soft drinks, which are also a major source of the drug. This is particularly true for children and adolescents, who often consume large quantities of soft drinks virtually every day.

A BRIEF HISTORY OF SOFT DRINKS

It could perhaps be argued that Hippocrates planted the first seeds of the soft-drink industry when he wrote that mineral waters might bring health benefits. However, he and other ancient Greeks and Romans used them, instead, for relaxation and bathing. Indeed, it was centuries later that the term "soda water" was coined in 1798. The first patent for imitation mineral waters was issued in 1810, and they came to be considered the "health drinks" of the 19th century. By the 1830s, pharmacists were experimenting with adding such ingredients as barks and flowers to enhance these perceived benefits, and the result was the first series of flavored sodas, including root beer, lemon, and ginger ale. Root beer was first produced for wide public sale, primarily in soda fountains, in 1876 and cola in 1881. In 1885, Charles Aderton introduced Dr. Pepper; in 1886, John Pemberton invented Coca-Cola,™ and, in 1898, Caleb Bradham formulated Pepsi-Cola.™ By the early 1920s, soft drinks were sold in six-packs for home consumption and in automatic vending machines.

SOFT-DRINK PRODUCTION

From 1970 to 1997, production of regular, sweetened soft drinks in the United States increased from 22.2 to 41.4 gallons per person per year, and the production of diet soft drinks increased from 2.1 to 11.6 gallons per person per year. These amounts mean that the annual per capita supply of 12-ounce soft drinks in the United States is equivalent to 442 regular and 124 diet drinks: a cumulative total of 566 cans of soft drinks per person each year (Nestle, 2000). Converted to gallons, the average American's 566-can soft-drink consumption totals 53 gallons per year, supporting a $60 billion industry that uses 12 billion gallons of water and employs 183,000 people nationally, most of them in the 500 bottling plants that dot the country, each producing 2000 soft drinks per minute (NSDA, 2006).

Contents

Regular soft drinks contain 90% and diet sodas 99% water. Carbon dioxide is dissolved in the water to enhance the flavor of the soft drink and provide its characteristic "bubbly" quality. It is typically the last ingredient added to soft drinks during manufacture. The term "soda" derives from the fact that carbon dioxide was originally made from sodium salts. The flavor of soft drink comes from formulas carefully guarded by the major manufacturers that consist of mixtures of natural oils and extracts, spices, herbs, and artificial flavorings. Food color is added to provide the desired hue, and acidulants, such as citric and phosphoric acid, are added to preserve the soda and give it a tart quality.

Sweeteners for regular soft drinks include sucrose and high-fructose corn syrup and make up 7 to 14% of soft-drink ingredients other than water. The principal sweeteners in diet sodas are aspartame (sold under the brand name NutriSweet) and sucralose (Splenda). The former has been in use since 1983 and is added at the rate of 15 mg per ounce. Sucralose was approved in 1998 and is 600 times sweeter than sugar. Other sweeteners include Acesulfame K (Sunnett), which is 200 times sweeter than sugar, and saccharin, which is 300 times sweeter. More sweeteners are currently in safety evaluation trials, including alitame, which is actually 2,000 times as sweet as sugar (NSDA, 2006). A final ingredient—our principal interest here—is caffeine. Caffeine is used in soft drinks because its bitter taste quality may actually enhance other flavors, but primarily because it provides the arousing effects that many drinkers desire. In fact, the manufacturers of Coca-Cola recognized the sales value of this quality even when Coke was in its infancy. At that time, however, the arousal agent in Coke was not caffeine but cocaine!

Caffeine Content

Use of *Cola acuminata*, the cola nut, during the manufacturing of soft drinks is partially responsible for the presence of natural caffeine in the final product. However, 95% of the caffeine in most soft drinks is added (Institute of Food Technologists' Expert Panel on Food Safety and Nutrition, 1983). Ounce for ounce, soft drinks are considerably lower in caffeine content than coffee or tea. This is, in part, because U.S. regulations restrict caffeine content of sodas to a maximum of 6 mg/ounce or 72 mg per 12-oz beverage. The two major colas, Coca-Cola and Pepsi-Cola, are among the lowest in caffeine content, with 45.6 and 37.2 mg/12 oz, respectively.

Among soft drinks sold in the United States, Jolt pushes the federal limit with 71.2 mg and Royal Crown's RC Edge is a close second with 70.2 mg. Mountain Dew (55 mg) and Surge (54 mg) are among those in a middle group. However, a caffeine-free version of Mountain Dew is now available. A number of soft drinks, including Coke and Pepsi and their diet versions, also have caffeine-free forms. Indeed, the advent of the caffeine-free soft drinks originated with increasing public concern over the health effects of caffeine. Table 2.13 shows the amount of caffeine found in common soft drinks.

ENERGY DRINKS: THE NEWEST TREND

Energy drinks are the most recent addition to the major sources of caffeine consumed. Typically, energy drinks are similar to traditional soft drinks, with three exceptions: they generally taste less sweet than soft drinks, generally have less carbonation than soft drinks, and often contain other stimulant drugs in addition to caffeine.

TABLE 2.13
Amount of Caffeine in 12 oz (333 ml) of Common Soft Drinks

Source	Caffeine (mg)	Source	Caffeine (mg)
Barq's	22	Ruby Red Squirt	39
Diet Barq's	0	Sun Drop	63
Cherry Coca-Cola	34	Diet Sun Drop	69
Coca-Cola Classic	34	Sunkist Orange Soda	41
Diet Coke	45	Tahitian Treat	<1
Diet Coke with Splenda	34	Mountain Dew	55
Coca-Cola Zero	34	Diet Mountain Dew	55
Coca-Cola C2	34	Pepsi-Cola	37
Mello Yello	51	Diet Pepsi-Cola	36
Diet Mr. Pibb	40	Pepsi One	55
TAB	47	Wild Cherry Pepsi	38
Vanilla Coke	34	Diet Wild Cherry Pepsi	36
Diet Vanilla Coke	45	AMP Energy Drink (8 oz)	75
Vault	70	Royal Crown Cola	43.2
A&W Crème Soda	29		
Diet A&W Crème Soda	22		
Dr. Pepper	41		
Diet Dr. Pepper	41		
IBC Cherry Cola	23		

Source: Adapted from NSDA. Retrieved March 13, 2006, from http://www.ameribev.org/.

HISTORY

Although the consumption of energy drinks has only recently become widespread, such drinks have a lengthy history, originating in the United Kingdom when the pharmaceutical giant Beecham (later of SmithKlineBeecham and eventually GlaxoSmithKline) first sold their *Lucozade* energy drink in 1938. Although the per capita consumption of energy drinks has been increasing, it is still low in the U.K. when compared with coffee and tea. The Japanese energy-drink market leader, Lipovitan, has been around since 1962 and currently has sales of 2 million bottles a day (Pharmiweb.com, 2006).

The overwhelming popularity of energy drinks in Japan and other Southeast Asian countries prompted Austrian businessman Dietrich Mateschitz to formulate and launch his Red Bull drink in Austria in 1987. Currently, Austria has one of the highest per-capita rates of energy-drink consumption, averaging approximately 3 L per capita annually. Red Bull was introduced into the United States in 1997, and approximately 300 drinks are available on shelves today (Corazza, 2006). With about 80 mg of caffeine in an 8-oz can, Red Bull was the first energy drink to see widespread consumption in Europe and North America.

In 1984, as an international marketing director for a German household-products company called Blendax (which was later bought by the American giant Proctor & Gamble), Mateschitz traveled to Thailand, where he met a Blendax licensee named Chaleo Yoovidhya. Yoovidhya sold a tonic drink, which he called Krating Daeng ("red water buffalo"), in his Thai pharmacies. Realizing the potential for this drink in Western markets, Mateschitz developed a partnership with Yoodihvya and, for the next 3 years, Mateschitz worked with the drink formula and developed a marketing strategy. Finally, in 1987 Red Bull was released in the Western market. For Western marketing purposes, Mateschitz decided to add carbonation and package Red Bull in a slim blue-and-silver can (Dolan, 2006).

PRODUCTION TRENDS

Following the drink's approval, Red Bull began to show up in retail outlets and bars across Austria. It soon spread to Hungary and the United Kingdom and, in 1994, entered the German market, where the drink became so popular that the company could not meet the demand of nearly 1 million cans a day. Sales doubled to 2 million cans the second year and doubled again to 4 million cans in 1996, its third year on the German market (Dolan, 2006). In some countries, Red Bull dominates with an 80% market share. Currently, it commands a 47% share of the U.S. energy-drink market, with sales growing annually at 40%. In 2005, 700 million cans of Red Bull were sold in the United States, and projected sales in 2006 were 1 billion cans (Dolan).

The energy-drink industry is not dominated by large companies, as seen in the soft-drink industry (and as will be seen later, the chocolate-candy industry), but instead is characterized by stiff competition among an increasing number of smaller companies, all catering to a very select consumer base. However, this has not stopped the major soft-drink companies, Pepsi and Coca-Cola, from attempting to enter the energy-drink industry. Pepsi produces SoBE Adrenaline Rush and AMP Energy Drink (a reformulation of Mountain Dew in energy-drink form). Coke produces a similar energy drink called Full Throttle. Sports bars have also recently started carrying Budweiser's B^E (Bud Energy), an energy-drink beer. As the major soft-drink manufacturers increase their production of energy drinks, it will be interesting to note whether the FDA decides to regulate energy-drink caffeine levels as it does those for soft drinks.

As a whole, the energy-drink industry caters to a younger market. The primary target for the majority of energy-drink companies is male teenagers and people in their 20s. Many energy-drink companies are also directing their products at very specific groups of consumers, such as extreme-sports enthusiasts, video-game players, and hip-hop fans. Advertising for most of these energy drinks has been limited to television ads. However, a number of energy-drink manufacturers also sponsor extreme events and publicity stunts to promote awareness of their product to the desired consumer group; other energy-drink companies rely on celebrity endorsements (Fact Expert, 2006).

CONTENTS AND CONCERNS

The caffeine levels in energy drinks range from 30 mg/250 ml to 150 mg/250 ml, depending on the brand. Red Bull, with 80 mg of caffeine, has more than double the dose found in the larger Coke serving (Dolan, 2006). This high caffeine content of some energy drinks relative to other foods and beverages containing caffeine is of concern. Due to the high caffeine levels of energy drinks, some authorities recommend that young children, people with heart disease, pregnant women (especially during the first 3 months of pregnancy), and those who are sensitive to caffeine avoid them.

What makes these energy drinks different from other sources of caffeine, such as soft drinks, tea, or coffee, is the content of stimulating herbal ingredients, such as taurine, guarana, and glucoronalactone. Some medical professionals believe that glucoranalactone is structurally similar to the popular club drug GHB (gamo hydroxy butyrate), a chemical solvent and dietary supplement popular for its relaxing and euphoric properties (Moffett, 2006). According to Project GHB, a Website dedicated to spreading awareness about the dangers of this drug, GHB overdoses have surpassed Ecstasy overdoses. Red Bull has 600 mg of glucoronalactone in one can; by comparison, a liter of wine has only 20 mg. Taurine is an amino acid found in the heart, brain, muscles, blood cells, and retina, and most energy drinks have 1000 mg of taurine per can; a typical diet rich in meat provides at most 40 to 400 mg of taurine a day. What concerns medical experts most about energy drinks is the combination of high caffeine levels and these unresearched herbal ingredients (Moffett).

Red Bull has been linked to deaths in Ireland, Australia, and Sweden. Of the three deaths documented in Sweden, one individual had consumed Red Bull shortly after exercising and the other two mixed alcohol with Red Bull. The multiple-stimulant cocktail found in energy drinks may raise heart rate and blood pressure more so than caffeine alone and may cause abnormal heart rhythms and stroke in older persons, resulting in death (Corazza, 2006). Important for future empirical research will be the derivation of a formula to measure the total stimulant load of the combination of caffeine and these herbal ingredients, perhaps derived from their overall effect on the reticular activating system. According to a 2004 Higher Education Center Study (Kapner, 2004), the stimulating effect of energy drinks mixed with alcohol can deceive people into believing that they are less intoxicated than they actually are, leading to the possibility of overconsumption, alcohol poisoning, or driving under the influence of alcohol.

Two other common ingredients of energy drinks also have raised concerns. Many energy drinks are sweetened with high-fructose corn syrup, which has been linked to increases in obesity and diabetes. They also contain citric acid, which can lead to tooth decay and heightened sensitivity. A study by the Academy of General Dentistry (AGD) found that energy drinks are more damaging to dental enamel than colas because they contain higher levels of citric acid (AGD.org). However, as of the publication date of this book, we are aware of no legislation passed to limit levels of citric acid (or that of caffeine, as mentioned previously) in energy drinks.

CHOCOLATE: "DIAMOND OF DESSERTS"

It is the rare man, woman, or child who does not at least occasionally delight in a savory chocolate mousse pie, the dense pleasure of a brownie, the unique sweetness of a chocolate bar, or the cool, smooth bliss of chocolate ice cream. The early Mayan and Aztec cultures called the cocoa plant *Theobroma cacao*, meaning "food of the gods" (Sweet Seductions Chocolatier, 2001). Indeed, chocolate—in all its various incarnations—has long been touted as the diamond of desserts, the gold of candies, and a fare fit for kings and queens. At the same time, it is a common source of calories and guilt— the bane of the dieter's existence.

HISTORY OF CHOCOLATE

Although the exact time and place at which chocolate appeared is unknown, it seems that the manufacture of chocolate originated between 3,000 and 4,000 years ago in Central America and the Amazon basin of South America; from there, it has spread across the world (Coe & Coe, 1996; Malgieri, 1998; The Chocolate Room, 2006). For centuries, it was used primarily as a beverage. It was not until the 19th century that chocolate in bars and other candy forms was introduced (Malgieri). The ancient Olmec civilization of Mexico was the first to process cocoa beans into a hot beverage. The Maya, Toltec, and Aztec peoples also adopted the use of cocoa. The Aztecs used chocolate in their religious rituals and used cocoa beans as a form of currency (Coe & Coe). By the fourth century, A.D., chocolate had gained importance in the Mayan culture as a highly desired food, and cocoa pods symbolized fertility.

By 1200 A.D., the Aztec culture virtually worshiped the cocoa tree, believing that the god Quetzalcoatl had descended to Earth, bringing the tree from paradise. However, he later lost his powers at the hands of another god and was relegated to returning to Earth only every 52 years. It happened that 1519, a year in which Quetzalcoatl was expected to return, was the year in which the Spanish explorer Cortez arrived. He was mistaken for the god and given hot cocoa to drink. He also discovered that the beans were often used as currency, a practice eventually used in Spain as well (Coe & Coe, 1996).

Cortez returned to Spain with cocoa beans, as had Columbus in 1502, and cocoa soon became a favorite drink, not only because of its flavor, but also because of the arousing effects it produced when consumed in large quantities. By the end of the 16th century, cocoa beans were being exported to Spain. During the 17th century, French and Italian missionaries brought cocoa with them to their home countries. Cocoa may have entered Great Britain via pirates, who, in the mid-16th century, raided Spanish ships returning from the Americas. Chocolate was approved by Pope Pius V in 1569 and became very popular in the French court of the 1600s under Louis XIV. It soon came into favor among the wealthy throughout Europe and eventually reached the general population. Cocoa drinking spread across Europe throughout the 18th century, and chocolate began to be used in making desserts. By 1755, American colonists had discovered chocolate, and the first U.S. chocolate factory opened in New England in 1765.

The origins of modern chocolate trace back to 19th century Holland, when Conrad van Houten developed a method of processing cocoa with alkali in 1828. Alkali processing gives cocoa powder a darker color and milder flavor. Later innovations in chocolate production came from Switzerland. Swiss chocolatier Daniel Peter developed milk chocolate in 1875; in 1879, fellow Swiss Rudolphe Lindt developed the process of conching cocoa powder (see later discussion) to make chocolate smoother (Coe & Coe, 1996). The next development in chocolate production was tempering, developed by fellow Swiss Gene Tobler. Tempering cocoa powder refers to blending the powder with cocoa butter to give the chocolate a richer taste. Prior to Tobler, another Swiss chocolatier named Daniel Peter had blended cocoa powder with Henri Nestle's dry milk powder to make "milk chocolate," which also had a richer taste.

Later, during World War I, the U.S. Army saw value in the energizing properties of chocolate and procured 20- to 40-pound blocks of it for distribution to the doughboys in Europe. It was this practice more than anything else that bolstered the chocolate industry in the United States because the soldiers came home wanting more chocolate and touting its virtues to others (Brenner, 1999).

The U.S. chocolate industry contributed much to the further development, refinement, and variety of chocolate. However, many of the developments remain trade secrets to this day. The U.S. chocolate candy market is dominated by two large companies—M&M/Mars and Hershey's—that collectively account for two thirds of domestic chocolate sales. These companies, founded by Forrest Mars and Milton Hershey, respectively, remain family run (M&M/Mars remains family owned; Hershey is now publicly owned, but remains family run) and both are highly secretive. Because the majority of these companies' secrets of chocolate production could not be protected by law, they maintain strict control over their manufacturing secrets, thus resembling the scenario of recluse chocolatier Willy Wonka in Roald Dahl's tale, "Charlie and the Chocolate Factory." Thus, little is known about the exact production of the majority of chocolate candy today (Brenner, 1999).

Milton Hershey founded Hershey's Chocolate Company in 1894. Hershey was the owner of Lancaster Caramel Company and produced caramels. However, after seeing the manufacture of chocolate at the 1893 World's Fair, he decided to enter the chocolate business. Chocolatiers had spent centuries attempting to produce milk chocolate, and Daniel Peter had only succeeded in using powdered milk. To this day, milk chocolate uses real milk (Hershey's contribution) as well as cocoa butter (Tobler's contribution) (Coe & Coe, 1996).

Forrest Mars founded M&M, Ltd., in 1940, using chocolate and equipment received from Hershey. Mars had already created the successful Mars Bar, but he wanted to develop a new chocolate candy and needed Hershey's connections to succeed. He was able to convince Hershey's president, William Murrie, that Murrie's name should go down in chocolate history. Murrie had been president of Hershey's for 50 years, but would never see his name on a product. Thus, Mars convinced him, to create a new candy called M&M, for Murrie & Mars. The "Murrie" in M&M actually referred to William Murrie's son, Charles, who was Mars's 20% partner in the new venture. The success of M&Ms made Mars Hershey's only serious competitor in an industry over which Hershey would have otherwise held a virtual monopoly. To this day, representatives from the two companies are said to communicate as little as possible with each other, stockholders, or the press, despite the fact that Hershey's is now publicly owned (Brenner, 1999).

GROWING AND PROCESSING CHOCOLATES

Theobroma cacao, the cocoa tree, belongs to the family Sterculiaceae. It was initially cultivated in areas of South America and arrived in Europe in the 16th century.

However, it is now found primarily in western Africa. The cacao tree, with its glossy leaves and small, pink flowers, grows to a height of 20 feet. If carefully protected and cultivated, this delicate tree will begin to produce fruit in its fifth year. It may then yield several harvests per year, but only 30 of about 6,000 blossoms produce the 12-inch pods containing the almond-shaped seeds that we call cocoa beans.

The tree *Theobroma cacao* is the single species responsible for cocoa powder and cocoa butter. *Cacao* is one of approximately 20 species in the *Theobroma* (Greek for "food of the gods") genus, but it is one of only two edible species in the genus. The other species, *Theobroma bicolor*, is used to make a beverage consumed in Central America, but it does not share the popularity of chocolate. Cacao trees today are grown around the world (including Africa, the Caribbean, Hawaii, South America, and the South Pacific), but only within 20° north and south of the equator. This is because the tree requires high temperatures, high humidity, and insects called midges, which pollinate the trees. Although *Theobroma* produces tufts of flowers all over its trunk and branches, only a small percentage of them produce fruit. Nonetheless, *Theobroma* flowers produce fruit throughout the year, not just during a limited growing season.

Cocoa powder is the basis for the various forms of chocolate with which we are all familiar, and the contents of many of these are partially regulated by law. In the United States, semisweet chocolate must contain a minimum of 35% chocolate liquor, and milk chocolate must be at least 10% chocolate liquor and 12% whole milk. White chocolate contains cocoa butter but no cocoa solids (Brenner, 1999). *Ganache* is a mixture of chocolate and hot cream that is often used as a filling in gourmet chocolate cakes; *couverture* contains at least 32% cocoa butter and is used by professionals as the thin, shiny chocolate coating on fruits and as the shell of gourmet filled chocolates.

To produce chocolate from cocoa beans, the fruits are split with a machete and the beans removed. These beans are allowed to ferment in covered piles on the ground. The goal of fermentation is the germination of the beans, which occurs at approximately 120°F. Germination causes the familiar chocolate flavor to develop. Following germination, the beans are uncovered and spread in the sunlight to dry out and halt the fermentation process. The next step in chocolate production is roasting, which may occur at the growing site or the factory where chocolate will be produced. Following roasting, the now papery husks are removed, which usually occurs through crushing cocoa beans into smaller pieces, called nibs, and allowing the husks to be removed and discarded easily (Coe & Coe, 1996).

The nibs are then crushed into "chocolate liquor," which is actually a solid at room temperature. For this reason, chocolate liquor is also known as "chocolate solids" and is sold directly to the public as unsweetened baking chocolate. Cocoa butter can be extracted from chocolate liquor for use in the production of chocolate candy or added to cosmetics, lotions, or sunblock. Following the removal of cocoa butter from chocolate liquor, the remaining dry cakes can be crushed to form cocoa powder. If alkali treatment occurs at this stage, the cocoa powder may be sold as "alkalized cocoa" or "Dutch processed cocoa."

Chocolate candy is made by not extracting cocoa butter from the chocolate liquor nibs, but instead adding sugar and vanilla to the nibs. Lecithin is then added

TABLE 2.14
Amount of Caffeine in Chocolate Sources

Source	Caffeine (mg)
Baking chocolate, unsweetened (1 oz–28 g)	57
Baker's baking chocolate, German sweet (1 oz–28 g)	8
Baker's baking chocolate, semisweet (1 oz–28 g)	13
Baker's chocolate chips, semisweet (1/4 c–43 g)	13
Baker's chocolate chips, German sweet (1/4 c–43 g)	15
Cadbury's chocolate bar (1 oz–8 g)	15
Milk chocolate bar (1/4 oz–7 g)	3–10
White chocolate bar (1/4 oz–7 g)	2–4
Dark chocolate bar (1/4 oz–7 g)	28
Chocolate milk, bought from store (8 oz–224 g)	8
Chocolate milk, made from mix (8 oz–224 g)	2–7
Chocolate syrup (2 T)	5
Cocoa (hot chocolate), made from mix with water or milk	4–6

Source: Adapted from Jean, A. T., Pennington, A. D. B., & Church, H. N. (1998). *Bowes & Church's food values of portions commonly used* (17th ed.). Philadelphia: Lippincott.

to emulsify the chocolate and thus keep it from separating. For the production of high-quality chocolate, extra cocoa butter is added at this stage. After all the ingredients are added, the chocolate mixture is conched, a process of rolling the cocoa between granite rollers that may last for several days. Conching decreases the bitterness and gives the chocolate a smoother taste and texture. Following conching, the chocolate must be tempered, a process that causes its molecules to retain their original shape following cooling. After the chocolate is tempered, it may be poured into molds and shaped into candy bars or other products (Coe & Coe, 1996).

CAFFEINE CONTENT

Because caffeine occurs naturally in cocoa beans, it is found in all chocolate products. Table 2.14 lists some of these products and their caffeine contents. Because many people eat chocolate in large quantities, it is clearly a dietary source of caffeine, though a much smaller source than coffee or tea. Due to the secrecy of the two major chocolate manufacturers, data on the levels of caffeine in chocolate products are limited (Barone & Roberts, 1984).

MEDICATIONS: CAFFEINE AS A MEDICINE

Caffeine is also an ingredient in many medications, including stimulants, diet aids, painkillers, and cold remedies. The largest amounts of caffeine are found in drugs sold specifically as stimulants intended to produce alertness and reduce feelings of

---

TABLE 2.15
Amount of Caffeine in a Variety of Medications

Over-the-counter medications	mg
Alka-Seltzer Morning Relief	65
Anacin Extra Strength	32
Anacin Pain Reliever	32
Cope Analgesic Pain Reliever	32
Excedrin Extra Strength	65
Excedrin Migraine	65
Excedrin Tension Headache	65
Goody's Extra Strength Headache Powders	32.5
Midol Maximum Strength	60
NoDoz Maximum Strength	200
Vanquish Extra-Strength Pain Reliever	33
Prescription medications	
Darvan Compound-65 Pulvule	32.4
Fiorecet	40
Fiorinal capsule	40
Fiorinal tablet	40
Hycomine compound tablet	30
Migranal (per ml)	10

Source: Adapted from *Harvard women's health watch* (2004).

---

fatigue. NoDoz and Vivarin are common examples of such medications. Caffeine is also used in diet aids to increase metabolism and suppress appetite and in pain medications to increase the overall effectiveness of a basic analgesic, such as aspirin. Table 2.15 shows the amount of caffeine in each of a number of nonprescription and prescription medications.

CONCLUSIONS

Activation of the central nervous system, resulting in increased arousal and accompanying alertness, can be accomplished in many ways—through intense exercise; strong stimuli, such as bright lights and loud sounds; anxiety-producing thoughts; and painful experiences, to name a few. However, perhaps the single most common source of intentional arousal incrementation is caffeine. It is found in a number of sources, including coffee, tea, soft drinks, energy drinks, chocolate, and certain medications, and its worldwide annual consumption reaches into the millions of tons. The remainder of this book provides an in-depth examination of caffeine from its processing in the body and impact on neurophysiological substrates to its effects on health in such areas as cardiovascular functioning, fertility, mood, and performance.

REFERENCES

AATea.com. (2001) Retrieved November 21, 2001, from www.aatea.com/white_tea_info.htm.

Academy of General Dentistry. New study indicates that popular sports beverages cause more irreversible damage to teeth than soda. http://www.agd.org/.

Arabee Coffee (2006). Retrieved June 30, 2006 from http://www.arabree.coffee.com/articles.cfm? AID = 7.

Barone, J. J., & Roberts, H. (1984). Human consumption of caffeine. In P. B. Dews (Ed.), *Caffeine: Perspectives from recent research*. Berlin: Springer–Verlag.

Brenner, J. G. (1999). The emperors of chocolate: Inside the secret world of Hershey and Mars. New York: Random House.

Bunker, M. L., & McWilliams, M. (1979). Sources of caffeine in common beverages. *Journal of the American Dietician, 74*, 28–32.

The Chocolate Room. Retrieved February 17, 2006, from http://www.thechocolateroom.com/functions. htm.

CNN Food. Retrieved March 13, 2006, from http://www.cnn.com/HEALTH/indepth.food/beverages/tea/.

Coe, S. D., & Coe, M. D. (1996). *The true history of chocolate*. New York: Thames & Hudson.

Coffee FAQ. (2006a). Retrieved February 17, 2006, from http://coffeefaq.com/caffaq.html.

Coffee FAQ. (2006b). Retrieved February 17, 2006, from http://coffeefaq.com/coffaq9.htm.

Coffee Research. Retrieved on March 13, 2006, from http://www.coffeeresearch.org/.

Community Integrated Pest Management. http://www.communityipm.org/.

Corazza, R. (2006). Energy drinks: The new coffee? *Idsnews*. http://www.idsnews.com.

Dolan. (March, 2005). The soda with buzz. *Forbes Magazine*. http://www.forbes.com.

Dufour, P. S. (1685). *Traitez noveaux & curieux du café, du the et du chocolate*. Lyons: Chez Jean Girin & B. Riviere.

European Fair Trade Association (2006). Retrieved June 30, 2006 from http://www.eftafairtrade.org/.

Every, A. H. (2001). The history of tea. Retrieved November 21, 2001, from http://hub-uk.com/interesting/teahistory.htm.

Fact Expert. (2006). Retrieved February 17, 2006, from http://energydrinks.factexpert.com/882-energy-drink-industry.php.

FAO. (2006a). Retrieved February 17, 2006, from http://www.fao.org/DOCREP/003/X6939E/X6939e02.htm.

FAO. (2006b). Retrieved February 17, 2006, from http://www.fao.org/newsroom/en/news/2005/105404/.

Garattini, S. (1993). *Caffeine, coffee, and health. Monographs of the Mario Negri Institute for Pharmacological Research*, Milan. New York: Raven Press.

Gepts, P. (2002). The crop of the day: Tea, *Camellia sinensis*. Retrieved February 17, 2006, from http://www.agronomy.ucdavis.edu/gepts/pb143/CROP/Tea/Tea.htm.

Goodman, L. E. (1992). *Avicenna*. London: Routledge.

Hawaiian Agricultural Products. (http://hawaiianagriculturalproducts.com/).

Hu, S. Y. (1979). The botany of Yaupon. In C. M. Hudson (Ed.), *Black drink*. Athens: University of Georgia Press.

Hudson, C. M. (1979). Introduction. In C. M. Hudson (Ed.), *Black drink.* Athens: University of Georgia Press.

ICO. (2006). Retrieved February 17, 2006, from http://www.ico.org/caffeine.asp.

In Pursuit of Tea. (2006). Retrieved February 17, 2006, from http://www.inpursuitoftea.com/category_s/25.htm.

Institute of Food Technologists Expert Panel of Food Safety and Nutrition. (1983).

James, J. E. (1997). *Understanding caffeine.* Thousand Oaks, CA: Sage Publications.

Jean, A. T., Pennington, A. D. B., & Church, H. N. (1998). *Bowes & Church's food values of portions commonly used* (17th ed.). Philadelphia: Lippincott.

Kaldi Coffee. (2006). Retrieved February 17, 2006, from http://www.kaldi.com.au/.

Kapner, D. (April 2004). Ephedra and energy drinks on college campuses. U.S. Department of Education. http://www.edc.org.

Lee, S., & Levine, J. (2000). How about a nice $10 cuppa tea? *Forbes, 166,* 362.

Lipton Tea Company. (2006). Retrieved February 17, 2006, from http://www.lipton.tea.com.

Malgieri, N. (1998). *Chocolate: From simple cookies to extravagant showstoppers.* New York: HarperCollins Publishers.

Moffett, E. (2006). In the Red: Energy drinks and alcohol. Is it all a big mix-up? *The NU Comment.* Retrieved June 30, 2006 from http://www.nucomment.com.

National Geographic Society. (2006). *African Origins.* Retrieved February 17, 2006, from http://www.nationalgeographic.com/coffee/legend1.html.

NCAUSA. (2006a). Retrieved February 17, 2006, from http://www.ncausa.org/i4a/pages/index.cfm?pageid=68.

NCAUSA. (2006b). Retrieved February 17, 2006, from http://www.ncausa.org/i4a/pages/index.cfm?pageid=67.

Nescafe. (2006). Retrieved February 17, 2006, from http://www.nescafe.co.uk/coffee_world/origins/index.asp.

Nestle, Marion. (2000). Soft drink pouring rights: Marketing empty calories. *Public Health Reports 2000.* Oxford University Press.

NewCROP http://www.hort.purdue.edu/newcrop/default.html/.

North Coast Coffee. (2006). Retrieved February 17, 2006, from http://www.northcoastcoffee.com/ACKaldi.htm.

NSDA. (2006). Retrieved February 17, 2006, from http://www.ameribev.org/.

Owen, D. (2006). *Coffee and caffeine FAQ.* Retrieved on February 17, 2006, from http://72.14.203.104/search?q=cache:1v5Vl7Ia0zAJ:coffeefaq.com/coffaq.htm+Coffee+FAQ&hl=en&gl=us&ct=clnk&cd=2.

Pharmiweb.com. Energy drinks. http://www.pharmiweb.co.uk.

Rasmussen, W., & Rhinehart, R. (1998). *Tea basics: A quick & easy guide.* New York: John Wiley & Sons.

The Roast and Post Coffee Company. (2006). Retrieved February 17, 2006, from http://www.realcoffee.co.uk/Article.asp?Cat=History&Page=1.

Sally's Place. (2006). Retrieved February 17, 2006, from http://www.sallys-place.com/beverages/coffee/right_for_you.htm.

Smith, B. D., Osborne, A., Mann, M., Jones, H., & White, T. (2004). Arousal and behavior: Biopsychological effects of caffeine. In A. Nehlig (Ed.), *Coffee, tea, chocolate, and the brain* (pp. 35–52). Boca Raton, FL: CRC Press.

Spiller, G. A. (1998). *Caffeine.* New York: CRC Press.

Stashtea. (2006). Retrieved February 17, 2006, from http://www.stashtea.com/facts.htm.

Sweet Seductions Chocolatier. (2001). Retrieved December 18, 2001, from http://sweet-seductions.co.uk/info/beans/history.html.

Tea and Coffee. http://www.teaandcoffee.net/.

The Tea House. (2006). Retrieved February 17, 2006, from http://www.theteahouse.com/ topics.htm.

Ukers, W. H. (1935). *All about coffee.* New York: The Tea and Coffee Trade Journal Company.

USDA (United States Department of Agriculture). (2006). Retrieved February 17, 2006, from http://www.fas.usda.gov/htp/tropical/2005/12-05/december%202005%20text.pdf.

Wikipedia. (2006). Retrieved February 17, 2006, from http://en.wikipedia.org/wiki/Camellia.

3 Pharmacological Properties and Neurophsysiological Effects of Caffeine

Astrid Nehlig

CONTENTS

SUMMARY

At doses relevant to the general human consumption, caffeine exerts most of its pharmacological effects by acting as an antagonist at the level of adenosine A1 and A2a receptors. A1 receptors are widely distributed throughout the brain and inhibit the release of neurotransmitters; A2a receptors are mostly restricted to the striatum where they colocalize in a selective population of neurons with dopamine D2 receptors.

The functions most sensitive to low doses of caffeine are locomotor activity, sleep, and mood. At higher doses, caffeine may trigger anxiety, especially in a subset of sensitive individuals. Caffeine given acutely acts as a proconvulsant and chronic exposure to caffeine increases seizure threshold and has neuroprotective properties.

Such opposite effects between acute and chronic exposure to caffeine are also seen in models of ischemia, with the chronic treatment affording neuroprotective effects. Caffeine consumption delays or prevents the occurrence of Parkinson's disease and reinforces the efficiency of the classical dopaminergic treatment of the disease. Finally, the regular level of consumption of caffeine does not activate the brain structures involved in addiction and reward; rather, caffeine appears to be used by individuals to manage mood state, vigilance, and energy over the course of a day.

INTRODUCTION

Caffeine is the most widely consumed psychoactive substance in the world. More than 80% of the world's population, irrespective of age, gender, geography, or culture, consumes caffeine daily (Benowitz, 1990; James, 1991). The consumption of caffeine occurs in a variety of forms—that is, drinking coffee, tea, mate, or soft drinks, chewing cola nuts, consuming cocoa products, or taking over-the-counter pain or slimming medications. The mean daily caffeine consumption for adult consumers reaches 2.4 to 4.0 mg/kg in North America and the United Kingdom and up to 7.0 mg/kg in Scandinavia (Barone & Roberts, 1996; Debry, 1994; Viani, 1996). In Scandinavia, more than 80% of the caffeine consumed comes from coffee, while in the United Kingdom, 55% comes from tea and about 43% from coffee; the remaining 2% comes from cola drinks (Barone & Roberts). Among children under 18, the mean daily intake of caffeine is about 1.0 mg/kg in the United States and less than 2.5 mg/kg in Denmark (Barone & Roberts).

Mild positive subjective effects such as self-rated feelings of well-being, calmness, alertness, energy, and ability to concentrate occur at low to moderate doses of caffeine (50 to 300 mg, i.e., one to three cups of coffee) (Zwyghuizen–Doorenbos, Roehrs, Lipschutz, Timms, & Roth, 1990). At high doses (400 to 800 mg), rather negative feelings such as anxiety, nervousness, jitteriness, and insomnia are reported, especially in volunteers who are usually caffeine abstinent (Fredholm, Bättig, Holmen, Nehlig, & Zvartau, 1999; Lieberman, Wurtman, Emde, & Coviella, 1987). On the basis of recent data of the literature, the focus of this chapter will be to describe the pharmacological properties of caffeine underlying its mechanism of action and to detail some of the neurophysiological properties of the methylxanthine.

PHARMACOLOGICAL PROPERTIES OF CAFFEINE

Several biochemical mechanisms of action of caffeine have been described; in chronological order of their discovery, they are the release of intracellular calcium; inhibition of cyclic nucleotide phosphodiesterases; and, finally, antagonism at the level of adenosine receptors. The direct action of caffeine on the release of intracellular calcium, probably via an action at ryanodine receptors, occurs only at millimolar concentrations. Also, the inhibition of cyclic nucleotide phosphodiesterases needs rather high concentrations in the high micromolar to millimolar range that cannot be attained during normal caffeine consumption (Fredholm et al., 1999; Nehlig & Debry, 1994). The only mechanism of action of caffeine that is significantly affected at normal doses of human caffeine consumption is the antagonism at adenosine receptors (Fredholm, 1980, 1995).

REGULATION OF ADENOSINE CONCENTRATIONS IN THE BRAIN

If the consumption of caffeine is blocking the actions of endogenous adenosine at its receptors, it implies that adenosine must be present at levels high enough to activate adenosine receptors under basal conditions. Adenosine is a normal cellular constituent and its concentration is regulated by the balance of several enzymes (for review, see Fredholm, 1995, and Fredholm et al., 1999). Adenosine acts on four main subtypes of receptors—A1, A2a, A2b, and A3—that have been cloned and characterized in several species (Fredholm, et al., 1994; Fredholm, Chen, Cunha, et al., 2005). In humans and rats, the levels of the A3 receptor are low and this subtype is little affected by many methylxanthines, including caffeine (KDs of 80 and 190 μM in the human and rat brains, respectively).

However, these receptors may be involved in pathological situations leading to large release of adenosine such as ischemia or seizures. Likewise, the blockade of the A2b receptor requires amounts of caffeine higher than those found in normal caffeine consumption patterns. These receptors may be affected by endogenous adenosine and also caffeine under pathological conditions (Fredholm et al., 1999; Fredholm, Chen, Cunha, et al., 2005). Conversely, A1 and A2a receptors are activated at low basal conditions of adenosine and are likely to be major targets for caffeine.

Distribution and Properties of Adenosine A1 and A2a Receptors

A1 and A2a receptors are coupled to G-proteins. The A1 receptor is coupled to the pertussis toxin-sensitive G-proteins G_{i-1}, G_{i-2}, G_{i-3}, G_{o1}, and G_{o2}. Activation of A1 receptors leads to inhibition of adenylyl cyclase and of some types of voltage-sensitive Ca^{2+}-channels, such as the N- and Q-channels, and activation of several types of K^+-channels, phospholipase C, and phospholipase D that will cause a large variety of cellular effects. Conversely, A2a receptors are associated with G_s-proteins and their activation will induce activation of adenylyl cyclase and possibly of the L-type Ca^{2+}-channel (Fredholm et al., 1994, 1999; Fredholm, 1995). A recent study showed also the coupling of the A2a receptor with the Golf protein at the level of the striatum (Kull, Svenningsson, & Fredholm, 2000).

Adenosine A1 and A2a receptors have different regional distributions in the brain. A1 receptors are present in nearly all brain regions, with highest levels found in hippocampus, cerebral and cerebellar cortex, and certain thalamic nuclei and quite low levels in striatum (caudate-putamen and nucleus accumbens) (Goodman & Snyder, 1982; Fastbom, Pazos, & Palacios, 1987; Ochiishi et al., 1999). The corresponding mRNA is distributed partly in a different way (Mahan et al., 1991; Reppert, Weaver, Stehle, & Rivkees, 1991); this indicates that some A1 receptors are located on nerve terminals rather than on cell bodies (Johansson et al., 1993), thus mediating inhibition of transmitter release on neurons (Fredholm & Dunwiddie, 1988).

Finally, adenosine A1 receptors (negatively coupled to adenylyl cyclase) are colocalized with dopamine D1 receptors (positively coupled to adenylyl cyclase) in the neurons of the striatum that contain GABA, substance P, and dynorphin and project directly to the substantia nigra; this represents the anatomical basis of functional interactions between adenosine and dopamine (Ferré et al., 1997; Salmi, Chergui, & Fredholm, 2005). Thus, stimulation of adenosine A1 receptors blocks the stimulatory effect induced by dopamine D1 receptor agonists on behavior (Ferré, et al., 1994, 1998) and electroencephalographic (EEG) arousal (Popoli et al., 1996a). Conversely, blockade of adenosine A1 receptors potentiates the motor stimulation induced by a dopamine D1 receptor agonist (Popoli et al., 1996b).

Adenosine A2a receptors, both the protein and the gene, are found in neurons and some glial cells, mainly in the dorsal striatum, nucleus accumbens, globus pallidus, and olfactory tubercle (Jarvis & Williams, 1989; Svenningsson, Le Moine, et al., 1997). The A2a receptors (positively coupled to adenylyl cyclase) are mainly located in dopamine-rich regions and colocalize with dopamine D2 receptors (negatively coupled to adenylyl cyclase) in medium-size spiny neurons expressing GABA and enkephalin, which project to the globus pallidus. This colocalization is present in the dorsal striatum (Johansson et al., 1993; Schiffmann, Jacobs, & Vanderhaegen, 1991), nucleus accumbens, and olfactory tubercle (Svenningsson, Le Moine, et al., 1997).

Regulation of the activity of these neurons depends on the balance between A2a and D2 receptors. The two populations of receptors interact; for example, the activation of A2a receptors decreases the affinity of dopamine binding to D2 receptors (Ferré, von Euler, Johansson, Fredholm, & Fuxe, 1991). They also interact for the release of GABA; indeed, administration of dopamine in the striatum blocks the release of GABA in the globus pallidus (Ferré, O'Connor, Fuxe, & Ungerstedt, 1993) and this effect is reduced by endogenous adenosine.

Likewise, activation of A2a receptors stimulates GABA release from striatal slices (Mayfield, Suzuki, & Zahniser, 1993). Adenosine A2a receptors are also present in some cholinergic interneurons of the striatum (Preston et al., 2000). Stimulation of dopamine D1 receptors or adenosine A2a receptors and blockade of dopamine D2 receptors increase the protein kinase A (PKA)-dependent phosphorylation of DARPP-32 (dopamine- and cyclic AMP-regulated phosphoprotein of 32,000 kDa) that appears to be an important molecular target for integration of adenosine and dopamine signaling (Fredholm, Chen, Cunha, et al., 2005; Salmi et al., 2005).

Properties of Adenosine A1 and A2a Receptors and Actions of Caffeine on Adenosine Receptors

At the low concentrations reached after consumption of one or two cups of coffee, caffeine acts as a nonspecific antagonist of A1 and A2a adenosine receptors (Fredholm, 1995; Fredholm et al., 1999). Adenosine, by acting at the level of presynaptic A1 receptors, was first shown to inhibit the release of numerous neurotransmitters such as glutamate, GABA, acetylcholine, and monoamines. Adenosine acts more efficiently at the level of excitatory than inhibitory neurotransmission (Fredholm & Dunwiddie, 1988; Fredholm & Hedqvist, 1980). As a result of activation of adenosine A1 receptors (Dunwiddie, 1985), adenosine acts to decrease the rate of firing of central neurons (Phillis & Edstrom, 1976).

Recent studies confirmed that hyperactivity of glutamatergic fibers in the striatum promotes release of adenosine, which inhibits glutamatergic transmission. Such inhibition is lost in adenosine A1 receptor KO mice. Adenosine appears to depress synaptic transmission only via activation of A1 receptors (Fredholm, Chen, Masino, & Vaugeois, 2005; Salmi et al., 2005). The same mechanism of presynaptic blockade of glutamate release was confirmed in the hippocampus of mice in which A1 receptors were focally deleted in CA1 and CA3 (Scammel et al., 2003). Caffeine increases the turnover of monoamines such as serotonin, dopamine, and noradrenaline (Fernström & Fernström, 1984; Haldfield & Milio, 1989). Caffeine enhances also the firing rate of noradrenergic neurons of the locus coeruleus (Grant & Redmond, 1982) and of mesocortical cholinergic neurons (Rainnie, Grunze, McCarley, & Greene, 1994). These effects may reflect changes in the pattern of the EEG arousal induced by caffeine ingestion.

The affinity of caffeine is higher at the adenosine A2a receptor (2 and 8 μM in the human and rat brains, respectively) than at the A1 receptor (12 and 20 μM) (Fredholm et al., 1999). The action of caffeine on adenosine A2a receptors regulates dopaminergic transmission by caffeine (Salmi et al., 2005) and mediates most of its central effects (Svenningsson, Nomikos, & Fredholm, 1995; Svenningsson, Nomikos, Ongini, & Fredholm 1997). The effect of low doses of caffeine is restricted to the striatopallidal neurons that contain A2a receptors and is not present in striatonigral neurons that contain A1 receptors (Svenningsson, Nomikos et al., 1997). Conversely, high doses of caffeine induce expression of an immediate early gene, *c-fos*, in striatal neurons containing A1/D1 and those containing A2a/D2 receptors (Johansson, Lindström, & Fredholm, 1994). This confirms that, at high doses, caffeine acts on both types of adenosine receptors.

NEUROPHYSIOLOGICAL EFFECTS OF CAFFEINE

EFFECTS OF CAFFEINE ON LOCOMOTOR ACTIVITY

The effects of caffeine on locomotor activity have been reported for a long time and extensively studied (for review, see Nehlig, Daval, & Debry, 1992; Nehlig & Debry, 1994; and Fredholm et al., 1999). Locomotor activity mediated by the activity of the nigrostriatal dopaminergic system is very sensitive to caffeine, and functional activity in the striatum is increased by doses of caffeine as low as 1 mg/kg in the rat (Nehlig & Boyet, 2000). These very low doses are also able to modify the spontaneous electrical activity of striatal neurons (Hirsh, Forde, & Chou, 1982) and to induce dopamine release in this region (Okada, Mizuno, & Kaneko, 1996; Okada et al., 1997).

The effects of caffeine on spontaneous locomotor activity are biphasic. Low doses (1.5 to 20 mg/kg) increase the activity, but doses higher than 30 mg/kg decrease it (Nehlig et al., 1992; Nehlig & Debry, 1994). The increase in locomotor activity at low doses of caffeine depends upon inhibition of the adenosine A2a receptor. Indeed, administration of various selective A2a antagonists (El Yacoubi, Ledent, Ménard, et al., 2000; El Yacoubi, Ledent, Parmentier, Costentin, & Vaugeois, 2000a; Griebel, Misslin, & Vogel, 1991; Seale, Abla, Shamim, Carney, & Daly, 1988) increases locomotor activity, sometimes more efficiently than caffeine; adenosine A2a agonists depress locomotor activity (Nicojevic, Srages, Daly, & Jacobson, 1991). Likewise, A2a receptor KO mice exhibit a decrease in exploratory behavior (Ledent et al., 1997) and caffeine is unable to induce locomotor stimulant effects in these mice (Halldner et al., 2004), pointing to the critical role of A2a receptors in regulation of this function.

On the other hand, the selective A1 antagonist, DPCPX, does not affect (Griebel, Saffroy–Spitler, et al., 1991; Janusz & Berman, 1993) or decrease locomotor activity (El Yacoubi et al., 2000a), leading to the hypothesis that the motor depressant effect obtained at high doses of caffeine might be mediated by action at A1 receptors. Recent studies using adenosine A1 and/or A2a receptor KO mice showed that the A1 receptor seems rather to modulate the stimulatory effect of caffeine exerted via A2a blockade; the inhibitory effect of high doses of caffeine on locomotion is independent from the blockade of A1 or A2a adenosine receptors (Halldner et al., 2004) and possibly involves A3 receptors (Jacobson et al., 1993).

The close interaction between adenosine and dopamine neurotransmission in the striatonigral system has been mainly shown in studies on the rotation behavior induced by unilateral nigrostriatal dopamine denervation. Caffeine can induce con-traversive rotation in animals with unilateral nigrostriatal dopamine lesions, thus mimicking the effects of dopamine receptor agonists like apomorphine with a max-imum activity recorded at the dose of 30 to 50 mg/kg (Casas, Ferré, Cobos, Grau, & Jané, 1989a, b; Fredholm, Herrera–Marschitz, Jonzon, Lindström, & Ungerstedt, 1983; Garrett & Holtzman, 1994; Herrera–Marschitz, Casas, & Ungerstedt, 1988). This effect of caffeine is the consequence of adenosine receptor blockade.

Indeed, injection of an adenosine analog into the striatum induces rotation in the direction opposite (Brown, Gill, Evenden, Iversen, & Richardson, 1991; Green, Proudfit, & Yeung, 1982) to that induced by caffeine (Herrera–Marschitz et al., 1988; Josselyn & Beninger, 1991). Likewise, inhibitors of adenosine transport and ade-nosine deaminase that raise the brain level of adenosine reduce the rotation behavior induced by dopaminergic drugs (Fredholm et al., 1999).

EFFECTS OF CAFFEINE ON SLEEP

Hypnotic effects of adenosine are well documented. Adenosine accumulates in extracellular space during spontaneous and forced wakefulness and decreases during sleep (Porkka–Heiskanen et al., 1997; Porkka–Heiskanen, Strecker, & McCarley, 2000). Adenosine agonists and drugs that prevent adenosine elimination increase sleep and alter the EEG pattern (O'Connor, Stojanovic, & Radulovacki, 1991; Radulovacki, 1985) while caffeine has opposite effects (Yanik, Glaum, & Radulovacki, 1987; Porkka–Heiskanen, Alanko, Kalinchicuk, & Sternberg, 2002). Sleep is one of the functions most sensitive to ingestion of caffeine, which delays its onset (for review, see Snel, 1993, and Snel, Tieges, & Lorist, 2004).

The property of caffeine to increase wakefulness is one of the reasons why people consume daily caffeine and also represents one of the reasons why certain people limit ingestion of caffeine-containing drinks (Soroko, Chang, & Barrett–Connor, 1996). The natural daily pattern of caffeine consumption shows highest intake between 8:00 a.m. and 12:00 p.m., followed by a progressive decrease (Brice & Smith, 2002). The high sensitivity of sleep to caffeine is reflected by the selective increase in brain functional activity in the serotoninergic cell groupings, the dorsal and medial raphe nuclei that mediate sleep (Reinis & Goldman, 1982), which appears after a dose of 1 mg/kg caffeine in rats (Nehlig & Boyet, 2000).

These data are in accordance with the fact that caffeine increases the firing rate of noradrenergic neurons in the locus coeruleus (Grant & Redmond, 1982), thus affecting activity of mesocortical cholinergic neurons (Rainnie et al., 1994) and changing the pattern of EEG arousal. Likewise, caffeine reduces serotonin availability at postsynaptic receptor sites (Hirsh, 1984), which elicits a reduction in the sedative effects of the amine and affects sleep and motor functions (Gerson & Baldessarini, 1980; Jouvet, 1969). At low doses, caffeine lowers also electrical activity in the medial thalamus, which is an important site for arousal induced by caffeine (Chou, Forde, & Hirsh, 1980).

In humans, caffeine in doses as low as 100 mg (the content of one cup of coffee) taken at bedtime increases sleep latency and decreases the quality of sleep together with changes in the EEG pattern, especially during deep sleep (Landolt, Dijk, Gaus, & Borbely, 1995). Even morning caffeine can disturb sleep (Landolt, Werth, Borbely, & Dijk, 1995). However, the sleep-disturbing effects of caffeine do not seem to be different in normal or poor sleepers (Tiffin, Ashton, Marsh, & Kamali, 1995). The sleep EEG remains disturbed by caffeine usually during 3 to 4 h, which corresponds to the usual time of metabolism of the methylxanthine (Müller–Limmroth, 1972). Individuals whose sleep is mostly disturbed by caffeine could be those that metabolize the methylxanthine slowly (Levy & Zylber–Katz, 1983).

However, one recent study performed in real-life conditions reported that consumption of up to seven or eight cups of coffee (i.e., 600 mg caffeine daily) is not associated with a reduction in sleep time (Sanchez–Ortuno et al., 2005). More studies in real-life conditions are necessary to support these conclusions. Finally, slow-release 300-mg caffeine tablets given twice daily counteract deleterious consequences of sleep deprivation, increase intellectual performance, and maintain vigilance during continuous work that interferes with a normal sleep–wake rhythm (Beaumont et al., 2001).

It is widely accepted that activation of A1 and A2a adenosine receptors contributes to the capacity of adenosine to produce sedation or sleep (Porkka–Heiskanen et al., 1997, 2002; Radulovacki, 1985; Satoh, Matsumura, Suzuki, & Hayaishi, 1996). In rodents, adenosine analogs seem to facilitate sleep time in response to hypnotic drugs rather than to cause a direct deep hypnotic effect (Dunwiddie, 1985). Adenosine could rather act as a transient signal to go to sleep. Indeed, adenosine, its metabolizing enzymes, and receptors all undergo circadian rhythms (for review, see Fredholm et al., 1999) and are regulated by sleep. Adenosine levels increase in the cat forebrain during prolonged wakefulness and return to normal levels during sleep (Basheer, Porkka–Heiskanen, Strecker, Thakkar, & McCarley, 2000; Porkka–Heiskanen et al., 1997).

Adenosine A1 receptors may mostly act at the level of mesopontine cholinergic neurons under tonic adenosine A1 receptor control (Rainnie et al., 1994). Caffeine is known to increase dose-dependently the hippocampal and cortical level of acetylcholine (Carter, O'Connor, Carter, & Ungerstedt, 1995; Murray, Blaker, Cheney, & Costa, 1982); this mechanism most probably underlies the psychostim-ulant and awakening effects of caffeine (Carter et al., 1995). Injection of an A2a receptor agonist in the subarachnoid space underlying the basal forebrain has sleep-promoting effects and A2a antagonists attenuate sleep induced by prostaglandin D2 (Satoh et al., 1996; Satoh, Matsumura, & Hayaishi, 1998) and increase wakefulness and latency to REM sleep in rats, as the A1 antagonists also do (Bertorelli, Ferri, Adami, & Ongini, 1996). More recent studies on adenosine receptor KO mice reported that the arousal effect of caffeine depends on adenosine A2a receptors (Huang et al., 2005). The site of action of A2a receptors on sleep-promoting mech-anisms has been hypothesized to be the ventral nucleus accumbens and olfactory tubercle (Satoh et al., 1996).

EFFECTS OF CAFFEINE ON MOOD AND ANXIETY

Low doses of caffeine act positively on mood; subjects ingesting 20 to 200 mg of caffeine report that they feel energetic, imaginative, efficient, self-confident, alert, able to concentrate, and motivated to work (Casas, Ramos–Quiroga, Prat, & Qureshi, 2004; Griffiths et al., 1990; Griffiths & Mumford, 1995; Silverman, Mumford, & Griffiths, 1994). Positive effects of low doses of caffeine (40 to 60 mg) on perfor-mance and well-being may be more beneficial in situations of low arousal, such as the postlunch decrease in vigilance, the common cold (Smith, 1994; Smith, Rusted, Eaton–Williams, Savory, & Leathwood, 1990; Smith, Sturgess, & Gallagher, 1999; Smith, Thomas, Perry, & Whitney, 1997), and fatigue in drivers (Reyner & Horne, 2000) or during attention-requiring tasks (Lorist, Snel, Kok, & Mulder, 1994).

The alerting effects of caffeine are also able to reverse the deleterious effects of 36-h sleep deprivation (Patat et al., 2000), and moderate doses of caffeine were reported to improve mood state in U.S. Navy volunteers subjected to severe envi-ronmental stress and sleep deprivation (Lieberman, Tharion, Shukitt–Hale, Speckman, & Tulley, 2002). The latter two studies show that caffeine can improve mood even in adverse situations. Conversely, after high doses (400 to 600 mg), the effects of caffeine are rather negative (Loke, 1988; James, 1991) and, in a situation of free choice, subjects preferentially choose capsules containing 50, 100, or 200 mg of caffeine over those containing 400 mg while avoiding those containing 600 mg (Griffiths & Woodson, 1988a).

The influence of low doses of caffeine on mood correlates with the increase in cerebral functional activity recorded in the noradrenergic locus coeruleus and the serotoninergic median and dorsal raphe nuclei involved in regulation of wakefulness, mood, and well-being (Reinis & Goldman, 1982) after administration of 1 mg/kg of caffeine to rats (Nehlig & Boyet, 2000). Moreover, caffeine releases serotonin in limbic areas and dopamine in the cortex, an effect also obtained with antidepressants (Acquas, Tanda, & Di Chiara, 2002; Casas et al., 2004; Fredholm, 1995).

Caffeine has been reported to generate anxiety when absorbed in excessive amounts in the general population or in low doses in specifically sensitive individuals (for review, see Hughes, 1996). Individuals who do not consume caffeine or consume only low amounts appear to be more sensitive to caffeine's anxiogenic and psycho-stimulant effects than usual consumers (Uhde, 1990). The level of anxiety is also more markedly increased by caffeine in naturally anxious individuals or subjects suffering from panic attacks compared to the normal population (for review, see Nehlig & Debry, 1994). These individuals show the tendency to reduce or stop their caffeine intake because of the secondary unpleasant effects of the methylxanthine (Uhde, 1990), and their health status clearly improves after caffeine cessation (Bruce & Lader, 1989).

In sensitive subjects, panic attacks can occur after absorption of a single cup of coffee (80 to 110 mg of caffeine) (Uhde, 1988); however, in normal individuals, only caffeine doses higher than normal consumption levels can induce significant anxiogenic effects (James & Crosbie, 1987). The variable interindividual responses to the anxiogenic effects of caffeine relate to the polymorphism of the A2a receptor gene (Alsene, Deckert, Sand, & de Witt, 2003).The well-known effect of caffeine on anxiety correlates with significant increase in functional activity in the amygdala, a structure known to mediate fear and anxiety (Davis, 1992) after a moderate dose of caffeine in the rat (2.5 mg/kg) (Nehlig & Boyet, 2000).

In animals, caffeine has been shown to generate anxiety in mice and rats (for review, see Nehlig & Debry, 1994). The anxiogenic effect of caffeine could result from a simultaneous blockade of adenosine A1 and A2a receptors (Jain, Kemp, Adeyemo, Buchanan, & Stone, 1995), although some argue for a more prominent role of A2a receptors (Griebel, Saffroy–Spitter, et al., 1991; Imaizumi, Miyazaki, & Onodera, 1994). Indeed, A2a receptor KO mice were more anxious than their wild-type controls in two behavioral tests rating anxiety level (El Yacoubi, Ledent, Parmentier, Costentin, & Vaugeois, 2000b; Ledent et al., 1997). However, this elevated level of anxiety in A2a receptor KO mice could not be reproduced in a wild-type strain of mice administered A2a receptor antagonists (El Yacoubi et al., 2000b).

Data on adenosine A1 receptors are discordant. Although a preferential role of A1 receptors in modulation of anxiety was suggested (Florio, Prezioso, Papaioannou, & Bertua, 1998), A1 receptor agonists can be without effect (El Yacoubi et al., 2000b) or anxiolytic (Jain et al., 1995), depending on the strain of mice. Adenosine A1 receptor KO mice exhibit increased anxiety (Gimenez–Llort et al., 2002), which is consistent with the anxiogenic effects of high doses of caffeine expected to block most of both types of adenosine receptors; low doses block only A2a receptors (Fredholm et al., 1999). Thus, other mechanisms than the antagonism at adenosine receptors are likely to be involved in the anxiogenic effects of caffeine. The noradrenergic system is involved in this effect (Baldwin & File, 1989). High levels of caffeine can also decrease the binding of benzodiazepines, but this effect would not directly produce anxiety (Daly, 1993).

EFFECTS OF CAFFEINE ON DEPRESSION

The relationship between caffeine intake and depression remains a controversial issue. As described earlier, caffeine affects sleep and one of the major predictors for depression is sleep disorders (Chang, Ford, Mead, Cooper–Patrick, & Klag, 1997). However, it is not clear whether caffeine intake is related to depression; indeed, in one study, the relationship between poor sleep and depression remained after correction for caffeine intake (Chang et al., 1997); in another, there was a correlation between symptoms of depression and caffeine intake (Rihs, Muller, & Baumann, 1996).

Coffee drinking is negatively correlated with suicide (Kawachi, Willett, Colditz, Stampfer, & Speizer, 1996). However, it is not demonstrated yet whether caffeine exerts a direct effect on depressive symptoms including suicide or if depressive individuals spontaneously reduce their caffeine intake, as anxious subjects do. Moreover, in depressive patients, consumption of coffee may partly be used to counteract some side effects of medication such as dry mouth (Leviton, 1983; Stephenson, 1977).

Adenosinergic mechanisms may be involved in depression. Indeed, the A2a receptor is present mostly in the striatum in which it colocalizes with the dopamine D2 receptor. The antidepressant drugs most commonly used act at the level of the neuronal transporters of serotonin and dopamine (Richelson, 1994) and enhance the mesolimbic dopaminergic neurotransmission via D2 receptors (Willner, 1997). Because A2a and D2 receptors exert antagonistic effects at the level of the ventral striatum (Ferré, 1997), an antagonist of adenosine A2a receptors could exhibit antidepressant properties, as was shown for agonists of the D2 receptor (Mouret, Lemoine, & Minuit, 1987; Sitland–Marken, Wells, Froemming, Chu, & Brown, 1990).

In addition, A2a receptor KO mice have a tendency to escape more actively aversive situations than their wild-type controls (El Yacoubi et al., 2000a; Ledent et al., 1997). Similarly, adenosine A2a receptor antagonists increase mobility time in the forced swim test used in mice to test resignation and hence depressive behavior (Borsini, Lecci, Mancinelli, D'Aranno, & Meli, 1988; Duterte–Boucher, Leclère, Panissaud, & Costentin, 1988). Thus, adenosinergic mechanisms could be involved in symptoms of depression and adenosine A2a receptor antagonists might offer a novel approach to the treatment of depression.

CAFFEINE AND EPILEPTIC ACTIVITY

Seizures may be life-threatening events and represent a problem in clinical use of another methylxanthine, theophylline, in the treatment of asthma in epileptic patients. Indeed, high concentrations of theophylline cause hyperexcitability characterized by restlessness and tremor, and toxic levels are associated in some cases with focal and generalized seizures (Dunwiddie & Worth, 1982; Stone & Javid, 1980) and even difficult-to-treat status epilepticus (Oki et al., 1994; Shannon, 1993). Moreover, theophylline and caffeine in nonconvulsive doses prolong kindled seizures in rats (Albertson, Joy, & Stark, 1983; Dragunow, 1990), induce seizures in genetically epilepsy-prone rats (De Sarro, Grasso, Zappala, Nava, & De Sarro, 1997), and have proconvulsant effects on seizures induced by kainic acid, pentylenetetrazol, or pilocarpine (Ault et al., 1987; Cutrufo, Bortot, Giachetti, & Manzini, 1992; Turski et al., 1985). Likewise, caffeine has been used for a long time to lengthen seizures and improve the efficacy of electroconvulsive therapy (ECT) in severely depressed patients (Coffey, Figiel, Weiner, & Saunders, 1990; Hinckle, Coffey, Weiner, Cress, & Christison, 1987; Shapira et al., 1987).

Sensitivity to the proconvulsant effects of methylxanthines is inversely related to age, with higher sensitivity in young animals (Bernaskova & Mares, 2000; Yokohama, Onodera, Yagi, & Iinuma, 1997). In children with epilepsy, theophylline-induced convulsions are more frequent before than after the age of 1 year (Miura &

Kimura, 2000). A pivotal role in methylxanthine-induced seizures may be played by the balance between GABA and glutamate (Amabeoku, 1999; Corradetti, Lo Conte, Moroni, Passani, & Pepeu, 1984; De Sarro & De Sarro, 1991; Segev, Rehavi, & Rubistein, 1988). The convulsant action of methylxanthines may be linked to blockade of the effects of endogenous adenosine at presynaptic A1 receptors located on glutamatergic neurons, hence allowing larger release of the excitatory neurotransmitter, glutamate (Dunwiddie, 1980; Dunwiddie, Hoffer, & Fredholm, 1981; Salmi et al., 2005).

It has been suggested that adenosine may provide an inhibitory tone in the mammalian nervous system (for review, see Knutsen & Murray, 1997). Thus, adenosine could act as a potential endogenous anticonvulsant (Dragunow, 1986; Dragunow, Goddard, & Laverty, 1985). During epileptic seizures, large quantities of adenosine are released by cells surrounding the epileptic focus (Berman, Fredholm, Adén, & O'Connor, 2000; During & Spencer, 1992; Park, van Wylen, Rubio, & Berne, 1987; Winn, Welsch, Bryner, Rubio, & Berne, 1979; Winn, Welsch, Rubio, & Berne, 1980) that may contribute to termination of ongoing seizure activity as well as to the post-ictal refractory period (During & Spencer, 1992).

The most likely candidate for the antiepileptic effect of adenosine is the A1 receptor because of its known inhibitory activity on the release of neurotransmitters, especially excitatory transmitters whose release is increased during seizures (Fredholm & Hedqvist, 1980; Fredholm & Dunwiddie, 1988). Indeed, A1 receptor agonists reduce the seizures induced by chemical or electrical stimuli (Barraco, Swanson, Phillis, & Berman, 1984; Concas et al., 1993; De Sarro, De Sarro, Di Paola, & Bertorelli, 1999; Klitgaard, Knutsen, & Thomsen, 1993; Wiesner et al., 1999; Young & Dragunow, 1994; Zhang, Franklin, & Murray, 1994). In addition, adenosine is able to inhibit calcium fluxes and to open 4-aminopyridine-sensitive K^+-channels (Schubert, Heinemann, & Kolb, 1986; Schubert & Lee, 1986). Both of these actions would result in membrane hyperpolarization and increase in threshold for the activation of the glutamate NMDA receptor subtype.

Conversely, the literature concerning the role of the A2a receptor in epilepsy is more controversial and it is still not clear whether this receptor is involved in the regulation of convulsive seizures. A2a agonists may aggravate (De Sarro et al., 1999) or antagonize (von Lubitz, Paul, Carter, & Jacobson, 1993) seizures in rodents; A2a receptor antagonists have only a limited capacity to antagonize chemically induced seizures (Klitgaard et al., 1993). In fact, a low density of A2a receptors is found in the hippocampus and cortex (Cunha, Constantino, & Ribeiro, 1999; Rosin, Robeva, Woodward, Guyenet, & Linden, 1998) together with a high density of A1 receptors (Fastbom et al., 1987; Goodman & Snyder, 1982; Ochiishi et al., 1999).

In the hippocampus most often involved in seizure activity, localization of A1 and A2a receptors overlaps in the pyramidal layers of the CA1, CA2, and CA3 regions where they modulate excitability in opposite ways. For example, activation of the A2a receptor attenuates the capacity of an A1 agonist to lower hippocampal excitability (Cunha, Milusheva, Vizi, Ribeiro, & Sebastiao, 1994). Conversely, activation of adenosine A2a receptors can induce release of two excitatory neurotransmitters, acetylcholine and glutamate (Dunwiddie & Fredholm, 1997; Sebastiao & Ribeiro, 1996). These two transmitters are released during alcohol withdrawal

(Imperato, Dazzi, Carta, Colombo, & Biggio, 1998; Rossetti & Carboni, 1995), which leads to convulsive seizures; an A1 agonist (Concas, Cucchedu, Floris, Mascia, & Bioggio, 1994) or the deletion of the A2a receptor gene in mice (El Yacoubi et al., 2001) reduces alcohol withdrawal syndrome.

Finally, the role of the A3 adenosine receptor in seizures is unclear. A selective A3 receptor agonist, IB-MECA has neuroprotective properties against NMDA- and pentylenetetrazol-induced seizures (von Lubitz et al., 1995), but is entirely ineffective in ameliorating tonic convulsions induced by electroshocks (Jacobson, von Lubitz, Daly, & Fredholm, 1996). Thus, the role of adenosine during seizures appears to be more complex than its commonly accepted endogenous anticonvulsant effect mediated by the activation of A1 receptors.

ACUTE VERSUS CHRONIC CAFFEINE EFFECTS IN ISCHEMIA AND EPILEPSY

Acute administration of caffeine in the rat worsens ischemic damage consecutive to stroke (Dux, Fastbom, Ungerstedt, Rudolphi, & Fredholm, 1990; Rudolphi, Keil, & Grome, 1990; von Lubitz, Dambrosia, & Redmond, 1989), while a chronic exposure to the methylxanthine protects the brain from ischemic damage occurring in adult (Rudolphi, Keil, Fastbom, & Fredholm, 1989; Rudolphi et al., 1990; Sutherland et al., 1991) or neonatal rodents (Bona, Adén, Fredholm, & Hagberg, 1995). This effect could be reproduced by an adenosine A2a antagonist but not by an A1 antagonist (Bona, Adén, Gilland, Fredholm, & Hagberg, 1997). The extent of focal ischemic damage was also reduced in A2a receptor KO adult mice compared with wild-type animals, which suggests that A2a receptors play a prominent role in development of ischemic injury and demonstrates the potential for anatomical and functional neuroprotection against stroke by A2a receptor antagonists (Chen et al., 1999).

Conversely, in immature A2a receptor knockout mice, brain damage is aggravated after hypoxic ischemia, which suggests that A2a receptors play an important protective role in neonatal hypoxic-ischemic brain injury (Adén et al., 2003). In man, chronic caffeine consumption is inversely related to the risk of fatal and nonfatal strokes (Grobbee et al., 1990). In fact, one paper advised drinking enough coffee to allow an increase in the number of adenosine receptors, but also to stop drinking caffeine-containing beverages when a stroke occurs to prevent caffeine from inducing a blockade at the level of adenosine receptors (Longstreth & Nelson, 1992). The neuroprotective effect of methylxanthines against stroke-induced neuronal damage has been for many years attributed to increase in the number of adenosine receptors reported in numerous studies after chronic exposure to quite high doses of caffeine (for review, see Nehlig & Debry, 1994). However, using more realistic doses of caffeine given in drinking water and relevant to daily human consumption, more recent data showed no change in the density of adenosine A1 or A2a receptors after chronic caffeine exposure (Bona et al., 1995; Georgiev, Johansson, & Fredholm, 1993).

Adenosine has neuroprotective effects in situations of ischemia, both global and focal (Dragunow & Faull, 1988; Dux et al., 1990; Evans, Swann, & Meldrum, 1987; Marangos, von Lubitz, Daval, & Deckert, 1990; Miller & Hsu, 1992; Rudolphi, Schubert, Parkinson, & Fredholm, 1992; von Lubitz, Dambrosia, Kempski, &

Redmond, 1988). Extracellular concentration of adenosine increases rapidly during an episode of ischemia (Berne, Rubio, & Curnish, 1974; Hagberg et al., 1987) but the number of adenosine receptors decreases promptly (Adén, Lindström, Bona, Hagberg, & Fredholm, 1994; Lee, Tetzlaff, & Kreutzberg, 1986). Acute treatment with adenosine A1 receptor agonists protects neurons from injury induced by focal or global ischemia (Rudolphi et al., 1992). This acute treatment is effective even when administered up to 30 min postischemia (von Lubitz et al., 1989).

Conversely, a chronic treatment with an adenosine A1 agonist leads to damage and mortality significantly exceeding that of untreated animals (von Lubitz, Lin, Melman, et al., 1994). The effects of A2a receptors in ischemia are less clear and were only studied acutely. A2a agonists have no apparent effect on hippocampal damage (von Lubitz et al., 1995); A2a antagonists can reduce (Gao & Phillis, 1994) or not (von Lubitz et al., 1995) the extent of neuronal damage. The role of A3 receptors in ischemia is poorly understood (Jacobson et al., 1996). Acute preischemic stimulation of A3 receptors with agonists results in significant increase in morphological damage and mortality (Webb, Sills, Chovan, Peppard, & Francis, 1993), but chronic exposure to the A3 agonist reduces damage and mortality (von Lubitz, Lin, Popik, Carter, & Jacobson, 1994).

Concerning epilepsy, an acute exposure to methylxanthines worsens brain damage induced by seizures (Pinard, Riche, Puiroud, & Seylaz, 1990) and decreases the threshold to various convulsants (Albertson et al., 1983; Ault et al., 1987; Cutrufo et al., 1992; De Sarro et al., 1997; Dragunow, 1990; Turski et al., 1985). Conversely, as shown in ischemia, chronic treatment with caffeine or an adenosine A1 antagonist leads to decreased susceptibility to seizures (Georgiev et al., 1993; Johansson, Georgiev, Kuosmanen, & Fredholm, 1996; von Lubitz, et al., 1993; von Lubitz, Paul, Ji, Carter, & Jacobson, 1994). A chronic treatment with a low dose of caffeine protects also the hippocampus in a lesional model of temporal lobe epilepsy (Rigoulot, Leroy, Koning, Ferrandon, & Nehlig, 2003).

Conversely, chronic treatment with an adenosine A1 agonist, cyclopentyladenosine, results in pronounced increase in seizure-induced intensity and mortality (von Lubitz, Paul, et al., 1994). A chronic treatment with the A3 receptor agonist, IB-MECA, results in almost complete protection against NMDA-induced seizures and significant reduction of mortality after electroshock and pentylenetetrazol-induced seizures (von Lubitz et al., 1995). These effects occur without changes in the number of adenosine A1 receptors and are most markedly observed during ongoing treatment and not after (Georgiev et al., 1993). This effect may, however, involve an action at the A1 receptors because decreased susceptibility to seizures results also from chronic exposure to an adenosine A1 receptor antagonist (von Lubitz, Paul, et al., 1994). The exact mechanism has not been yet clarified.

Thus, upregulation of adenosine receptors does not appear to be necessary to allow chronic exposure to caffeine to exert neuroprotective or anticonvulsant effects. However, as suggested by Johansson et al. (1996), a primary effect on adenosine receptors triggered by the chronic exposure to caffeine could lead to adaptive changes in other transmission systems and/or in fundamental properties related to neuronal excitability, as reflected by a reduction in c-fos expression after seizures in animals treated with caffeine (Johansson et al., 1996). Among other mechanisms, the excitatory action of acetylcholine on cholinergic neurons is reduced (Lin & Phillis, 1990) and the coupling of receptors to G-proteins is altered by chronic caffeine treatment (Chen et al., 1999; Fastbom & Fredholm, 1990).

In addition, the psychostimulant effects of caffeine involve the phosphorylation of DARPP-32 (Fredholm, Chen, Cunha, et al., 2005). Thus, it is likely that the effects of chronic caffeine exposure in ischemia and epilepsy are mediated via a complex cascade of downstream reactions involving adenosine receptors, G-proteins, and DARPP-32 whose regulation might be altered with consequences on various neurotransmission systems, even in the absence of a change in the total number of adenosine receptors.

CAFFEINE AND PARKINSON'S DISEASE

Parkinson's disease is caused by severe degeneration of dopamine neurons in the substantia nigra, which leads to incapacity to control voluntary movements and tremor, akinesia, rigidity, and postural instability. It is presently treated by the precursor of dopamine, L-dopa, which is not very active on tremor, or dopamine D2 receptor agonists. These treatments lead to long-term complications, including loss of drug efficacy and dyskinesia (Marsden, 1990). Bromocriptine, a dopamine D2 receptor agonist, induces locomotor stimulation in rodents (Jackson et al., 1995) and is currently used alone or in combination with L-dopa to achieve greater effectiveness (Montastruc, Rascol, Senard, & Rascol, 1994; Nakanishi et al., 1992; Olsson, Rascol, Korten, Dupont, & Gauthier, 1989).

Likewise, experimental evidence suggests that the antiparkinsonian effects of dopamine agonists could be improved if an adenosine antagonist were used in a combined therapy. Indeed, in the rat model of unilateral lesion of striatal dopaminergic pathways by 6-hydroxydopamine (6-OHDA), the contralateral rotation induced by dopaminergic agonists is potentiated by acute treatment with caffeine or theophylline (Fredholm, Fuxe, & Agnati, 1976; Fredholm et al., 1983; Fuxe & Ungerstedt, 1974). Similar effects have been obtained using selective A2a receptor antagonists in the same model (Fenu, Pinna, Ongini, & Morelli, 1997; Jiang et al., 1993; Pinna, Di Chiara, Wardas, & Morelli, 1996).

In monkey and marmoset models of Parkinson's disease, administration of an A2a antagonist improves the antiparkinsonian activity of L-dopa (Kanda et al., 1998, 2000; Shimada et al., 1997). In human parkinsonian patients, use of adenosine antagonists such as methylxanthines has led to contradictory results. Some older studies report no change when caffeine is combined with L-dopa or bromocriptine (Kartzinel, Shoulson, & Clane, 1976; Shoulson & Chase, 1975), while a more recent one finds improvements in tremor, but only after prolonged treatment (Mally & Stone, 1994).

Although it is well recognized that methylxantines possess dopamine-like properties in animal models of parkinsonism (Casas et al., 1989a, b; Herrera–Marschitz et al., 1988), one of the major limitations for their use is the rapid tolerance to their dopamine agonist-like properties (Evans & Griffiths, 1992; Finn & Holtzman, 1987). However, several recent experimental data suggest that tolerance to caffeine-induced rotational behavior in rodents can be reversed if coadministered with substances like the cholinergic muscarinic receptor antagonist, scopolamine (Casas et al., 1999a), the dopamine D2 receptor agonist, bromocriptine (Casas et al., 1999b), or the mixed dopamine D1/D2 receptor agonist, pergolide (Prat et al., 2000). In fact, simultaneously to activation of the D2 receptors, a maximal activation of the D1 receptors may be necessary to prevent tolerance to caffeine in this rat model of Parkinson's disease (Casas et al., 2000). Thus, many experimental data suggest that methylxantines or A2a adenosine receptor antagonists could be introduced in the treatment of Parkinson's disease because tolerance to their effect can be counteracted.

Ahead of treatment, it has also been shown that caffeine consumption could delay onset or possible occurrence of Parkinson's disease. Epidemiological studies starting as early as 1968 reported that coffee intake is inversely related to the occurrence of Parkinson's disease (Benedetti et al., 2000; Fall, Frederikson, Axelson, & Granérus, 1999; Grandinetti, Morens, Reed, & MacEachem, 1994; Hellenbrand et al., 1996; Jimenez–Jimenez, Mateo, & Gimenez–Roldan, 1992; Nefzger, Quadfazel, & Karl, 1968; Ross et al., 2000; Tan et al., 2003). This effect is consistent in populations from all over the world. Only one study showed that the protective effect of coffee intake disappeared after adjustment for smoking (Grandinetti et al., 1994).

The inverse relation between caffeine intake and risk of Parkinson's disease was recently reported in large cohort studies including 8,004 to 88,565 participants studied over a duration of 10 to 30 years (Ascherio et al., 2001; Paganini–Hill, 2001; Ross et al., 2000; for review, see Schwarzschild & Ascherio, 2004). Most recent case-control studies also favored an inverse relationship between caffeine consumption and the incidence of Parkinson's disease (Fall et al., 1999; Hellenbrand et al., 1996; Hernán, Takkouche, Caarmaño–Isorna, & Gestal–Otero, 2002), with the exception of one study (Checkoway et al., 2002).

For example, the study from the Honolulu Heart Program reported that men who drank more than four cups of coffee a day were five times less likely to develop the disease than those who drank no coffee (Ross et al., 2000). This relationship is valid for caffeine from all sources. No other constituents of coffee like niacin, milk, or sugar are associated with the disease. It was suggested that an underlying preclinical olfactory deficit preventing the rewarding effects of the smell of coffee may exist among the population of future parkinsonians (Benedetti et al., 2000). However, recent data suggest that the progressive degeneration of the striatonigral neurons that underlies development of the disease has little effect on caffeine consumption (Schwarzschild & Ascherio, 2004).

The American Nurse's Health Study and Health Professionals Follow-up Study reported a clear inverse dose–response in men with a protective effect of coffee and tea and no protection from decaffeinated coffee. In women, the relationship has a U shape, with the highest for moderate caffeine consumption (Ascherio et al., 2001). Two more recent studies confirmed a protective role of caffeine consumption for postmenopausal women not using estrogen, but a reverse, deleterious fourfold increased risk for women who take estrogens and drink six or more cups of coffee daily (Ascherio et al., 2003, 2004). The reasons underlying this interaction are not clear.

The mechanism of action hypothesized concerns adenosine A2a receptors that are mainly the target of low doses of caffeine. A2a receptors are colocalized with dopamine D2 receptors in brain regions involved in control of locomotion. Blockade of A2a adenosine receptors increases locomotor activity via stimulation of dopamine D2 receptors. Thus, in animal models of Parkinson's disease, A2a receptor antagonists improve motor deficits (Kuwana et al., 1999).

Two human studies confirm these data. The use of theophylline, an A2a receptor antagonist associated or not with L-dopa, alleviated part of the motor symptoms of parkinsonian patients (Kostic, Svetel, Sternic, Dragosevic, & Przedborski, 1999; Mally & Stone, 1994). Furthermore, A2a receptor antagonists and D2 agonists possess neuroprotective properties (Chen et al., 2001; Iida et al., 1999) and their combined use could represent a future strategy for treatment of degeneration in Parkinson's disease. However, the efficacy of this type of combination needs to be confirmed further (for review, see Chen, 2003, and Schwarschild & Ascherio, 2004). Moreover, a recent study reported the potentiation of beneficial effects of combined inactivation of A2a and metabotropic subtype 5 glutamate receptors, supporting this pharmacological strategy as a promising anti-parkinsonian therapy (Coccurello, Breysse, & Amalric, 2004).

CAN CAFFEINE BE CONSIDERED A DRUG OF DEPENDENCE?

Caffeine has been shown to act as a mild reinforcer (i.e., maintaining its self-administration or being preferentially chosen over placebo)—although not consistently—in humans and animals (Griffiths & Mumford, 1996). At abrupt cessation, caffeine induces a withdrawal syndrome in a subset of sensitive individuals, about 11 to 22% of the population (Dews, O'Brien, & Bergman, 2002). This syndrome is mostly characterized by headaches, feelings of weakness, impaired concentration, fatigue, irritability, and withdrawal feelings (Griffiths et al., 1990; for review, see Nehlig, 1999, 2004). These symptoms usually start 12 to 24 h after caffeine cessation and reach a peak after 20 to 48 h. They never occur when caffeine consumption is progressively decreased. Therefore, the possible physical dependence on the methyxanthine has been considered for about two decades (Griffiths et al., 1990; Griffiths & Mumford, 1995, 1996; Griffiths & Woodson, 1988b; Holtzman, 1990; Strain, Mumford, Silverman, & Griffiths, 1994), but appears quite low compared to common drugs of abuse such as cocaine, amphetamine, morphine, and nicotine.

Drugs of abuse selectively activate the shell of the nucleus accumbens, which plays a critical role in drug dependence (Di Chiara, 1995; Self & Nestler, 1995). This nucleus is functionally and morphologically divided into a core and a shell part. The ventromedial shell part belongs to the mesolimbic dopaminergic system that originates in the ventral tegmental area and ends mainly in the frontal and prefrontal cortices. The shell of the nucleus accumbens plays a role in emotions, motivation, and reward functions; the laterodorsal core is thought to regulate somatomotor functions (Alheid & Heimer, 1988; Heimer, Zahm, Churchill, Kalivas, & Wohltmann, 1991).

Drugs of abuse specifically increase dopamine release and functional activity in the shell of the nucleus accumbens without affecting the core of the nucleus

(Orzi, Passarelli, La Riccia, Di Grezia, & Pontieri, 1996; Pontieri, Tanda, & Di Chiara, 1995; Pontieri, Tanda, Orzi, & Di Chiara, 1996; Porrino, Domer, Crane, & Sokoloff, 1988; Stein & Fuller, 1992). These drug-induced changes in the shell of the nucleus accumbens have been hypothesized to relate to the general abuse liability of these drugs independently from their specific mechanism of action (Orzi et al., 1996; Porrino et al., 1988).

In the structures mediating motor activity, sleep, and mood that are all very sensitive to the effects of caffeine, functional activity is significantly increased after a low dose of 1 mg/kg in the rat (Nehlig & Boyet, 2000). Conversely, at 1 and 2.5 mg/kg, caffeine does not induce any change in glucose utilization in any part of the mesolimbic dopaminergic system that mediates addiction and reward. At 5 mg/kg, methylxanthine increases functional activity in the ventral tegmental area, the site of origin of the mesolimbic dopamine cell bodies; other parts of the mesolimbic dopaminergic system, such as the shell of the nucleus accumbens and medial prefrontal cortex, are only activated after 10 mg/kg caffeine. Likewise 0.5 to 5 mg/kg caffeine do not trigger any release of dopamine in the shell of the nucleus accumbens (Acquas et al., 2002; Solinas et al., 2002); this is in contrast to what occurs with common drugs of abuse that, at low doses, induce dopamine release specifically in the shell compared to the core of the nucleus (Di Chiara & Imperato, 1988; Orzi et al., 1996; Pontieri et al., 1995, 1996).

The increase in functional activity and dopamine release in the shell of the nucleus accumbens occurs only after high doses of caffeine (at least 10 mg/kg) at which the methylxanthine also activates the core part of the same nucleus and induces widespread nonspecific metabolic increases in a majority of brain regions (Nehlig & Boyet, 2000; Solinas et al., 2002). The general activating effects of high doses of caffeine on brain functional activity are likely to reflect the numerous side and adverse effects of ingestion of such doses of the methylxanthine—that is, anxiety, nervousness, and dysphoria (James, 1991; Nehlig et al., 1992).

However, although high doses of caffeine appear to be able to activate the brain circuits of reward, this occurs in a nonspecific way. Low doses of caffeine reflecting the usual human level of consumption do not appear to be able to activate the shell of the nucleus accumbens. Conversely, caffeine triggers dopamine release in the sensitive locomotor region, the caudate nucleus (Okada et al., 1996, 1997), and induces also *c-fos* mRNA labeling only in the caudate nucleus. Amphetamine and cocaine label more the nucleus accumbens than the caudate nucleus (Johansson et al., 1994) and even more the shell than the core, especially cocaine (Graybiel, Moratalla, & Robertson, 1990).

The difference in the functional consequences of the psychostimulants cocaine and amphetamine on the one hand and caffeine on the other is most likely relevant to their respective mechanisms of action. Amphetamine and cocaine induce a release or inhibit the uptake of dopamine (McMillen, 1983), which will bind to D1 and D2 dopamine receptors in the striatum. At low doses, caffeine acts preferentially at the level of adenosine A2a receptors (Fredholm, 1995) mainly found in the striatum where they colocalize with dopamine D2 receptors. This adenosine A2–dopamine D2 interaction, which underlies most of the central actions of caffeine (Fuxe, Ferré, Zoli, & Agnati, 1998), explains the high sensitivity of functional activity in the striatum to caffeine (Nehlig & Boyet, 2000) as well as the specific caffeine-induced striatal expression of immediate early genes (Johansson et al., 1994; Svenningsson, Nomikos, & Fredholm, 1995; Svenningsson, Ström, Johanson, & Fredholm, 1995).

When circulating levels of caffeine increase, the methylxanthine binds also to adenosine A1 receptors (Fredholm, 1995) present in other neurons of the striatum in which they colocalize with D1 dopamine receptors. The higher doses of caffeine lead to expression of immediate early genes in A1–D1 and A2a–D2 neurons in the striatum (Johansson et al., 1994; Svenningsson, Nomikos, et al., 1995; Svenningsson, Ström, et al., 1995). In the present study, it appears that caffeine mimics the effects of amphetamine and cocaine by activating the brain reward pathways only at rather high doses (10 mg/kg), when binding to A1 adenosine receptors is already likely to occur.

However, at the latter dose, there is no specificity of response in the shell of the nucleus accumbens as reported with dopamine and cocaine (Orzi et al., 1996; Pontieri et al., 1995, 1996; Porrino et al., 1988; Stein & Fuller, 1992) because 10 mg/kg caffeine also trigger an increase in functional activity in the core of the nucleus accumbens, which is not involved in addiction and reward, as well as in most other brain regions. This generalized response most likely reflects the widespread distribution of adenosine A1 receptors that are participating in the brain's response to large doses of caffeine.

Thus, although caffeine acts as a psychostimulant and activates the dopaminergic system as amphetamine and cocaine do, the different substances lead to quite different effects on cerebral functional activity. In fact, caffeine appears to be used consciously or unconsciously to manage mood state and alleviate the adverse effects of caffeine deprivation (Phillips–Bute & Lane, 1998; Rogers & Dernoncourt, 1998). It must also be remembered that human caffeine consumption is fractioned over the day, but doses given in animal studies are usually injected as an intravenous or intraperitoneal bolus. Thus, data on the effects of increasing doses of caffeine on cerebral functional activity are rather in favor of caffeine acting as a positive rein-forcer at the doses reflecting the general human consumption and do not support participation of the brain circuitry of addiction and reward at low doses (one cup per day) of caffeine, as hypothesized in the study by Strain et al. (1994).

CONCLUSION

The evolution of recent animal research has moved from the use of high to low realistic doses of caffeine relevant to the daily human consumption. At these low doses, caffeine exerts most of its stimulatory effects via blockade of adenosine A2a and A1 receptors. Caffeine also interacts with dopamine receptors, but the mechanism is very different from that of drugs like amphetamine and cocaine. The functions most sensitive to caffeine appear to be locomotor activity, sleep, and mood; at doses relevant to human daily consumption, caffeine does not activate the brain circuit of addiction and reward.

Therapeutic use of caffeine or A2a receptor antagonists has already been tested in Parkinson's disease, for which coffee consumption prior to the disease delays or prevents the occurrence of symptoms. The mechanisms underlying the difference between acute and long-term effects of the methylxanthine in brain pathologies should be studied in more detail to allow induction of the adaptive changes that seem to be able to trigger neuroprotection.

REFERENCES

Acquas, E., Tanda, G., & Di Chiara, G. (2002). Differential effects of caffeine on dopamine and acetylcholine transmission in brain areas of drug-naive and caffeine-pretreated rats. *Neuropsychopharmacology, 27*, 182–193.

Adén, U., Halldner, L., Lagercrantz, H., Dalmau, I., Ledent, C., & Fredholm, B. B. (2003). Aggravated brain damage after hypoxic ischemia in immature adenosine A2a knock-out mice. *Stroke, 34*, 739–744.

Adén, U., Lindström, K., Bona, E., Hagberg, H., & Fredholm, B. B. (1994). Changes in adenosine receptors in the neonatal brain following hypoxic ischemia. *Molecular Brain Research, 23*, 354–358.

Albertson, T. E., Joy, R. M., & Stark, L. G. (1983). Caffeine modification of kindled amygdaloid seizures. *Pharmacology, Biochemistry and Behavior, 19*, 339–344.

Alheid, G. F., & Heimer, L. (1988). New perspectives in basal forebrain organization of special relevance for neuropsychiatric disorders; the striatopallidal, amygdaloid, and corticopetal components of the substantia innominata. *Neuroscience, 27*, 1–39.

Alsene, K., Deckert, J., Sand, P., & de Wit, H. (2003). Associations between A2a receptor gene polymorphisms and caffeine-induced anxiety. *Neuropsychopharmacology, 28*, 1694–1702.

Amabeoku, G. J. (1999). Gamma-aminobutyric acid and glutamic acid receptors may mediate theophylline-induced seizures in mice. *General Pharmacology, 32*, 365–372.

Ascherio, A., Chen, H., Schwarzschild, M. A., Zhang, S M., Colditz, G. A., & Speizer, F. E. (2003). Caffeine, postmenopausal estrogen, and risk of Parkinson's disease. *Neurology, 60*, 790–795.

Ascherio, A., Weisskopf, M. G., O'Reilly, E. J., McCullough, M. L., Calle, E. E., Rodriguez, C., & Thun, M. J. (2004). Coffee consumption, gender, and Parkinson's disease mortality in the cancer prevention study II cohort: The modifying effects of estrogen. *American Journal of Epidemiology, 160*, 977–984.

Ascherio, A., Zhang, S. M., Hernán, M. A., Kawachi, I., Colditz, G. A., Speizer, F. E., & Willett, W. C. (2001). Prospective study of caffeine consumption and risk of Parkinson's disease in men and women. *Annals of Neurology, 50*, 56–63.

Ault, B., Olney, M. A., Joyner, J. L., Boyer, C. E., Notrica, M. A., Soroko, F. E., & Wang, C. M. (1987). Proconvulsant actions of theophylline and caffeine in the hippocampus: implications for the management of temporal lobe epilepsy. *Brain Research, 426*, 93–102.

Baldwin, H. A., & File, S. E. (1989). Caffeine-induced anxiogenesis: the role of adenosine, benzodiazepine and noradrenergic receptors. *Pharmacology, Biochemistry and Behavior, 32*, 181–186.

Barone, J. J., & Roberts, H. R. (1996). Caffeine consumption. *Food and Chemical Toxicology, 34*, 119–126.

Barraco, R. A., Swanson, T. H., Phillis, J. W., & Berman, R. F. (1984). Anticonvulsant effects of adenosine analogues onamygdaloid-kindled seizures in rats. *Neuroscience Letters, 46*, 317–322.

Basheer, R., Porkka–Heiskanen, T., Strecker, R. E., Thakkar, M., & McCarley, R. W. (2000). Adenosine as a biological signal mediating sleepiness following prolonged wakefulness. *Biological Signals and Receptors, 9*, 319–327.

Beaumont, M., Batejat, D., Pierard, C., Coste, O., Doireau, P., Van Beers, P., Chauffard, F., Chassard, D., Enslen, M., Denis, J. B., & Lagarde, D. (2001). Slow release caffeine and prolonged (64-h) continuous wakefulness: effects on vigilance and cognitive performance. *Journal of Sleep Research, 10*, 265–276.

Benedetti, M. D., Bower, J. H., Maranganore, D. M., McDonnel, S. K., Peterson, B. J., Ahlsklog, J. E., Schaid, D. J., & Rocca, W. A. (2000). Smoking, alcohol, and coffee consumption preceding Parkinson's disease. *Neurology*, *55*, 1350–1358.

Benowitz, N. L. (1990). Clinical pharmacology of caffeine. *Annual Review of Medicine*, *41*, 277–288.

Berman, R. F., Fredholm, B. B., Adén, U., & O'Connor, W. T. (2000). Evidence for increased dorsal hippocampal adenosine release and metabolism during pharmacologically induced seizures. *Brain Research*, *872*, 44–53.

Bernášková, K., & Mareš, P. (2000). Proconvulsant effects of aminophylline on cortical epileptic afterdischarges varies during ontogeny. *Epilepsy Research*, *39*, 183–190.

Berne, R. N., Rubio, R., & Curnish, R. R. (1974). Release of adenosine from ischemic brain. *Circulation Research*, *35*, 262–271.

Bertorelli, R., Ferri, N., Adami, M., & Ongini, E. (1996). Effects of selective agonists and antagonists for A1 and A2A adenosine receptors on sleep-waking patterns in rats. *Drug Development Research*, *37*, 65–72.

Bona, E., Adén, U., Fredholm, B. B., & Hagberg, H. (1995). The effect of long term caffeine treatment on hypoxic-ischemic brain damage in the neonate. *Pediatric Research*, *38*, 312–318.

Bona, E., Adén, U., Gilland, E., Fredholm, B. B., & Hagberg, H. (1997). Neonatal cerebral hypoxia-ischemia: the effect of adenosine receptor antagonists. *Neuropharmacology*, *36*, 1327–1338.

Borsini, F., Lecci, A., Mancinelli, A., D'Aranno, V., & Meli, A. (1988). Stimulation of dopamine-D2 but not dopamine-D1 receptors reduces immobility time of rats in the forced swimming test: Implication for antidepressant activity. *European Journal of Pharmacology*, *148*, 301–307.

Brice, C. F., & Smith, A. (2002). Factors associated with caffeine consumption. *International Journal of Food Science and Nutrition*, *53*, 55–64.

Brown, S. J., Gill, S., Evenden, J. L., Iversen, S. D., & Richardson, P. J. (1991). Striatal A2 receptor regulates apomorphine-induced turning in rats with unilateral dopamine denervation. *Psychopharmacology Series (Berlin)*, *103*, 78–82.

Bruce, M. S., & Lader, M. (1989). Caffeine abstention in the management of anxiety disorders. *Psychological Medicine*, *19*, 211–214.

Carter, A. J., O'Connor, W. T., Carter, M. J., & Ungerstedt, U. (1995). Caffeine enhances acetylcholine release in the hippocampus *in vivo* by a selective interaction with adenosine A1-receptors. *Journal of Pharmacology and Experimental Therapeutics*, *273*, 637–642.

Casas, M., Ferré, S., Cobos, A., Grau, G. M., & Jané, F. (1989a). Relationship between rotational behavior induced by theophylline in 6-OHDA nigrostriatal denervated rats is dependent on the supersensitivity of striatal dopamine receptors. *Pharmacology, Biochemistry and Behavior*, *29*, 609–613.

Casas, M., Ferré, S., Cobos, A., Grau, G. M., & Jané, F. (1989b). Rotational behavior induced by apomorphine and caffeine in rats with unilateral lesion of the nigrostriatal pathway. *Neuropharmacology*, *28*, 407–409.

Casas, M., Prat, G., Robledo, P., Barbanoj, M., Kulisevsky, J., & Jané, F. (1999a). Scopolamine prevents tolerance to the effects of caffeine on rotational behavior in 6-hydroxydopamine denervated rats. *European Journal of Pharmacology*, *366*, 1–11.

Casas, M., Prat, G., Robledo, P., Barbanoj, M., Kulisevsky, J., & Jané, F. (1999b). Repeated coadministration of caffeine and bromocriptine prevents tolerance to the effects of caffeine in the turning behavior animal model. *Neurospychopharmacology*, *9*, 515–521.

Casas, M., Prat, G., Robledo, P., Barbanoj, M., Kulisevsky, J., & Jané, F. (2000). Lack of synergism between caffeine and SKF 38393 on rotational behavior in 6-hydroxydopamine-denervated rats. *European Journal of Pharmacology*, *396*, 93–99.

Casas, M., Ramos–Quiroga, J., Prat, G., & Qureshi, A. (2004). Effects of coffee and caffeine on mood and mood disorders. In A. Nehlig (Ed.) *Coffee, tea, chocolate and the brain* (pp. 73–83). Boca Raton, FL: CRC Press.

Chang, P. P., Ford, D. E., Mead, L. A., Cooper–Patrick, L., & Klag, M. L. (1997). Insomnia in young men and subsequent depression: The Johns Hopkins Precursors Study. *American Journal of Epidemiology, 146,* 105–114.

Checkoway, H., Powers, K., Smith–Weller, T., Franklin, G. M., Longstreth, W. T., & Swanson, P. D. (2002). Parkinson's disease risks associated with cigarette smoking, alcohol consumption, and caffeine intake. *American Journal of Epidemiology, 155,* 732–738.

Chen, J. F. (2003). The adenosine A(2A) receptor as an attractive target for Parkinson's disease treatment. *Drug News Perspectives, 16,* 597–604.

Chen, J.F., Huang, Z., Ma, J., Zhu, J., Moratalla, R., Standaert, D., et al (1999). A (2A) adenosine receptor deficiency attenuates brain injury induced by transient focal ischemaia in mice. *Jounal of Neuroscience, 19,* 1992–9200.

Chen, J. F., Xu, K., Petzer, J. P., Staal, R., Xu, Y. H., Beilstein, M., Sonsalla, P. K., Castagnoli, K., Castagnoli, N., Jr., & Schwarzschild, M. A. (2001). Neuroprotection by caffeine and A(2A) adenosine receptor inactivation in a model of Parkinson's disease. *Journal of Neuroscience, 21,* RC143.

Chou, D. T., Forde, J. H., & Hirsh, K. R. (1980). Unit activity in medial thalamus, comparative effects of caffeine and amphetamine. *Journal of Pharmacology and Experimental Therapeutics, 213,* 580–585.

Coccurello, R., Breysse, N., & Amalric, M. (2004). Simultaneous blockade of adenosine A2A and metabotropic glutamate mGlu5 receptors increase their efficacy in reversing Parkinsonian deficits in rats. *Neuropsychopharmacology, 29,* 1451–1461.

Coffey, C. E., Figiel, G. S., Weiner, R. D., & Saunders, W. B. (1990). Caffeine augmentation of ECT. *American Journal of Psychiatry, 147,* 579–585.

Concas, A., Cuccheddu, T., Floris, S., Mascia, M. P., & Biggio, G. (1994). 2-Chloro-N6-cyclopentyladenosine (CCPA), an adenosine A1 receptor agonist, suppresses ethanol withdrawal syndrome in rats. *Alcohol and Alcoholism, 29,* 261–264.

Concas, A., Santoro, G., Mascia, M. P., Maciocco, E., Dazzi, L., Ongini, E., & Biggio, G. (1993). Anticonvulsant doses of 2-chloro-N6-cyclopentyladenosine, an adenosine A1 receptor agonist, reduce GABAergic transmission in different areas of the mouse brain. *Journal of Pharmacology and Experimental Therapeutics, 267,* 844–851.

Corradetti, R., Lo Conte, R., Moroni, F., Passani, M. B., & Pepeu, G. (1984). Adenosine decreases aspartate and glutamate release from rat hippocampal slices. *European Journal of Pharmacology, 104,* 19–26.

Cunha, R. A., Constantino, M. D., & Ribeiro, J. A. (1999). G protein coupling of CGS 21680 binding sites in tha rat hippocampus and cortex is different from that of adenosine A_1 and striatal A_{2A} receptors. *Naunyn–Schmiedeberg's Archives of Pharmacology, 359,* 295–302.

Cunha, R. A., Milusheva, E., Vizi, E. S., Ribeiro, J. A., & Sebastiao, A. M. (1994). Excitatory and inhibitory effects of A1 and A2 adenosine receptor activation on the electrically evoked (^{3}H)acetylcholine release from different areas of the rat hippocampus. *Journal of Neurochemistry, 63,* 207–214.

Cutrufo, C., Bortot, L., Giachetti, A., & Manzini, S. (1992). Differential effects of various xanthines on pentylenetetrazol-induced seizures in rats: An EEG and behavioral study. *European Journal of Pharmacology, 222,* 1–6.

Daly, J. W. (1993). Mechanisms of action of caffeine. In S. Garattini (Ed.). *Coffee, caffeine and health* (pp. 97–150). New York: Raven Press.

Davis, M. (1992). The role of amygdala in fear and anxiety. *Annual Review of Neuroscience, 15,* 353–375.

Debry, G. (1994). *Coffee and health.* Paris: John Libbey.

De Sarro A., & De Sarro G. B. (1991). Responsiveness of genetically epilepsy-prone rats to aminophylline-induced seizures and interactions with quinolones. *Neuropharmacology, 30,* 169–176.

De Sarro, A., Grasso, S., Zappala, M., Nava, F., & De Sarro, G. B. (1997). Convulsant effects of some xanthine derivatives in genetically epilepsy-prone rats. *Naunyn–Schmiedeberg's Archives of Pharmacology, 356,* 48–55.

De Sarro, G. B., De Sarro, A., Di Paola, E. D., & Bertorelli, R. (1999). Effects of adenosine receptor agonists and antagonists on audiogenic seizure-sensible DBA/2 mice. *European Journal of Pharmacology, 371,* 137–145.

Dews, P. B., O'Brien, C. P., & Bergman, J. (2002). Caffeine: Behavioral effects of withdrawal and related issues. *Food and Chemical Toxicology, 40,* 1257–1261.

Di Chiara, G. (1995). The role of dopamine in drug abuse viewed from the perspective of its role in motivation. *Drug and Alcohol Dependence, 38,* 95–137.

Di Chiara, G., & Imperato, A. (1988). Drugs abused in humans preferentially increase synaptic dopamine concentrations in the mesolimbic system of freely moving rats. *Proceedings of the National Academy of Sciences of the USA, 85,* 5274–5278.

Dragunow, M. (1986). Adenosine: the brain's natural anticonvulsant? *Trends in Pharmacological Sciences, 7,* 128–130.

Dragunow, M. (1990). Adenosine receptor antagonism accounts for the seizure-prolonging effects of aminophylline. *Pharmacology, Biochemistry and Behavior, 36,* 751–755.

Dragunow, M., & Faull, R. (1988) Neuroprotective effects of adenosine. *Trends in Pharmacological Sciences, 9,* 193–194.

Dragunow, M., Goddard, G. V., & Laverty, R. (1985). Is adenosine an endogenous anticonvulsant? *Epilepsia, 26,* 480–487.

Dunwiddie, T. V. (1980). Endogenously released adenosine regulates excitability in the in vitro hippocampus. *Epilepsia, 21,* 541–548.

Dunwiddie, T. V. (1985). The physiological role of adenosine in the central nervous system. *International Reviews of Neurobiology, 27,* 63–139.

Dunwiddie, T. V., & Fredholm, B. B. (1997). Adenosine modulation. In K. A. Jacobson & M. F. Jarvis (Eds.), *Purinergic approaches in experimental therapeutics* (pp. 359–382). New York: Wiley–Liss.

Dunwiddie, T. V., & Worth, T. (1982). Sedative and anticonvulsant effects of adenosine analogs in mouse and rat. *Journal of Pharmacology and Experimental Therapeutics, 220,* 70–76.

Dunwiddie, T. V., Hoffer, B. J., & Fredholm, B. B. (1981). Alkylxanthines elevate hippocampal excitability. Evidence for a role of endogenous adenosine. *Naunyn–Schmiedeberg's Archives of Pharmacology, 316,* 326–330.

During, M. J., & Spencer, D. D. (1992). Adenosine: A potential mediator of seizure arrest and postictal refractorisness. *Annals of Neurology, 32,* 618–624.

Duterte-Boucher, D., Leclère, J. F., Panissaud, C., & Costentin, J. (1988). Acute effects of direct dopamine agonists in the mouse behavioral despair test. *European Journal of Pharmacology, 154,* 185–190.

Dux, E., Fastbom, J., Ungerstedt, U., Rudolphi, K., & Fredholm, B. B. (1990). Protective effects of adenosine and a novel xanthine derivative propentofylline on the cell damage after bilateral carotid occlusion in the gerbil hippocampus. *Brain Research, 516,* 248–256.

El Yacoubi, M., Ledent, C., Ménard, J. F., Parmentier, M., Costentin, J., & Vaugeois, J. M. (2000). SCH 58261 and ZM 241385 differentially prevent the motor effects of CGS 21680 in mice: Evidence for a functional "atypical" adenosine A_{2A} receptor. *European Journal of Pharmacology, 401,* 63–77.

El Yacoubi, M., Ledent, C., Parmentier, M., Costentin, J., & Vaugeois, J. M. (2000a). The stimulant effects of caffeine on locomotor behaviour in mice are mediated through its blockade of adenosine A_{2A} receptors. *British Journal of Pharmacology*, *129*, 1465–1473.

El Yacoubi, M., Ledent, C., Parmentier, M., Costentin, J., & Vaugeois, J. M. (2000b). The anxiogenic-like effects of caffeine in two experimental procedures measuring anxiety in the mouse is not shared by selective adenosine A_{2A} receptor antagonists. *Psychopharmacology*, *148*, 153–163.

El Yacoubi, M., Ledent, C., Parmentier, M., Daoust, M., Costentin, J., & Vaugeois, J. M. (2001). Absence of the adenosine A_{2A} receptor or its chronic blockade decrease ethanol withdrawal-induced seizures in mice. *Neuropharmacology*, *40*, 424–432.

Evans, M. C., Swan, J. H., & Meldrum, B. S. (1987). An adenosine analogue, 2-chloroadenosine, protects against long-term development of ischemic cell loss in the rat. *Neuroscience Letters*, *83*, 287–292.

Evans, S. M., & Griffiths, R. R. (1992). Caffeine tolerance and choice in humans. *Psychopharmacology*, *108*, 51–59.

Fall, P. A., Frederikson, M., Axelson, O., & Granérus, A. K. (1999). Nutritional and occupational factors influencing the risk of Parkinson's disease: a case-control study in southeastern Sweden. *Movement Disorders*, *14*, 28–37.

Fastbom, J., & Fredholm, B. B. (1990). Effects of long-term theophylline treatment on adenosine A_1-receptors in rat brain: Autoradiographic evidence for increased receptor number and altered coupling to G-proteins. *Brain Research*, *507*, 195–199.

Fastbom, J., Pazos, A., & Palacios, J. M. (1987). The distribution of adenosine A1 receptors and 5'-nucleotidase in the brain of some commonly used experimental animals. *Neuroscience*, *22*, 813–826.

Fenu, S., Pinna, A., Ongini, E., & Morelli, M. (1997). Adenosine A2A receptor antagonism potentiates L-DOPA-induced turning behavior and c-fos expression in 6-hydroxy-dopamine-lesioned rats. *European Journal of Pharmacology*, *321*, 143–147.

Fernström, J. D., & Fernström, M. H. (1984). Effects of caffeine on monoamine neurotransmitters in the central and peripheral nervous system. In P. B. Dews (Ed.), *Caffeine: Perspectives from recent research* (pp. 107–118). Heidelberg: Springer–Verlag.

Ferré, S. (1997). Adenosine-dopamine interactions in the ventral striatum. Implications for the treatment of schizophrenia. *Psychopharmacology*, *133*, 107–120.

Ferré, S., Fredholm, B. B., Morelli, M., Popoli, P., & Fuxe, K. (1997). Adenosine-dopamine receptor-receptor interactions as an integrative mechanism in the basal ganglia. *Trends in Neuroscience*, *20*, 482–487.

Ferré, S., O'Connor, W. T., Fuxe, K., & Ungerstedt, U. (1993). The striatopallidal neuron: a main locus for adenosine-dopamine interactions in the brain. *Journal of Neuroscience*, *13*, 5402–5406.

Ferré, S., Popoli, P., Gimenez–Llort, L., Finnman, U. B., Martinez, E., Scotti de Carolis, A., & Fuxe, K. (1994). Postsynaptic antagonistic interaction between adenosine A1 and dopamine D1 receptors. *NeuroReport*, *6*, 73–76.

Ferré, S., Torvinen, M., Antoniou, K., Irenius, E., Civelli, O., Arenas, E., Fredholm, B. B., & Fuxe, K. (1998). Adenosine A1 receptor-mediated modulation of dopamine D1 receptors in stably cotransfected fibroblast cells. *Journal of Biological Chemistry*, *273*, 4718–4724.

Ferré, S., von Euler, G., Johansson, B., Fredholm, B. B., & Fuxe, K. (1991). Stimulation of high-affinity adenosine A2 receptors decreases the affinity of dopamine D2 receptors in rat striatal membranes. *Proceedings of the National Academy of Sciences of the USA*, *88*, 7238–7241.

Finn, I. B., & Holtzman, S. G. (1987). Pharmacological specificity of tolerance to caffeine-induced stimulation of locomotor activity. *Psychopharmacology, 93,* 428–434.

Florio, C., Prezioso, A., Papaioannou, A., & Bertua, R. (1998). Adenosine A1 receptors modulate anxiety in CD1 mice. *Psychopharmacology, 136,* 311–319.

Fredholm, B. B. (1980). Are methylxanthine effects due to antagonism of endogenous adenosine? *Trends in Pharmacological Sciences, 1,* 129–132.

Fredholm, B. B. (1995). Astra Award lecture. Adenosine, adenosine receptors and the actions of caffeine. *Pharmacology and Toxicology, 76,* 93–101.

Fredholm, B. B., Abbracchio, M. P., Burnstock, G., Daly, J. W., Harden, T. K., Jacobson, K. A., Leff, P., & Williams, M. (1994). Nomenclature and classification of purinoceptors. *Pharmacological Reviews, 46,* 143–156.

Fredholm, B. B., Bättig, K., Holmen, J., Nehlig, A., & Zvartau, E. E. (1999). Actions of caffeine in the brain with special reference to factors that contribute to its widespread use. *Pharmacological Reviews, 51,* 83–133.

Fredholm, B. B., Chen, J. F., Cunha, R. A., Svenningson, P., & Vaugeois, J. M. (2005). Adenosine and brain function. *International Review of Neurobiology, 63,* 191–270.

Fredholm, B. B., Chen, J. F., Masino, S. A., & Vaugeois, J. M. (2005). Actions of adenosine at its receptors in the CNS: Insights from knockouts and drugs. *Annual Review of Phramacology & Toxicology, 63,* 191–270.

Fredholm, B. B., & Dunwiddie, T. V. (1988). How does adenosine inhibit transmitter release? *Trends in Pharmacological Sciences, 9,* 130–134.

Fredholm, B. B., Fuxe, K., & Agnati, L. (1976). Effect of some phosphodiesterase inhibitors on central dopamine mechanisms. *European Journal of Pharmacology, 38,* 31–38.

Fredholm, B. B., & Hedqvist, P. (1980). Modulation of neurotransmission by purine nucleotides and nucleosides. *Biochemical Pharmacology, 29,* 1635–1643.

Fredholm, B. B., Herrera–Marschitz, M., Jonzon, B., Lindström, K., & Ungerstedt, U. (1983). On the mechanism by which methylxanthines enhance apomorphine-induced rotation behavior in the rat. *Pharmacology, Biochemistry and Behavior, 19,* 535–541.

Fuxe, K., Ferré, S., Zoli, M., & Agnati, L. F. (1998). Integrated events in central dopamine transmission as analyzed at multiple levels. Evidence for intramembrane adenosine A_{2A}/dopamine D_2 and adenosine A_1/dopamine D_1 receptor interactions in the basal ganglia. *Brain Research Reviews, 26,* 258–273.

Fuxe, K., & Ungerstedt, U. (1974). Action of caffeine and theophylline on supersensitive receptors: considerable enhancement of receptor response to treatment with L-dopa and dopamine receptor agonists. *Medical Biology, 52,* 48–54.

Gao, Y., & Phillis, J. W. (1994). CGS 15943, an adenosine A2 receptor antagonist, reduces cerebral ischemic injury in the Mongolian gerbil. *Life Sciences, 55,* 61–65.

Garrett, B. E., & Hotzman, S. G. (1994). D1 and D2 dopamine receptor antagonists block caffeine-induced stimulation of locomotor activity in rats. *Pharmacology, Biochemistry and Behavior, 47,* 89–94.

Georgiev, V., Johansson, B., & Fredholm, B. B. (1993). Long-term treatment leads to a decreased susceptibility to NMDA-induced clonic seizures in mice without changes in adenosine A_1 receptor number. *Brain Research, 612,* 271–277.

Gerson, S. C., & Baldessarini, R. J. (1980). Motor effects of serotonin in the central nervous system. *Life Sciences, 27,* 1435–1451.

Gimenez–Llort, L., Fernandez–Terruel, A., Escorihuela, R. M., Fredholm, B. B., Tobena, A., Pekny, M., & Johansson, B. (2002). Mice lacking the adenosine A1 receptor are anxious and aggressive, but are normal learners with reduced muscle strength and survival rate. *European Journal of Neuroscience, 16,* 547–550.

Goodman, R. R., & Snyder, S. H. (1982). Autoradiographic localization of adenosine receptor in rat brain using (^{3}H)cyclohexyladenosine. *Journal of Neuroscience, 2,* 1230–1241.

Grandinetti, A., Morens, D., Reed, D., & MacEachem, D. (1994). Prospective study of cigarette smoking and the risk of developing idiopathic Parkinson's disease. *American Journal of Epidemiology, 139,* 1129–1138.

Grant, S. J., & Redmond, D. E., Jr. (1982). Methylxanthine activation of noradrenergic unit activity and reversal by clonidine. *European Journal of Pharmacology, 85,* 105–109.

Graybiel, A. M., Moratalla, R., & Robertson, H. A. (1990). Amphetamine and cocaine induce drug-specific activation of the *c-fos* gene in striosome-matrix compartments and limbic subdivisions of the striatum. *Proceedings of the National Academy of Sciences of the USA, 87,* 6912–6916.

Green, R. D., Proudfit, H. K., & Yeung, S. M. (1982). Modulation of striatal dopaminergic function by local injection of 5′-N-ethylcarboxamide adenosine. *Science, 218,* 58–61.

Griebel, G., Misslin, R., & Vogel, E. (1991). Behavioral effects of selective A2 adenosine receptor antagonists, CGS 21197 and CGS 22706, in mice. *NeuroReport, 2,* 139–140.

Griebel, G., Saffroy–Spittler, M., Misslin, R., Remmy, D., Vogel, E., & Bourguignon, J. J. (1991). Comparison of the behavioral effects of an adenosine A1/A2-receptor antagonist, CGS 15943A, and an A1-selective antagonist, DPCPX. *Psychopharmacology, 103,* 541–544.

Griffiths, R. R., Evans, S. M., Heishman, S. J., Preston, K. L., Sannerud, C. A., Wolf, B., & Woodson P. P. (1990). Low-dose caffeine physical dependence in humans. *Journal of Pharmacology and Experimental Therapeutics, 255,* 1123–1132.

Griffiths, R. R., & Mumford, G. K. (1995). Caffeine—A drug of abuse? In F. E. Bloom & D. J. Kupfer (Eds.), *Psychopharmacology. The fourth generation of progress* (pp. 1699–1713). New York: Raven Press.

Griffiths, R. R., & Mumford, G. K. (1996). Caffeine reinforcement, discrimination, tolerance and physical dependence in laboratory animals and humans. In C. R. Schuster & M. J. Kuhar (Eds.), *Handbook of experimental pharmacology* (Vol. 118, pp. 315–341). Heidelberg: Springer–Verlag.

Griffiths, R. R., & Woodson, P. P. (1988a). Reinforcing effects of caffeine in humans. *Journal of Pharmacology and Experimental Therapeutics, 246,* 21–29.

Griffiths, R. R., & Woodson, P. P. (1988b). Caffeine physical dependence, a review of human and laboratory animal studies. *Psychopharmacology, 94,* 437–451.

Grobbee, D. E., Rimm, E. B., Giovannucci, E., Colditz, G., Stampfer, M., & Willet, W. (1990). Coffee, caffeine, and cardiovascular disease in men. *New England Journal of Medicine, 323,* 1026–1032.

Hagberg, H., Andersson, P., Lacarewicz, J., Jacobson, I., Butcher, S., & Sandberg, M. (1987). Extracellular adenosine, inosine, hypoxanthine, and xanthine in relation to tissue nucleotides and purines in rat striatum during transient ischemia. *Journal of Neurochemistry, 49,* 227–231.

Haldfield, M. G., & Milo, C. (1989). Caffeine and regional brain monoamine utilization in mice. *Life Sciences, 45,* 2637–2644.

Halldner, L., Adén, U., Dahlberg, V., Johansson, B., Ledent, C., & Fredholm, B. B. (2004). The adenosine A1 receptor contributes to the stimulatory, but not the inhibitory effect of caffeine on locomotion: A study in mice lacking A1 and A2A adenosine receptors. *Neuropharmacology, 46,* 1008–1017.

Heimer, L., Zahm, D. S., Churchill, L., Kalivas, P. W., & Wohltmann, C. (1991). Specificity in the projection patterns of accumbal core and shell in the rat. *Neuroscience, 41,* 89–125.

Hellenbrand, W., Seidler, A., Boeing, H., Robra, B. P., Vieregge, P., Nischan, P., Joerg, J., Oertel, W. H., Schneider, E., & Ulm, G. (1996). Diet and Parkinson's disease. II: A possible role for the past intake of specific nutrients: Results from a self-administered food-frequency questionnaire in a case-control study. *Neurology, 47*, 644–650.

Hernán, M. A., Takkouche, B., Caamaño–Isorna, F., & Gestal–Otero, J. J. (2002). A meta-analysis of coffee drinking, cigarette smoking, and the risk of Parkinson's disease. *Annals of Neurology, 52*, 276–284.

Herrera–Marschitz, M., Casas, M., & Ungerstedt, U. (1988). Caffeine produces contralateral rotation in rats with unilateral dopamine denervation: comparisons with apomorphine-induced responses. *Psychopharmacology, 94*, 38–45.

Hinckle, P. E., Coffey, C. E., Weiner, R. D., Cress, M., & Christison, C. (1987). Use of caffeine to lengthen seizures in ECT. *American Journal of Psychiatry, 144*, 1143–1148.

Hirsh, K. (1984). Central nervous system pharmacology of the dietary methylxanthines. In G. A. Spiller (Ed.), *The methylxanthine beverages and food, chemistry, consumption and health effects* (pp. 235–301). New York: Alan Liss.

Hirsh, K., Forde, J., & Chou, D. T. (1982). Effects of caffeine and amphetamine SO_4 on single unit activity in the caudate nucleus. *Society for Neuroscience Abstracts, 8*, 898.

Holtzman, S. G. (1990). Caffeine as a model drug of abuse. *Trends in Pharmacological Sciences, 11*, 355–356.

Huang, Z. L., Qu, W. M., Eguchi, N., Chen, J. F., Schwarzschild, M. A., Fredholm, B. B., Urade, Y., & Hayaishi, O. (2005). Adenosine A2A, but not A1 receptors mediate the arousal effect of caffeine. *Nature Neuroscience*, online publication doi:10.1038/nn1491.

Hughes, R. N. (1996). Drugs that induce anxiety: Caffeine. *New Zealand Journal of Psychology, 25*, 36–42.

Iida, M., Miyazaki, I., Tanaka, K., Kabuto, H., Iwato–Ichikawa, E., & Ogawa, N. (1999). Dopamine D2 receptor-mediated antioxydant and neuroprotective effects of ropinirole, a dopamine agonist. *Brain Research, 838*, 51–59.

Imaizumi, M., Miyazaki, S., & Onodera, K. (1994). Effects of xanthine derivatives in a light/dark test in mice and the contribution of adenosine receptors. *Methods and Findings in Experimental and Clinical Pharmacology, 16*, 639–644.

Imperato, A., Dazzi, L., Carta, G., Colombo, G., & Biggio, G. (1998). Rapid increase in basal acetylcholine release in the hippocampus of freely moving rats induced by withdrawal from long-term ethanol intoxication. *Brain Research, 784*, 347–350.

Jackson, D. M., Mohell, N., Georgiev, J., Bengtsson, A., Larsson, L. G., Magnusson, O., & Ross, S. B. (1995). Time course of bromocriptine-induced excitation in the rat: behavioral and biochemical studies. *Naunyn–Schmiedeberg's Archives of Pharmacology, 351*, 146–155.

Jacobson, K. A., Nikodijevic, O., Shi, D., Gallo–Rodriguez, C., Olah, M. E., Stiles, G. L., & Daly, J. W. (1993). A role for central A_3-adenosine receptors. Mediation of behavioral depressant effects. *FEBS Letters, 336*, 57–60.

Jacobson, K. A., von Lubitz, D. K. J. E., Daly, J. W., & Fredholm, B. B. (1996). Adenosine receptor ligands: Differences with acute versus chronic treatment. *Trends in Pharmacological Sciences, 17*, 108–113.

Jain, N., Kemp, N., Adeyemo, O., Buchanan, P., & Stone, T. W. (1995). Anxiolytic activity of adenosine receptor activation in mice. *British Journal of Pharmacology, 116*, 2127–2133.

James, J. E. (1991). *Caffeine and health.* London: Academic Press.

James, J. E., & Crosbie, J. (1987). Somatic and psychological health implications in heavy caffeine use. *British Journal of Addiction, 82*, 503–509.

Janusz, C., & Berman, R. F. (1993). Adenosinergic modulation of the EEG and locomotor effects of the A2 agonist, CGS 21680. *Pharmacology, Biochemistry and Behavior, 45*, 913–919.

Jarvis, M. F., & Williams, M. (1989). Direct autoradiographic localization of adenosine A2 receptors in the rat brain using the A2-selective agonist, (^{3}H)CGS 21680. *European Journal of Pharmacology, 168*, 243–246.

Jiang, H., Jackson–Lewis, V., Muthane, U., Dollison, A., Ferreira, M., Espinosa, A., Parsons, B., & Przedborski, S. (1993). Adenosine receptor antagonists potentiate dopamine receptor agonist-induced rotational behavior in 6-hydroxydopamine-lesioned rats. *Brain Research, 613*, 347–351.

Jimenez–Jimenez, F. J., Mateo, D., & Gimenez–Roldan, S. (1992). Permorbid smoking, alcohol consumption, and coffee drinking habits in Parkinson's disease: A case-control study. *Movement Disorders, 7*, 339–344.

Johansson, B., Ahlberg, S., van der Ploeg, I., Brené, S., Lindenfors, N., Persson, H., & Fredholm, B. B. (1993). Effect of long term caffeine treatment on A1 and A2 ade-nosine receptor binding and on mRNA levels in rat brain. *Naunyn–Schmiedeberg's Archives of Pharmacology, 347*, 407–414.

Johansson, B., Georgiev, V., Kuosmanen, T., & Fredholm, B. B. (1996). Long-term treatment with some methylxanthines decreases the susceptibility to bicuculline- and pentylentetrazol-induced seizures in mice. Relationship to *c-fos* expression and receptor binding. *European Journal of Neuroscience, 295*, 147–154.

Johansson, B., Lindström, K., & Fredholm, B. B. (1994). Differences in the regional and cellular localization of c-fos messenger RNA induced by amphetamine, cocaine and caffeine in the rat. *Neuroscience, 8*, 2447–2458.

Josselyn, S. A., & Beninger, R. J. (1991). Behavioral effects of intrastriatal caffeine mediated by adenosinergic modulation of dopamine. *Pharmacology, Biochemistry and Behavior, 39*, 97–103.

Jouvet, M. (1969). Biogenic amines and the states of sleep. *Science, 163*, 32–41.

Kanda, T., Jackson, M. J., Smith, L. A., Pearce, R. K. B., Nakamura, J., Kase, H., Kuwana, Y., & Jenner, P. (1998). Adenosine A_{2A} antagonist: a novel antiparkinsonian agent that does not provoke dyskinesia in parkinsonian monkeys. *Annals of Neurology, 43*, 507–513.

Kanda, T., Jackson, M. J., Smith, L. A., Pearce, R. K. B., Nakamura, J., Kase, H., Kuwana, Y., & Jenner, P. (2000). Combined use of the adenosine A_{2A} antagonist KW-6002 with L-DOPA or with selective D1 or D2 dopamine agonists increases antiparkinsonian activity but not dyskinesia in MPTP-treated monkeys. *Experimental Neurology, 162*, 321–327.

Kartzinel, R., Shoulson, I., & Clane, D. B. (1976). Studies with bromocriptine: III. Concom-itant administration of caffeine to patients with idiopathic parkinsonism. *Neurology, 26*, 741–743.

Kawachi, I., Willett, W. C., Colditz, G. A., Stampfer, M. J., & Speizer, F. E. (1996). A prospective study of coffee drinking and suicide in women. *Archives of Internal Medicine, 156*, 521–525.

Klitgaard, H., Knutsen, L. J. S., & Thomsen, C. (1993). Contrasting effects of adenosine A1 and A2 receptor ligands in different chemoconvulsive rodent models. *European Journal of Pharmacology, 242*, 221–228.

Knutsen, L. J. S., & Murray, T. F. (1997). Adenosine and ATP in epilepsy. In K. A. Jacobson & M. J. Jarvis (Eds.), *Purinergic approaches in experimental therapeutics* (pp. 423–447). New York: Wiley–Liss.

Kostic, V. S., Svetel, M., Sternic, N., Dragosevic, N. & Przedborski, S. (1999). Theophylline increases "on" time in advanced parkinsonian patients. *Neurology, 52*, 1916.

Kull, B., Svenningson, P., & Fredholm, B. B. (2000). Adenosine A(2A) receptors are colocalized with and activate g(olf) in rat striatum. *Molecular Pharmacology, 58,* 771–777.

Kuwana, Y., Shiozaki, S., Kanda, T., Kurokawa, M., Koga, K., Ochi, M., Ikeda, K., Kase, H., Jackson, M. J., Smith, L. A., Pearce, R. K., & Penner, P. G. (1999). Antiparkinsonian activity of adenosine A2A antagonists in experimental models. *Advances in Neurology, 80,* 121–123.

Landolt, H. P., Dijk, D. J., Gaus, S. E., & Borbely, A. A. (1995). Caffeine reduces low-frequency delta activity in the human sleep EEG. *Neuropsychopharmacology, 12,* 229–238.

Landolt, H. P., Werth, E., Borbely, A. A., & Dijk, D. J. (1995). Caffeine intake (200 mg) in the morning affects human sleep and EEG power spectra at night. *Brain Research, 675,* 67–74.

Ledent, C., Vaugeois, J. M., Schiffmann, S. N., Pedrazzini, T., El Yacoubi, M., Vanderhaegen, J. J., Costentin, J., Heath, J. K., Vassart, G., & Parmentier, M. (1997). Aggressiveness, hypoalgesia, and high blood pressure in mice lacking the adenosine A_{2A} receptor. *Nature, 388,* 674–678.

Lee, K. S., Tetzlaff, W., & Kreutzberg, G. W. (1986). Rapid downregulation of hippocampal adenosine receptors following brief anoxia. *Brain Research, 380,* 155–158.

Leviton, A. (1983). Biological effects of caffeine. Behavioral effects. *Food Technology, 37,* 44–47.

Levy, M., & Zylber–Katz, E. (1983). Caffeine metabolism and coffee-attributed sleep disturbances. *Clinical Pharmacology and Therapeutics, 33,* 770–775.

Lieberman, H. R., Tharion, W. J., Shukitt–Hale, B., Speckman, K. L., & Tulley, R. (2002). Effects of caffeine, sleep loss, and stress on cognitive performance and mood during U.S. Navy SEAL training. *Psychopharmacology, 164,* 250–261.

Lieberman, H. R., Wurtman, R. J., Emde, G. G., & Coviella, I. L. G. (1987). The effects of caffeine and aspirin on mood and performance. *Journal of Clinical Pharmacology, 7,* 315–320.

Lin, Y., & Phillis, J. W. (1990). Chronic caffeine exposure reduces the excitant action of acetylcholine on cerebral cortical neurons. *Brain Research, 524,* 316–318.

Loke, W. H. (1988). Effects of caffeine on mood and memory. *Physiology and Behavior, 44,* 376–382.

Longstreth, W. T., & Nelson, M. (1992). Caffeine and stroke (letter). *Stroke, 23,* 117.

Lorist, M. M., Snel, J., Kok, A., & Mulder, G. (1994). Influence of caffeine on selective attention in well-rested and fatigued subjects. *Psychophysiology, 31,* 525–534.

Mahan, L. C., McVittie, L. D., Smyk–Randall, E. M., Nakata, H., Monsma, F. J., Jr., Gerfen, C. R., & Sibley, D. R. (1991). Cloning and expression of an A1 adenosine receptor from rat brain. *Molecular Pharmacology, 40,* 1–7.

Mally, J., & Stone, T. W. (1994). The effect of theophylline on parkinsonian symptoms. *Journal of Pharmacy and Pharmacology, 46,* 515–517.

Marangos, P. J., von Lubitz, D. K. J. E., Daval, J. L., & Deckert, J. (1990). Adenosine: Its relevance to the treatment of brain ischemia and trauma. *Progress in Clinical Research, 361,* 331–349.

Marsden, C. D. (1990). Parkinson's disease. *Lancet, 335,* 948–952.

Mayfield, R. D., Suzuki, F., & Zahniser, N. R. (1993). Adenosine A2a receptor modulation of electrically evoked endogenous GABA release from slices of rat globus pallidus. *Journal of Neurochemistry, 60,* 2334–2337.

McMillen, B. A. (1983). CNS stimulants, two distinct mechanisms of action for amphetamine-like drugs. *Trends in Pharmacological Sciences, 4,* 429–432.

Miller, L. P., & Hsu, C. (1992). Therapeutic potential of adenosine receptor activation in ischemic brain injury. *Journal of Neurotrauma, 9*, 563–577.

Miura, T., & Kimura, K. (2000). Theophylline-induced convulsions in children with epilepsy. *Pediatrics, 105*, 920.

Montastruc, J. L., Rascol, O., Senard, J. M., & Rascol, A. A. (1994). Randomized controlled study comparing bromocriptine to which levodopa was later added, with levodopa alone in previously untreated patients with Parkinson's disease. *Journal of Neurology, Neurosurgery and Psychiatry, 57*, 1034–1038.

Mouret, J., Lemoine, P., & Minuit, M. P. (1987). Marqueurs polygraphiques, cliniques et thérapeutiques des dépressions dopamine dépendantes. *Comptes-Rendus de l'Académie des Sciences, Paris, Série 3, 305*, 301–306.

Müller–Limmroth, W. (1972). Der Einfluss von coffeinhaltigem und coffeinfreiem Kaffee auf den Schlaf des Menschen. *Zeitschrift für Ernährungswissenschaft, 14*, Suppl 14, 46–53.

Murray, T. F., Blaker, W. D., Cheney, D. L., & Costa. E. (1982). Inhibition of acetylcholine turnover rate in rat hippocampus and cortex by intraventricular injection of adenosine analogs. *Journal of Pharmacology & Experimental Therapy, 222*, 550–554.

Nakanishi, T., Iwata, M., Goto, I., Kanazawa, I., Kowa, H., Mannen, T., Mizuno, Y., Nishitani, H., Ogawa, N., Tkahashi, A., Tashiro, K., Toghi, H., & Yanagisawa, N. (1992). Nation-wide collaborative study on the long-term effects of bromocriptine in the treatment of Parkinsonian patients. *European Neurology, 32*, 9–22.

Nefzger, M. D., Quadfasel, F. A., & Karl, V. C. (1968). A retrospective study of smoking in Parkinson's disease. *American Journal of Epidemiology, 88*, 149–158.

Nehlig, A. (1999). Are we dependent on coffee and caffeine? A review on human and animal data. *Neuroscience and Biobehavioral Reviews, 23*, 563–576.

Nehlig, A. (2004). Dependence upon coffee and caffeine: An update. In A. Nehlig (Ed.), *Coffee, tea, chocolate and the brain* (pp. 133–146). Boca Raton, FL: CRC Press.

Nehlig, A., & Boyet, S. (2000). Dose–response study of caffeine effects on cerebral functional activity with a specific focus on dependence. *Brain Research, 858*, 71–77.

Nehlig, A., Daval, J. L., & Debry, G. (1992). Caffeine and the central nervous system: mechanisms of action, biochemical, metabolic and psychostimulant effects. *Brain Research Reviews, 17*, 139–170.

Nehlig, A., & Debry, G. (1994). Effects of coffee on the central nervous system. In G. Debry (Ed.), *Coffee and health* (pp. 157–249). Paris: John Libbey.

Nikojevic, O., Sarges, R., Daly, J. W., & Jacobson, K. A. (1991). Behavioral effects of A_1- and A_2-selective adenosine agonists and antagonists: evidence for synergism and antagonism. *Journal of Pharmacology and Experimental Therapeutics, 259*, 286–294.

Ochiishi, T., Chen, L., Yukawa, A., Saitoh, Y., Sekino, Y., Arai, T., Nakata, H., & Miyamoto, H. (1999). Cellular localization of adenosine A1 receptors in rat forebrain: immuno-histochemical analysis using adenosine A1 receptor-specific monoclonal antibody. *Journal of Comparative Neurology, 411*, 301–316.

O'Connor, S. D., Stojanovic, M., & Radulovacki, M. (1991). The effect of soluflazine on sleep in rats. *Neuropharmacology, 30*, 671–674.

Okada, M., Kiryu, K., Kawata, Y., Mizuno, K., Wada, K., Tasaki, H., & Kaneko, S. (1997). Determination of the effects of caffeine and carbamazepine on striatal dopamine release by *in vivo* microdialysis. *European Journal of Pharmacology, 321*, 181–188.

Okada, M., Mizuno, K., & Kaneko, S. (1996). Adenosine A1 and A2 receptors modulate extracellular dopamine levels in rat striatum. *Neuroscience Letters, 212*, 53–56.

Oki, J., Yamamoto, M., Yanagawa, J., Ikeda, K., Taketazu, M., & Miyamota, A. (1994). Theophylline-induced seizures in a 6-month-old girl. Serum and cerebrospinal fluid levels. *Brain & Development*, *16*, 162–164.

Olsson, J. E., Rascol, A., Korten, J. J., Dupont, E., & Gauthier, G. (1989). Early treatment with a combination of bromocriptine and levodopa compared with levodopa mono-therapy in the treatment of Parkinson's disease. *Current Therapeutic Research*, *46*, 1002–1014.

Orzi, F., Passarelli, F., La Riccia, M., Di Grezia, R., & Pontieri, F. E. (1996). Intravenous morphine increases glucose utilization in the shell of the rat nucleus accumbens. *European Journal of Pharmacology*, *302*, 49–51.

Paganini–Hill, A. (2001). Risk factors for Parkinson's disease: The leisure world cohort study. *Neuroepidemiology*, *20*, 118–124.

Park, T. S., Van Wylen, D. G. L., Rubio, R., & Berne, R. M. (1987). Interstitial fluid adenosine analogs on amygdala, hippocampus and caudate nucleus kindled seizures. *Epilepsia*, *28*, 658–666.

Patat, A., Rosenzweig, P., Enslen, M., Trocherie, S., Miget, N., Bozon, M. C., Allain, H., & Gandon, J. M. (2000). Effects of a new slow release formulation of caffeine on EEG, psychomotor and cognitive functions in sleep-deprived subjects. *Human Psychopharmacology, Clinical and Experimental*, *15*, 153–170.

Phillips–Bute, B. G., & Lane, J. D. (1998). Caffeine withdrawal symptoms following brief caffeine deprivation. *Physiology and Behavior*, *63*, 35–39.

Phillis, J. W., & Edstrom, J. P. (1976). Effects of adenosine analogis on rat cerebral cortical neurons. *Life Science*, *19*, 1041–1053.

Pinard, E., Riche, D., Puiroud, S., & Seylaz, J. (1990). Theophylline reduces cerebral hyperemia and enhances brain damage induced by seizures. *Brain Research*, *511*, 303–309.

Pinna, A., Di Chiara, G., Wardas, J., & Morelli, M. (1996). Blockade of A2a adenosine receptors positively modulates turning behavior and *c-fos* expression induced by D1 agonists in dopamine-denervated rats. *Journal of Neuroscience*, *8*, 1176–1181.

Pontieri, F. E., Tanda, G., & Di Chiara, G. (1995). Intravenous cocaine, morphine, and amphetamine preferentially increase extracellular dopamine in the "shell" as compared with the "core" of the rat nucleus accumbens. *Proceedings of the National Academy of Sciences of the USA*, *92*, 12304–12308.

Pontieri, F. E., Tanda, G., Orzi, F., & Di Chiara, G. (1996). Effects of nicotine on the nucleus accumbens and similarity to those of addictive drugs. *Nature*, *382*, 255–257.

Popoli, P., Ferré, S., Pezzola, A., Reggio, R., DeCarolis, A. S., & Fuxe, K. (1996a). Stimulation of adenosine A1 receptors prevents the EEG arousal due to dopamine D-1 receptor activation in rabbits. *European Journal of Pharmacology*, *305*, 123–126.

Popoli, P., Gimenez–Llort, L., Pezzola, A., Reggio, R., Martinez, E., Fuxe, K., & Ferré, S. (1996b). Adenosine A1 receptor blockade selectively potentiates the motor effects induced by dopamine D1 receptor stimulation in rodents. *Neuroscience Letters*, *218*, 209–213.

Porkka–Hieskanen, T., Alanko, L., Kalinchuk, L., & Sternberg, D. (2002). Adenosine and sleep. *Sleep Medicine Reviews*, *6*, 321–332.

Porkka–Hieskanen, T., Strecker, R. E., & McCarley, R. W. (2000). Brain site specificity of extracellular concentration changes during sleep deprivation and spontaneous sleep: An *in vivo* microdialysis study. *Neuroscience*, *99*, 507–517.

Porkka–Hieskanen, T., Strecker, R. E., Thakkar, M., Bjorkum, A. A., Greene, R. W., & McCarley, R. W. (1997). Adenosine: A mediator of the sleep-inducing effects of prolonged wakefulness. *Science*, *276*, 1265–1268.

Porrino, L. J., Domer, F. R., Crane, A. M., & Sokoloff, L. (1988). Selective alterations in cerebral metabolism within the mesocorticolimbic dopaminergic system produced by acute cocaine administration in rats. *Neuropsychopharmacology, 1*, 109–118.

Prat, G., Robledo, P., Rubio, A., Barbanoj, M., Jané, F., & Casas, M. (2000). Effects of subchronic treatment with pergolide and caffeine on contralateral rotational behavior in unilateral 6-hydroxydopamine-denervated rats. *Brain Research, 868*, 376–379.

Preston, Z., Lee, K., Widdowson, L., Freeman, T. C., Dixon, A. K., & Richardson, P. J. (2000). Adenosine receptor expression and function in rat striatal cholinergic interneurons. *British Journal of Pharmacology, 130*, 886–890.

Radulovacki, M. (1985). Role of adenosine in sleep in rats. *Review of Clinical and Basic Pharmacology, 5*, 327–339.

Rainnie, D. G., Grunze, H. C., McCarley, R. W., & Greene, R. W. (1994). Adenosine inhibition of mesopontine cholinergic neurons: Implications for EEG arousal. *Science, 263*, 689–692.

Reinis, S., & Goldman, J. M. (1982). *The chemistry of behavior. A molecular approach to neuronal plasticity.* New York: Plenum Press.

Reppert, S. M., Weaver, D. R., Stehle, J. H., & Rivkees, S. A. (1991). Molecular cloning and characterization of a rat A1-adenosine receptor that is widely expressed in brain and spinal cord. *Molecular Endocrinology, 5*, 1037–1048.

Reyner, L. A., & Horne, J. A. (2000). Early morning driver sleepiness: Effectiveness of 200 mg caffeine. *Psychobiology, 37*, 251–256.

Richelson, E. (1994). Pharmacology of antidepressants—Characteristics of the ideal drug. *Mayo Clinic Proceedings, 69*, 1069–1081.

Rigoulot, M. A., Leroy, C., Koning, E., Ferrandon, A., & Nehlig, A. (2003). A chronic low-dose caffeine exposure protects against hippocampal damage but not against the occurrence of epilepsy in the lithium-pilocarpine model in the rat. *Epilepsia, 44*, 529–535.

Rihs, M., Muller, C., & Baumann, P. (1996). Caffeine consumption in hospitalized psychiatric patients. *European Archives of Psychiatry and Clinical Neuroscience, 246*, 83–92.

Rogers, P. J., & Dernoncourt, C. (1998). Regular caffeine consumption, a balance of adverse and beneficial effects for mood and psychomotor performance. *Pharmacology, Biochemistry and Behavior, 59*, 1039–1045.

Rosin, D. L., Robeva, A., Woodard, R. L., Guyenet, P. G., & Linden, J. (1998). Immunohistochemical localization of adenosine A2A receptors in the rat central nervous system. *Journal of Comparative Neurology, 401*, 163–186.

Ross, G. W., Abbott, R. D., Petrovitch, H., Morens, D. M., Grandinetti, A., Tung, K. H., Tanner, C. M., Masaki, K. H., Blanchette, P. L., Curb, J. D., Popper, J. S., & White, L. R. (2000). Association of coffee and caffeine intake with the risk of Parkinson disease. *JAMA, 283*, 2674–2679.

Rossetti, Z. L., & Carboni, S. (1995). Ethanol withdrawal is associated with increased extracellular glutamate in the rat striatum. *European Journal of Pharmacology, 283*, 177–183.

Rudolphi, K. A., Keil, M., Fastbom, J., & Fredholm, B. B. (1989). Ischaemic damage in gerbil hippocampus is reduced following upregulation of adenosine (A1) receptors by caffeine treatment. *Neuroscience Letters, 103*, 275–280.

Rudolphi, K. A., Keil, M., & Grome, J. J. (1990). Adenosine—A pharmacological concept for the treatment of cerebral ischemia? In J. Krieglstein & H. Oberpichler (Eds.) *Pharmacology of Cerebral Ischemia* (pp. 439–448). Stuttgart: Wissenschaftliche Verlagsgesselschaft mbH.

Rudolphi, K. A., Schubert, P., Parkinson, F. E., & Fredholm, B. B. (1992). Neuroprotective role of adenosine in cerebral ischemia. *Trends in Pharmacological Sciences, 13,* 439–445.

Salmi, P., Chergui, K., & Fredholm, B. B. (2005). Adenosine-dopamine interactions revealed in knockout mice. *Journal of Molecular Neuroscience, 26,* 239–244.

Sanchez–Ortuno, M., Moore, N., Taillard, J., Valtat, C. Léger, D., Bioulac, B. & Philip, P. (2005). Sleep duration and caffeine consumption in a French middle-aged working population. *Sleep Medicine, 6,* 247–251.

Satoh, S., Matsumura, H., & Hayaishi, O. (1998). Involvement of adenosine A2a receptor in sleep promotion. *European Journal of Pharmacology, 351,* 155–162.

Satoh, S., Matsumura, H., Suzuki, F., & Hayaishi, O. (1996). Promotion of sleep mediated by the A2a-adenosine receptor and possible involvement of this receptor in the sleep induced by prostaglandin D2 in rats. *Proceedings of the National Academy of Sciences of the USA, 93,* 5980–5984.

Scammell, T. E., Arrigoni, E., Thompson, M. A., Ronan, P. J., Saper, C. B., & Greene, R. W. (2003). Focal deletion of the adenosine A1 receptor in adult mice using an adeno-associated viral vector. *Journal of Neuroscience, 23,* 5762–5770.

Schiffmann, S. N., Jacobs, O., & Vanderhaegen, J. J. (1991). Striatal restricted adenosine A2 receptor (RDC8) is expressed by enkephalin but not by substance P neurons: an *in situ* hybridization histochemistry study. *Journal of Neurochemistry, 57,* 1062–1067.

Schubert, P., Heinemann, U., & Kolb, R. (1986). Differential effects of adenosine on pre- and postsynaptic calcium fluxes. *Brain Research, 376,* 382–386.

Schubert, P., & Lee, K. S. (1986). Non-synaptic modulation of repetitive firing by adenosine is antagonized by 4-aminopyridine in rat hippocampal slice. *Neuroscience Letters, 67,* 334–338.

Schwarzschild, M. A., & Ascherio, A. (2004). Caffeine and Parkinson's disease. In A. Nehlig (Ed.), *Coffee, tea, chocolate and the brain* (pp. 147–163). Boca Raton, FL: CRC Press.

Seale, T. W., Abla, K. A., Shamim, M. T., Carney, J. M., & Daly, J. W. (1988). 3,7-Dimethyl-1-propargylxanthine: A potent and selective *in vivo* antagonist of adenosine analogs. *Life Sciences, 43,* 1671–1684.

Sebastiao, A. M., & Ribeiro, J. A. (1996). Adenosine A2 receptor-mediated excitatory actions on the nervous system. *Progress in Neurobiology, 48,* 167–189.

Segev, S., Rehavi, M., & Rubistein, E. (1988). Quinolones, theophylline and diclofenac interactions with the γ-aminobutyric acid receptor. *Antimicrobial Agents Chemotherapy, 32,* 1624–1626.

Self, D. W., & Nestler, E. J. (1995). Molecular mechanisms of drug reinforcement and addiction, *Annual Review of Neuroscience, 18,* 463–495.

Shannon, M. (1993). Predictors of major toxicity after theophylline overdose. *Annals of Internal Medicine, 119,* 1161–1167.

Shapira, B., Lerer, B., Gilboa, D., Drexler, H., Kugelmass, S., & Calev, A. (1987). Facilitation of ECT by caffeine pretreatment. *American Journal of Psychiatry, 144,* 1199–1202.

Shimada, J., Koike, N., Nonaka, H., Shiozaki, S., Yanagawa, K., Kanda, T., Kobayashi, H., Ichimura, M., Nakamura, J., Kase, H., & Suzuki, F. (1997). (E)-1,3-Diethyl-8-(3,4-dimethoxystyryl)-7-methylxanthine: A potent adenosine A2 antagonist with anticataleptic activity. *Bioorganic and Medicinal Chemistry Letters, 7,* 2349–2352.

Shoulson, Y., & Chase, T. (1975). Caffeine and the antiparkinsonian response to levodopa or piribidil. *Neurology, 25,* 722–724.

Silverman, K., Mumford, G. K., & Griffiths R. R. (1994). Enhancing caffeine reinforcement by behavioral requirements following drug ingestion. *Psychopharmacology, 114,* 424–432.

Sitland–Marken, P. A., Wells, B. G., Froemming, J. H., Chu, C. C., & Brown, C. S. (1990). Psychiatric applications of bromocriptine therapy. *Journal of Clinical Psychiatry*, *51*, 68–82.

Smith, A. (1994). Caffeine, performance, mood and states of reduced alertness. *Pharmacopsychoecologia*, *7*, 75–86.

Smith, A., Sturgess, W., & Gallagher, J. (1999). Effects of a low dose of caffeine given in different drinks on mood and performance. *Human Psychopharmacology, Clinical and Experimental*, *14*, 473–482.

Smith, A., Thomas, M., Perry, K., & Withney, H. (1997). Caffeine and the common cold. *Journal of Psychopharmacology*, *11*, 319–324.

Smith, A. P., Rusted, J. M., Eaton–Williams, P., Savory, M., & Leathwood, P. (1990). Effects of caffeine given before and after lunch on sustained attention. *Neuropsychobiology*, *23*, 160–163.

Snel, J. (1993). Coffee and caffeine: sleep and wakefulness. In S. Garattini (Ed.), *Coffee, caffeine and health* (pp. 255–290). New York: Raven Press.

Snel, J., Tieges, Z., & Lorist, M. M. (2004). Effects of caffeine on sleep and wakefulness: an update. In A. Nehlig (Ed.), *Coffee, tea, chocolate and the brain* (pp. 13–33). Boca Raton, FL: CRC Press.

Solinas, M., Ferré, S., You, Z. B., Karcz–Kubicha, M., Popoli, P. & Goldberg, S. R. (2002). Caffeine induces dopamine and glutamate release in the shell of the nucleus accumbens. *Journal of Neuroscience*, *22*, 6321–6324.

Soroko, S., Chang, J., & Barrett–Connor, E. (1996). Reasons for changing caffeinated coffee consumption: The Rancho Bernardo Study. *Journal of the American College of Nutrition*, *15*, 97–101.

Stein, E. A., & Fuller, S. A. (1992). Selective effects of cocaine on regional cerebral blood flow in the rat. *Journal of Pharmacology and Experimental Therapeutics*, *262*, 327–334.

Stephenson, P. E. (1977). Physiologic and psychotropic effects of caffeine on man. *Journal of the American Dietetic Association*, *71*, 240–247.

Stone, W. E., & Javid, M. J. (1980). Aminophylline and imidazole as convulsants. *Archives Internationales de Pharmacodynamie*, *248*, 120–131.

Strain, E. C., Mumford, G. K., Silverman, K., & Griffiths, R. R. (1994). Caffeine dependence syndrome. Evidence from case histories and experimental evaluations. *JAMA*, *272*, 1043–1048.

Sutherland, G. R., Peeling, J., Lesiuk, H. J., Brownstone, R. M., Rydzy, M., Saunders, J. K., & Geiger, J. D. (1991). The effects of caffeine on ischemic cerebral injury as determined by magnetic resonance imaging and histopathology. *Neuroscience*, *42*, 171–182.

Svenningsson, P., Le Moine, C., Kull, B., Sunahara, R., Bloch, B., & Fredholm, B. B. (1997). Cellular expression of adenosine A2A receptor messenger RNA in the rat central nervous system with special reference to dopamine innervated areas. *Neuroscience*, *80*, 1171–1185.

Svenningsson, P., Nomikos, G. G., & Fredholm, B. B. (1995). Biphasic changes in locomotor behavior and in expression of mRNA for NGFI-A and NGFI-B in rat striatum following acute caffeine administration. *Journal of Neuroscience*, *15*, 7612–7624.

Svenningsson, P., Nomikos, G. G., Ongini, E., & Fredholm, B. B. (1997). Antagonism of adenosine A2A receptors underlies the behavioral activating effect of caffeine and is associated with reduced expression of messenger RNA for NGFI-A and NGFI-B in caudate-putamen and nucleus accumbens. *Neuroscience*, *79*, 753–764.

Svenningsson, P., Ström, A., Johansson, B., & Fredholm, B. B. (1995). Increased expression of c-jun, junB, AP-1, and preproenkephalin mRNA in rat striatum following a single injection of caffeine. *Journal of Neuroscience, 15*, 3583–3593.

Tan, E. K., Tan, C., Fook–Chong, S. M., Lum, S. Y., Chai, A., Chung, H., Shen, H., Zhao, Y., Teoh, M. L., Yih, Y., Pavanni, R., Chandran, V. R., & Wong, M. C. (2003). Dose-dependent protective effect of coffee, tea, and smoking in Parkinson's disease: A study in ethnic Chinese. *Journal of Neurological Sciences, 216*, 163–167.

Tiffin, P., Ashton, H., Marsh, R., & Kamali, F. (1995). Pharmacokinetic and pharmacodynamic responses to caffeine in poor and normal sleepers. *Psychopharmacology, 121*, 494–502.

Turski, W. A., Cavalheiro, E. A., Ikonomidou, C., Mello, L. E., Bortolotto, Z. A., & Turski, L. (1985). Effects of aminophylline and 2-chloroadenosine on seizures produced by pilocarpine in rats: Morphological and electroencephalographic correlates. *Brain Research, 361*, 309–323.

Uhde, T. W. (1988). Caffeine: Practical facts for the psychiatrist. In P. P. Roy–Byrne (Ed.), *Anxiety: new research findings for the clinician* (pp. 73–98). Washington, D.C.: American Psychiatric Press.

Uhde, T. W. (1990). Caffeine provocation of panic: A focus on biological mechanisms. In J. C. Ballenger (Ed.), *Neurobiology of panic disorders* (pp. 219–242). New York: Alan Liss.

Viani, R. (1996). Caffeine consumption. *Proceedings of the Caffeine Workshop,* Thai FDA and ILSI, Bangkok.

von Lubitz, D. K. J. E., Carter, M., Deutsch, S. I., Lin, R. C., Mastropaolo, J., Meshulam, Y., & Jacobson, K. A. (1995). The effects of adenosine A3 receptor stimulation on seizures in mice. *European Journal of Pharmacology, 275*, 23–29.

von Lubitz, D. K. J. E., Dambrosia, J. M., Kempski, O., & Redmond, D. J. (1988). Cyclohexyl adenosine protects against neuronal death following ischemia in the CA1 region of gerbil hippocampus. *Stroke, 19*, 1133–1139.

von Lubitz, D. K. J. E., Dambrosia, J. M., & Redmond, D. J. (1989). Protective effects of cyclohexyl adenosine in treatment of cerebral ischemia in gerbils. *Neuroscience, 30*, 451–462.

von Lubitz, D. K. J. E., Lin, R. C., Melman, N., Ji, X. D., Carter, M. F., & Jacobson, K. A. (1994). Chronic administration of selective adenosine A1 receptor agonist or antagonist in cerebral ischemia. *European Journal of Pharmacology, 256*, 161–167.

von Lubitz, D. K. J. E., Lin, R. C. S., Popik, P., Carter, M. F., & Jacobson, K. A. (1994). Adenosine A3 receptor stimulation and cerebral ischemia. *European Journal of Pharmacology, 263*, 59–67.

von Lubitz, D. K. J. E., Paul, I. A., Carter, M., & Jacobson, K. A. (1993). Effects of N^6 cyclopentyl adenosine and 8-cyclopentyl-1,3-dipropylxanthine on N-methyl-D-aspartate induced seizures in mice. *European Journal of Pharmacology, 249*, 265–270.

von Lubitz, D. K. J. E., Paul, I. A., Ji, X. D., Carter, M. F., & Jacobson, K. A. (1994). Chronic adenosine A1 receptor agonist and antagonist: effect on receptor density and N-methyl-D-aspartate induced seizures in mice. *European Journal of Pharmacology, 253*, 95–99.

Webb, R. L., Sills, M. A., Chovan, J. P., Peppard, J. V., & Francis, J. E. (1993). Development of tolerance to the antihypertensive effects of highly selective adenosine A2a agonists upon chronic administration. *Journal of Pharmacology and Experimental Therapeutics, 267*, 287–295.

Wiesner, J. B., Ugarkar, B. G., Castellino, A. J., Barankiewicz, J., Dumas, D. P., Gruber, H. E., Foster, A. C., & Erion, M. D. (1999). Adenosine kinase inhibitors as a novel approach to anticonvulsant therapy. *Journal of Pharmacology and Experimental Therapeutics, 289,* 1669–1677.

Willner, P. (1997). The mesolimbic dopamine system as a target for rapid antidepressant action. *International Clinical Psychopharmacology, 12,* Suppl 3, S7–S14.

Winn, H. R., Welsh, J. E., Bryner, C., Rubio, R., & Berne, R. M. (1979). Brain adenosine production during the initial 60 seconds of bicuculline seizures in rats. *Acta Neurologica Scandinavica, 72,* 536–537.

Winn, H. R., Welsh, J. E., Rubio, R., & Berne, R. M. (1980). Changes in brain adenosine during bicuculline-induced seizures in rats: Effects of hypoxia and altered systemic blood pressure. *Circulation Research, 47,* 868–877.

Yanik, G., Glaum, S., & Radulovacki, M. (1987). The dose–response effects of caffeine on sleep in rats. *Brain Research, 403,* 177–180.

Yokohama, H., Onodera, K., Yagi, T., & Iinuma, K. (1997). Therapeutic doses of theophylline exert proconvulsant effects in developing mice. *Brain & Development, 19,* 403–407.

Young, D., & Dragunow, M. (1994). Status epilepticus may be caused by loss of adenosine anticonvulsant mechanisms. *Neuroscience, 58,* 245–261.

Zhang, G., Franklin, P. H., & Murray, T. F. (1994). Activation of adenosine A_1 receptors underlies anticonvulsant effect of CGS 21680. *European Journal of Pharmacology, 255,* 239–243.

Zwyghuizen–Doorenbos, A., Roehrs, T. A., Lipschutz, L., Timms, V., & Roth, T. (1990). The effects of caffeine on alertness. *Psychopharmacology, 100,* 36–39.

Section II

Cardiovascular Effects

4 Acute Cardiovascular Effects of Caffeine: Hemodynamics and Heart Function

Barry D. Smith and Katherine Aldridge

CONTENTS

INTRODUCTION

In 2005, Kerrigan and Lindsey reported two cases of fatal caffeine overdose. Femoral blood contained 192 mg/L of the drug in one patient and 567 mg/L in the other. In another case, a 41-year-old woman who presented with multisystem failure, including heart failure, 3 hours following ingestion of 50 g of caffeine, survived after heroic measures were taken (Holstege et al., 2003). Although such cases of severe caffeine intoxication are rare, they do demonstrate the toxic potential of this almost universally consumed drug. Indeed, it can produce extreme tachycardia, atrial and ventricular arrhythmias, convulsions, and coma (Cannon, Cooke, & McCarthy, 2001).

The toxic potential of caffeine is further extended by virtue of the fact that it can interact with a variety of prescription and nonprescription drugs. Such pharmacokinetic interactions arise from the fact that caffeine is metabolized through the cytochrome P450 system—primarily by the polycyclic aromatic hydrocarbon-inducible CYP-450 isoenzyme, CYP1A2. This same enzyme is inhibited by such drugs as quinolones, antipsychotics, bronchodilators, and anti arrhythmics. As a result, caffeine may increase serum concentrations of other drugs, again with potentially toxic results (Carrillo & Benitez, 2000).

In this chapter, we focus on the effects of acute doses of caffeine on the cardiovascular system, emphasizing the immediate impact on hemodynamics and heart function and implications of these short-term changes for potential long-term effects of the drug. Some of the likely implications are straightforward. However, others are not obvious, and it is important not to make leaps of faith in cases where simple logic might suggest a particular long-term impact.

AROUSAL EFFECTS AND THEIR IMPLICATIONS

The acute cardiovascular effects of caffeine are related to and, to some extent, stem from the arousal properties of the drug, which are well-demonstrated. Caffeine, for example, increases skin conductance level (SCL) and reduces EEG power in the alpha band (Barry et al., 2005). Along similar lines, other studies show that it raises blood pressure and decreases P300 latencies (Deslandes et al., 2005). All of these effects are consistent with increased general arousal, which may also have an impact on several heart-function parameters. These include heart rate (HR), heart rate variability (HRV), arrhythmias, and aortic stiffness. We will examine each of these and also some potentially positive effects of caffeine on exercise performance and endurance.

HEART RATE

Because most myocardial perfusion occurs during diastole, it is no surprise that chronically elevated heart rate is associated with cardiovascular and all-cause mortality. In one recent study, it was found that those with HRs of 83 bpm or greater were at significantly higher risk for cardiovascular mortality as well as total mortality (Diaz, Bourassa, Guertin, & Tardif, 2005). More generally, 32 of 38 published studies have reported these associations, with hazard ratios of 1.3 to 1.7 for cardiovascular mortality and 1.9 to 2.0 for all-cause mortality (Palatini, Benetos, & Julius, 2006). The relationship is stronger in males than in females, but is present in both sexes.

Chronically elevated HR is typically linked with patterns of blood flow associated with the long-term development of atherosclerotic plaques, and this may be the major pathogenic mechanism underlying the association (Bassioumy et al., 2002). Further support for this observation is seen in treatment regimens that lower HR, thereby reducing ischemia and lowering the risk of myocardial infarction (MI) (Danchin & Aly, 2004).

Caffeine is known to increase arousal (Barry et al., 2005), so it is reasonable to ask whether or not it consistently increases HR and, if so, whether or not it may contribute to atherosclerosis. There is little doubt that lifestyle factors can affect HR, and many tend to assume that caffeine consumption, as one factor, increases it (Stolarz et al., 2003). However, studies conducted to date do not, on the whole, support this hypothesis. In one recent investigation, participants performed a mental stress task after first consuming a triple espresso. Results did show a caffeine-induced increase in HR, but only in those who did not habitually drink coffee. In addition, it was found that an intravenous bolus of 250 mg of caffeine produced no HR increase at all (Sudano et al., 2005).

Other studies show no effect of caffeine under resting conditions (Schutte, Huisman, Van Rooyen, Oosthuizen, & Herling, 2003) or during exercise following sleep deprivation (McLellan, Bell, & Kamunori, 2004). Still others report that caffeine actually lowers HR in a dose–response fashion (Quinlan et al., 2000), a finding that appears to be particularly true for habitual nonusers (Berry, Richards, & Newman, 2003).

HEART RATE VARIABILITY

A second noninvasive index of cardiovascular risk is heart rate variability (HRV). Prone and ambulatory electrocardiographic studies have demonstrated that HRV is associated with myocardial anomalies and with risk for cardiovascular morbidity and mortality. One study, for example, showed that an HRV measure based on the Haar wavelet transform significantly differentiates between patients with known coronary artery disease (CAD) and normal controls (Pawlak–Bus et al., 2005). Another investigation employed ambulatory electrocardiography to assess HRV over a 24-h period. It was found that long-term HRV correlated with left ventricular ejection fraction and left ventricular diastolic dimension, which are established indices of severity of myocardial dysfunction and cardiac mortality (Minamihaba, Yamaki, Tomoike, & Kubota, 2003). Daniel Roach and his colleagues conclude, with other investigators, that reduced HRV is associated with heart failure and mortality (Roach, Wilson, Ritchie, & Sheldon, 2004).

Factors contributing to complex variations in heart rate are not yet well understood. However, some progress has been made, and some evidence indicates a genetic predisposition. Subjects in the Framingham Heart Study underwent Holter monitoring, and a power spectral analysis of HRV was performed in order to derive quantitative phenotypic markers. Results showed that a substantial proportion of the variance in HRV is genetic (Singh, Larson, O'Donnell, & Levy, 2001). A second Framingham study employed 24-h ambulatory cardiography to obtain HRV data from 725 subjects in 230 families. Using a 10-cm genome-wide scan, investigators found that specific genes on chromosomes 2 and 15 are associated with HRV, further supporting its genetic basis (Singh et al., 2002).

In addition to the genetic factor, it seems clear that a variety of environmental pathogens likely also contribute to HRV and the associated cardiac risk. In fact, a study of over 800 people, the European Project on Genes in Hypertension (EPOGH), provides support for the hypothesis that lifestyle factors do contribute some variance (Stolarz et al., 2003). More generally, such factors may include smoking, excessive alcohol consumption, diets high in calories or transfats, chronic insomnia, lack of aerobic exercise, and arousal agents like ephedrine and caffeine. Studies of the possible association between the latter drug and HRV are thus far few in number, but some preliminary findings are available.

In one investigation, HRV was measured at rest and then again after exercise. It was found that caffeine increased variability under resting conditions, but decreased it after exercise (Yeragani, Krishnon, Engels, & Greteneck, 2005). A second study used the time-stretch model of QT variability to examine the effects of caffeine during sleep. Subjects were given 400 mg caffeine or a placebo 30 min prior to going to bed. Results showed that the drug increased HRV during sleep (Bonnet, Tamcer, Unde, & Yergani, 2005). Results of studies like these suggest that caffeine may increase HRV, and others are beginning to show that the drug may, in fact, decrease cardiac risk under some conditions. One investigation examined HRV in diabetic patients, who are at increased risk of autonomic failure and sudden cardiac death, and in healthy controls. It was found that caffeine differentially affected HRV at baseline in diabetics as compared with controls (Richardson et al., 2004). The authors conclude that a modest amount of caffeine (250 mg twice daily in this study) may actually improve autonomic function and reduce the risk of cardiac events in at-risk populations with abnormal HRV.

Literature concerned with the caffeine–HRV risk relationship is thus far sparse, but already we are seeing that it is complex. Further studies of the impact of caffeine on HRV should address such issues as the proportion of variance accounted for by caffeine, differential role of the drug in varied patient and normal populations, and interaction of caffeine with such other lifestyle factors as smoking and diet.

ARRHYTHMIAS, MORTALITY, AND CAFFEINE

Atrial fibrillation, the most common sustained cardiac arrhythmia, is a serious risk factor for ischemic stroke (Go, Fang, & Singer, 2005) and contributes substantially to cardiac morbidity and mortality (Nattel & Opie, 2006). However, ventricular arrhythmias present an even greater cardiac risk. When ventricular tachycardia (VT) degenerates to ventricular arrhythmia (VA), sudden cardiac death (SCD) results, unless immediate intervention is successful. In some cases, SCD results from a channelopathy, an inherited primary electrical disorder. When the channelopathy produces cathecholaminergic polymorphic ventricular tachycardia or when Wolff–Parkinson–White (WPW) syndrome is present, SCD may result (Sarkozy & Brugada, 2005). Similarly, commotio cordis can result in death when a strong, nonpenetrating blow to the chest, particularly during repolarization (Link, 2003), produces immediate ventricular fibrillation (VF) (Geddes & Roeder, 2005).

Apart from such relatively rare instances, SCD is most likely to occur in patients with recent MIs and in those with cardiomyopathy (Reddy, Tandon, & Stafford, 1999) or congestive heart failure. In the latter case, death is due to SCD in about half of all patients (Ebinger, Krishnan, & Schuger, 2005). Apart from myocardial scar, current thinking suggests that many of these deaths involve abnormal calcium handling, ionic imbalances, neurohormonal anomalies, and potassium current disturbances (Rubart & Zipes, 2005).

When commotio cordis is the cause of SCD, other factors are not known to be involved. However, in all other instances, including those involving chemical imbalances or anomalies, with or without a genetic predisposition, a variety of influences may be involved in arrhythmias. Some of these factors may be arrhythmogenic and others antiarrhythmogenic. One class of substances that has received attention as potential contributors to arrhythmia is stimulants. Although much of the research effort has been devoted to cocaine (Egred & Davis, 2005), which is known to foster microangiopathy and hypertrophy with prolonged use (Karch, 2005), several recent studies have looked at the role of caffeine.

Cannon and colleagues (2001) report the case of a 25-year-old woman who consumed a guarana energy drink high in caffeine and went into intractable ventricular fibrillation. She had pre-existing mitral valve prolapse, but such cases do raise the question of whether or not caffeine may induce VF, at least in patients with certain existing cardiac anomalies. A study in which caffeine was injected into dogs appears to confirm this danger. A high dose of the drug induced VT, multifocal ventricular premature contractions (VPC), and atrial fibrillation (Mehta et al., 1997). Similar results are seen in some studies of mouse hearts (Balasubramaniam, Chawla, Grace, & Huang, 2005). However, there are few studies in humans and a more general association between caffeine and VT or VF has not been established.

One relevant study involved patients with histories of VT or VF. Ventricular stimulation was employed to induce VT with or without caffeine. It was found that the drug did not increase VT inducibility, even in this patient group (Chelsky et al., 1990). A second study, involving young, healthy volunteers, showed that caffeine actually optimized heart rhythm and enhanced parasympathotonia (Baida Mastiagina, Mastiagina, & Arushanian, 2005). Although caution is certainly warranted, thus far no clear evidence suggests that caffeine contributes to ventricular arrhythmias.

With regard to atrial fibrillation, research suggests that its development may be, in part, due to upregulation of calcium (CA2+) release from the sarcoplasmic reticulum (Hove–Madsen et al., 2004). Moreover, spontaneous release of CA2+ can produce after-depolarizations, which can, in turn, trigger the arrhythmia. If caffeine contributes to this process, it may induce episodes of fibrillation in patients with established AF. However, literature concerned with the caffeine–AF association provides mixed and complex results.

A survey study asked 100 patients with AF what triggered episodes of fibrillation. The most common reported causes were stress, physical exertion, and fatigue. However, 25% said that caffeine was one trigger. Similarly, a second study showed that high coffee consumption was associated with an increased risk of episodes of atrial fibrillation in patients with extant disorders (Mattioli, Bonatti, Monopol, Zennato, & Mattioli, 2005). On the other hand, data from over 47,000 participants in the Danish Diet, Cancer, and Health Study showed no association between AF or atrial flutter and caffeine consumption (Frost & Vestergaard, 2005).

Two final investigations examined the effects of caffeine in healthy volunteers on P-wave or QRS complex duration, both associated with AF. In the first, it was found that caffeine induced a small but statistically significant prolongation of the QRS complex, which the authors conclude would be unlikely to cause AF in those with healthy hearts (Donnerstein, Zhu, Samson, Bender, & Goldberg, 1998). In the second study, a 400-mg dose of caffeine had no effect on P-wave duration, P-wave maximum duration, or P-wave dispersion, suggesting that it would be unlikely to produce VT (which is also associated with P-wave duration) or AF (Caron, Song, Ammar, Kluger, & White, 2001). This small part of the literature, as a whole, suggests that there may be some risk that caffeine can induce episodes of AF in patients with an established disorder, but it is unlikely to produce the arrhythmia in healthy individuals. However, much more research is needed before firm conclusions can be drawn.

ARTERIAL STIFFNESS AND CAFFEINE

Any increase in arterial stiffness elevates central arterial pressure, with a resulting increase in cardiac workload and myocardial demand. It is therefore not surprising that arterial stiffness is associated with left ventricular hypertrophy, decreased myocardial perfusion, and hypertension (Vlachopoulos, Aznaouridis, & Stefanadis, 2005). Confirming these observations, investigators in the Rotterdam Study assessed CHD risk factors in 2885 subjects. They found that aortic pulse wave velocity, a measure of arterial stiffness, was associated with increased risk for coronary heart disease (CHD) and stroke (Mattace–Raso et al., 2006). The question we raise here is whether or not caffeine consumption increases arterial stiffness or aortic pulse wave reflection. Methods for measurement of these cardiovascular parameters are mixed, and there has been a call for standardization of measurement (Van Bortel et al., 2002). However, results relating to caffeine have been quite consistent (Papaioannou, Karatzis, Papmichael, & Lekakis, 2005).

The major contributors to this literature thus far have been the Vlachoupoulos group at the Athens Medical School. In a series of recent studies, they have consistently confirmed an association between caffeine and aortic stiffness and wave reflection. In one investigation, they showed that administration of 250 mg caffeine to 20 healthy volunteers produced an increase in aortic stiffness and wave reflection (Vlachopoulos, Hirata, & O'Rourke, 2003). In a second study, caffeine alone and smoking alone each increased aortic pulse wave velocity, and the two combined had a synergistic effect (Vlachopoulos et al., 2004). In a third study, it was found that habitual coffee consumption contributes to increases in aortic stiffness and wave reflection (Vlachopoulos, Panagiotakos, Ioakeimidis, Dima, & Stefandis, 2005).

Other studies from this group have also supported these associations (Vlachopoulos, Aznaouridis, & Stefanadis, 2005; Vlachopoulos, Dima, et al., 2005). On a more positive note, they have found that one caffeine source—dark chocolate (100 g)—decreased wave reflections, though it had no effect on aortic stiffness (Vlachopoulos, Aznaourdis, Alexopoulos, et al., 2005).

One investigation from another laboratory is consistent with the Vlachopoulos findings. In a small study of seven healthy volunteers, Mahmud and Feely (2001) administered 150 mg caffeine or a placebo. They measured aortic stiffness, using carotid-femoral pulse wave velocity, and arterial wave reflection, using applanation tonometry. Results showed that caffeine increased stiffness and wave reflection.

Based on research to date, it appears that caffeine may contribute to arterial stiffness and wave reflection. However, there are thus far relatively few studies, and most have examined only the effects of acute caffeine consumption, so further research is certainly warranted. Moreover, the mechanisms through which caffeine might operate to affect these arterial parameters need to be determined, and the effects of other stimulants should also be examined.

POSSIBLE BENEFICIAL EFFECTS OF CAFFEINE

Some work suggests that acute doses of caffeine may have beneficial effects. In particular, it may have ergogenic effects on exercise and its perception. In one study, participants engaged in a forced march, with sleep loss, and also ran on a treadmill to exhaustion. Results showed that caffeine maintained physical performance, even with sleep loss, and that time to exhaustion increased by 25% under influence of the drug (McLellan et al., 2004). A second study similarly showed that caffeine increased the time to exhaustion on an exercise bicycle ride (Bell & McLellan, 2003).

The same effect has been demonstrated in some sports. In particular, Birnbaum and Herbst (2004) report a modest ergogenic effect of caffeine and improved respiratory efficiency in cross-country runners. Finally, one study suggests that the drug may be beneficial in older exercisers. Men and women aged 70 or older engaged in physical exercise with and without caffeine. It was found that the drug increased cycling and arm flexion duration and reduced the perception that the exercise was tiring (Norager, Jensen, Madison, & Laurberg, 2005).

The potential importance of these studies, particularly the latter one, lies in the fact that exercise has been shown to improve myocardial flow reserve (Goldspink, 2005), protect against CHD (Duvernoy, Martin, Briesmiester, Muzik, & Mosca, 2006), and decrease mortality rates in elderly populations (Hanna & Wegger, 2005). Moreover, vigorous exercise is associated with greater cardioprotective benefits than is moderate exercise (Swain & Franklin, 2006). Thus, caffeine may contribute to the aerobic exercise benefit in the elderly by increasing exercise intensity. However, this remains a hypothesis pending further research directly addressing long-term outcomes when the drug is administered prior to exercise. In addition, the dose–response relationship will need to be examined, and it will be necessary to assess the cost/benefit ratio.

CONCLUSIONS

We have examined the effects of acute doses of caffeine on several major cardiovascular variables in an effort to better understand short-term impact and long-term implications. It is well established that caffeine does have an arousal effect, consistently producing increases in such common arousal indicators as electrodermal activity, EEG, and blood pressure. The question is whether the arousal properties of the drug or, more generally, the physiological changes it produces contribute to cardiovascular morbidity and mortality.

Studies show that chronic high heart rate is associated with atherosclerosis and cardiac mortality. However, studies show that caffeine, in normal doses, does not increase HR, or perhaps only in those who are not habitual users, and may even lower HR in some patient groups. If the drug does not affect HR in habitual users, it is clearly not, in this regard, a danger. The contribution of caffeine to heart rate variability is thus far unclear. Some studies suggest that the drug increases HRV under resting and sleep conditions, and some evidence indicates a protective effect through increasing this important cardiac prognostic indicator. However, much more research is needed.

A third concern has been with the possible role of caffeine in ventricular tachycardia, which can deteriorate to ventricular fibrillation. Here, the few available studies support the hypothesis that the drug has no deleterious effect. Similar findings are seen in the case of atrial fibrillation. Although 25% of AF patients reported in one survey study that caffeine triggers fibrillation episodes, most studies find that caffeine does not contribute to the development of AF or initiation of episodes.

The same cannot be said for the concept of arterial stiffness, including aortic stiffness. There is considerable evidence that increased arterial stiffness is associated with cardiovascular anomalies, CHD, and mortality. Moreover, it appears that caffeine may, in fact, be a contributing factor, with acute and habitual consumption tending to increase stiffness. Most of the relevant studies have thus far involved one laboratory and need to be confirmed in others. Moreover, considerable additional work must be done to understand more fully the impact of caffeine on this cardiovascular parameter.

Despite the possible deleterious effect of caffeine in furthering arterial stiffness, some studies suggest that the drug may also, indirectly, improve heart function and potentially reduce morbidity and mortality. In particular, caffeine improves physical exercise endurance, duration, and performance, as well as the perception of the exercise, in young and elderly populations. Because there is a dose–response relationship between duration and intensity of exercise and its cardioprotective value, the drug may actually increase heart health. However, this observation comes from a very small part of the literature, and considerable additional research will be needed to confirm it.

This chapter has focused primarily on the acute effects of caffeine on cardiovascular parameters, except blood pressure, which is addressed in chapter 6 in this volume. The next chapter reviews the extensive literature concerned with the possible role of caffeine in coronary heart disease.

REFERENCES

Baida Mastiagina, O. A., Mastiagina, S. S., & Arashanian, E. B. (2005). The role of timing factors for the effect of caffeine on heart rhythm variability in healthy humans. *Eksperimental'naia I klinicheskaia farmakologiia, 68*, 20–22.

Balasubramaniam, R., Chawla, S., Grace, A. A., & Huang, C. L. (2005). Caffeine-induced arrhythmias in murine hearts parallel changes in cellular Ca(2+) homeostasis. *American Journal of Physiology: Heart & Circulatory Physiology, 289*, H1584–1593.

Barry, R. J., Rushby, J. A., Wallace, M. J., Clarke, A. R., Johnstone, S. J., & Zlojutro, I. (2005). Caffeine effects on resting-state arousal. *Clinical Neurphysiology, 116*, 2693–2700.

Bassioumy, M., Zarins, C.K., Lee, D.C., Skelly, C.L., Fortunato, J.E., & Glagov, S. (2006). Diurnal heart rate reactivity: A predictor of severity of experimental coronary and carotid atherosclerosis. *Journal of Cardiovascular Research, 9*, 331–338.

Bell, D. G., & McLellan, T. M. (2003). Effects of repeated caffeine ingestion on repeated exhaustive exercise endurance. *Medicine & Science in Sports & Exercise, 35*, 1348–1354.

Berry, N. M., Richards, C. A., & Newman, D. G. (2003). The effect of caffeine on the cardiovascular responses to head-up tilt. *Aviation & Space Environmental Medicine, 74*, 725–730.

Birnbaum, L. J., & Herbst, J. D. (2004). Physiologic effects of caffeine on cross-country runners. *Journal of Strength & Conditioning Research, 18*, 463–465.

Bonnet, M., Tancer, M., Unde, T., & Yeragani, V. K. (2005). Effects of caffeine on heart rate and QT variability during sleep. *Depression & Anxiety, 22*, 150–155.

Cannon, M. E., Cooke, C. T., & McCarthy, J. S. (2001). Caffeine-induced cardiac arrhythmia: An unrecognized danger of health food products. *Medical Journal of Australia, 174,* 520–521.

Caron, M. F., Song, J., Ammar, R., Kluger, J., & White, C. M. (2001). An evaluation of the change in electrocardiographic P-wave variables after acute caffeine ingestion in normal volunteers. *Clinical Pharmacy & Therapeutics, 26,* 145–148.

Carrillo, J. A., & Benitez, J. (2000). Clinically significant pharmacokinetic interactions between dietary caffeine and medications. *Clinical Pharmacokinetics, 39,* 127–153.

Chelsky, L. B., Carter, J. E., Griffith, K., Kron, J., McClelland, J. H., & McAnulty, J. H. (1990). Caffeine and ventricular arrhythmias: an electrophysiological approach. *JAMA, 264,* 2236–2240.

Danchin, N., & Aly, S. (2004). Heart rate reduction: A potential target for the treatment of myocardial ischemia. *Therapie, 59,* 511–515.

Deslandes, A. C., Viega, H., Cagy, M., Piedade, R., Pompu, F., & Riberio, P. (2005). Effect of caffeine on the electrophysiological, cognitive and motor responses of the central nervous system. *Brazilian Journal of Medical and Biological Research, 38,* 1077–1086.

Diaz, A., Bourassa, M. G., Guertin, M. C., & Tardif, J. C. (2005). Long-term prognostic value of resting heart rate in patients with suspected or proven coronary artery disease. *European Heart Journal, 26,* 967–974.

Donnerstein, R. L., Zhu, D., Samson, R., Bender, A. M., & Goldberg, S. J. (1998). Acute effects of caffeine ingestion on signal averaged electrocardiograms. *American Heart Journal, 136,* 643–646.

Duvernoy, C. S., Martin, J. W., Briesmiester, K., Muzik, O., & Mosca, L. (2006). Self-reported physical activity and myocardial flow reserve in postmenopausal women at risk for cardiovascular disease. *Journal of Women's Health, 15,* 45–50

Ebinger, A. W., Krishnan, S., & Schuger, C. D. (2005). Mechanisms of ventricular arrhythmias in heart failure. *Current Heart Failure Report, 2,* 111–117.

Egred, M., & Davis, G. K. (2005). Cocaine and the heart. *Postgraudate Medical Journal, 81,* 568–571.

Frost, L., & Vestergaard, P. (2005). Caffeine and risk of atrial fibrillation or flutter: The Danish Diet, Cancer and Health Study. *American Journal of Clinical Nutrition, 81,* 578–582.

Geddes, L. A., & Roeder, R. A. (2005). Evolution of our knowledge of sudden death due to conmotis cordis. *American Journal of Emergency Medicine, 23,* 67–75.

Go, A. S., Fang, M. C., & Singer, D. E. (2005). Antithrombotic therapy for stroke prevention in atrial fibrillation. *Progress in Cardiovascular Disease, 48,* 108–124.

Goldspink, D. F. (2005). Aging and activity: The effects on the functional reserve capacities of the heart & vascular smooth and skeletal muscles. *Ergonomics, 48,* 1334–1351.

Hanna, I.C., & Wegger, N. K. (2005). Secondary prevention of coronary diseases in elderly patients. *American Family Physician, 71,* 289–296.

Holstege, C. P., Hunter, Y., Baer, A. B., Savory, J., Bruns, D. E., & Boyd, J. C. (2003). Massive caffeine overdose requiring vasopressin infusion and hemodialysis. *Journal of Toxicology, Clinical Toxicology, 41,* 1003–1007.

Hove–Madsen, L., Llach, A., Bayes–Genis, A., Roura, S., Rodriquez Font, E., Aris, A., et al. (2004). Atrial fibrillation is associated with increased spontaneous calcium release from the sacroplasmic reticulum in human atrial myocytes. *Circulation, 110,* 1358–1363.

Karch, S. B. (2005). Cocaine cardiovascular toxicity. *Southern Medical Journal, 98,* 794–799.

Kerrigan, S., & Lindsey, T. (2005). Fatal caffeine overdose: Two case reports. *Forensic Science International, 153,* 67–69.

Link, M. S. (2003). Mechanical induced sudden death in chest wall impact (commotio cordis). *Progress in Biophysics and Molecular Biology, 82,* 175–186.

Mahmud, A., & Feely, J. (2001). Acute effect of caffeine on arterial stiffness and aortic pressure waveform. *Hypertension, 38,* 227–231.

Mattace–Raso, F. U., van der Cammen, T. J., Jnetsch, A. M., van der Meiracker, A. H., Schalekamp, M. A., Hofman, A., et al. (2006). Arterial stiffness as the candidate underlying mechanism for postural blood pressure changes and orthostatic hypertension in older adults in Rotterdam Study. *Journal of Hypertension, 24,* 339–344.

Mattioli, A. V., Bonatti, S., Monopol, D., Zennaro, M., & Mattioli, G. (2005). Influences of regression of left ventricular hypertrophy on left atrial size and function in patients with moderate hypertension. *Blood Pressure, 14,* 273–344.

McLellan, T. M., Bell, D. G., & Kamunori, G. H. (2004). Caffeine improves physical performance during the 24 h of active wakefulness. *Aviation, Space, & Environmental Medicine, 75,* 666–672.

Mehta, S. K., Super, D. M., Salvator, A., Fradley, L. G., Connuck, D., & Kaufman, E. S. (1997). Heart rate variability by triangular index in infants exposed prenatally to cocaine. *Annals of Noninvasive Electrocardiology, 7,* 374–378.

Minamihaba, O., Yamaki, M., Tomoike, H., & Kubota, I. (2003). Severity in myocardial dysfunction contributed to long-term fluctuation of heart rate, rather than short term fluctuations. *Annals of Noninvasive Electrocardiology, 8,* 132–138.

Nattel, S., & Opie, L. H. (2006). Controversies in atrial fibrillation. *Lancet, 367,* 262–272.

Norager, C. B., Jensen, M. D., Madsen, M. R., & Laurberg, S. (2005). Caffeine improves endurance in 75-year-old citizens: A randomized, double-blind, placebo-controlled cross over study. *Journal of Applied Physiology, 99,* 2302–2306.

Palatini, P., Benetos, A., & Julius S. (2006). Impact on increased heart rate on clinical outcome in hypertension: Implications for antihypertensive drug therapy. *Drugs, 66,* 133–144.

Papaioannou, T. G., Karatzi, K., Karatzis, E., Papamichael, C., & Lekakis, J. P. (2005). Acute effects of caffeine on arterial stiffness, wave reflections, and central aortic pressures. *American Journal of Hypertension, 18,* 129–136.

Pawlak–Bus, K., Kolodziejczyk–Feliksik, M., Kramer, L., Nikisch E., Maczko, J., & Siminiak, T. (2005). The Allen factor: A new model of mathematical interpretation of heart rate variability in stable coronary artery disease. Preliminary report. *Kardiologia Polska, 63,* 125–132.

Quinlan, P. T., Lane, J., Moore, K. L., Aspen, J., Rycroft, J. A., & O'Brien, D. C. (2000). The acute physiological and mood effects of tea and coffee: The role of caffeine level. *Pharmacology, Biochemistry, and Behavior, 66,* 19–28.

Reddy, P. C., Tandon, N., & Stafford, P. R. (1999). Ventricualar tachycardia and sudden cardiac death. *Journal of Louisiana State Medical Society, 151,* 281–287.

Richardson, T., Rozkovec, A., Thomas, P., Ryder, J., Meckes, C,. & Kerr, D. (2004). Influence of caffeine on heart rate variability in patients with long standing type 1 diabetes. *Diabetes Care, 27,* 1127–1131.

Roach, D., Wilson, W., Ritchie, D., & Sheldon, R. (2004). Dissection of long-range heart rate variability: Controlled indication of prognostic measures by activity in the laboratory. *Journal of the American College of Cardiology, 43,* 2271–2277.

Rubart, M., & Zipes, D. P. (2005). Mechanisms of sudden cardiac death. *Journal of Clinical Investigation, 115,* 2305–2315.

Sarkozy, A., & Brugada, P. (2005). Sudden cardiac death: What is inside out genes. *Canadian Journal of Cardiology, 21,* 1099, 1110.

Schutte, A. F., Huisman, H. W., Van Rooyen, J. M., Oosthuizen, W., & Herling, J. C. (2003). Sensitivity of the Finometer device in detecting acute and medium-term changes in cardiovascular function. *Blood Pressure Monitor, 8,* 195–201.

Singh, J. P., Larson, M. G., O'Donnell, C. J., & Levy, D. (2001). Genetic factors contribute to the variance in frequency domain measures of heart rate variability. *Autonomic Neuroscience: Basic & Clinical, 90,* 122–126.

Singh, J. P., Larson, M. G., O'Donnell, C. J., Tsuji, H., Corey, D., & Levy, D. (2002). Genome scan linkage results for heart rate variability (the Framingham Heart Study). *American Journal of Cardiology, 90,* 1290–1293.

Stolarz, K., Staessen, J. A., Kuznesova, T., Tikhonoff, V., State, D., Babeanus, S., et al. (2003). Host and environmental determinants of heart rate and heart rate variability in four European populations. *Journal of Hypertension, 21,* 525–535.

Sudano, I., Spieker, L., Binggeli, C., Ruschizka, F., Luscher, T.F., Noll, et al. (2005). Coffee blunts mental stress-induced blood pressure increase in habitual but not in nonhabitual coffee drinkers. *Hypertension, 46,* 521–526.

Swain, D. P., & Franklin, B. A. (2006). Comparison of cardioprotective benefits of vigorous versus moderate intensity aerobic exercise. *American Journal of Cardiology, 97,* 141–147.

Van Bortel, L. M., Duprez, D., Starmans–Kool, M. J., Safar, M. E., Giannattasio, C., Cockcroft, J., et al. (2002). Clinical applications of arterial stiffness, Task Force III: Recommendations for user procedures. *American Journal of Hypertension, 15,* 445–452.

Vlachopoulos, C., Aznaoauridis, K., Alexopoulos, N., Economou, E., Andreadou, I., & Stefanadis, C. (2005). Effect of dark chocolate on arterial function in health individuals. *American Journal of Hypertension, 18,* 785–791.

Vlachopoulos, C., Aznaouridis, K., & Stefanadis, C. (2005). Clinical appraisal of arterial stiffness: The Argonauts in front of the Golden Fleece. *Heart, 9.*

Vlachopoulos, C., Dima, I., Aznaouridis, K., Vasliadou, C., Ioakeimidis, N., Aggeli, C., et al. (2005). Acute systemic inflammation increases arterial stiffness and decreases wave reflections in healthy individuals. *Circulation, 112,* 2193–2200.

Vlachopoulos, C., Hirata K., & O'Rourke, M. F. (2003). Effect of sildenafil on arterial stiffness and wave reflection. *Vascular Medicine, 8,* 243–248.

Vlachopoulos, C., Kosmopoulou, F., Panagiotakos, D., Ioakeimidis, N., Alexopoulos, Pitsavos, C., et al. (2004). Smoking and caffeine have a synergistic detrimental effect on aortic stiffness and wave reflections. *Journal of the American College of Cardiology, 44,* 1911–1917.

Vlachopoulos, C., Panagiotakos, D., Ioakeimidis, N., Dima, I., & Stefandis, C. (2005). Chronic coffee consumption has a detrimental effect on aortic stiffness and wave reflections. *American Journal of Clinical Nutrition, 81,* 1307–1312.

Yeragani, V. K., Krishnan, S., Engles, H. J., & Gretebeck, R. (2005). Effects of caffeine on linear and nonlinear measures of heart rate variability before and after exercise. *Depression & Anxiety, 21,* 130–134.

in Africa. In: Handbook of psychology of investigating the mind in Africa. In press.

Nsamenang, A. B. (ed.) (1992). Human development in cultural context: A third world perspective. Newbury Park, CA: Sage Publications.

5 The Multifactorial Model of Cardiovascular Pathology: Is Caffeine Pathogenic in Coronary Heart Disease?

Barry D. Smith, Radha Gholkar, Mark Mann, and Nancy Toward

CONTENTS

The role of caffeine consumption in coronary heart disease (CHD) and related conditions has long been debated. Early studies suggested a clear causal role, which quickly came into question when additional research was done, and studies completed within the past 2 years continue to yield mixed results. One thing that does seem clear is that if the consumption of caffeine or coffee exerts an impact on CHD, it does so within the framework of a multifactorial causal model. To better understand the complex findings concerned with the effects of caffeine and coffee on the cardiovascular system, we will therefore attempt to place the relevant findings in the context of that larger causal model.

THE HISTORICAL CONTEXT

At the dawn of the 20th century, the primary causes of death were pneumonia, influenza, and tuberculosis—all infectious diseases for which there were no effective preventative measures, treatments, or cures (Centers for Disease Control [CDC], 1999). Antibiotics had not yet been developed, and vaccines were in their infancy. Life expectancy at birth was only 47 in the United States, in part because these diseases could kill at virtually any age (CDC, 1999). It is notable that these killer diseases of the early 20th century and of earlier centuries were difficult for the individual to prevent or treat. Lifestyle factors thus had very little influence on mortality. However, as scientific research in medicine improved, that picture soon began to change.

In 1796, Edward Jenner performed his historic first vaccination against smallpox on an 8-year-old boy; over the next hundred years, Robert Koch and others demonstrated the microbial causes of disease. Armed with this information, French chemist Louis Pasteur, in the late 19th century, developed the rabies vaccine, which was soon followed by one for bubonic plague and, in the 1920s, vaccines against diphtheria, pertussis, tuberculosis, and tetanus. As these latter were being developed, Alexander Fleming, working in his laboratory at St. Mary's Hospital in London in 1928, discovered that penicillin mold growing in one of his petri dishes had killed numerous staph bacteria. Although penicillin would not be widely used until World

War II, the era of antibiotics had begun. Numerous other antibiotics were soon in development; at the same time, virologists continued to tackle one disease after another, producing vaccines for viral and bacterial disorders.

One result of these scientific advances was a dramatic change in the profile of fatal human diseases. Fewer people would die of the complications that can occur when the streptococcus bacillus that causes simple "strep" sore throat invades the heart, kidneys, and other major organ systems. Similarly, antibiotics could effectively treat tuberculosis, and increasingly effective vaccines helped to prevent influenza and a host of other dangerous viral diseases, as well as bacterial forms of pneumonia and other disorders.

With these important medical developments, life expectancy has gradually risen to 77.6 years in the United States (Hoyert, Kung, & B. Smith, 2005). Like taxes, however, death is certain, and new primary causes of mortality were inevitable. Living to more advanced ages means dying of disorders that tend to develop over longer periods of time and therefore to depend far more on lifestyle factors. Such slowly progressing disorders include heart disease, cancer, and stroke, the three principal causes of death in Western societies today (Hoyert et al., 2005). It is also notable that two of the three are cardiovascular disorders.

In the United States, 1 in every 2.6 deaths (38%) is the result of cardiovascular disease. In fact, over 70 million people were estimated to have cardiovascular disease in 2002, and over 900,000 died of the disease in that year. Of these deaths, nearly 500,000 were in women (American Heart Association, 2005). Coronary heart disease remains the leading cause of death in the United States and worldwide (Hoyert et al., 2005). However, according to the American Cancer Society, cancer surpassed heart disease as the leading cause of death in people under the age of 85 when data were aggregated by age (Jemal et al., 2005). This discrepancy can be explained by the method of aggregation employed by the ACS and the delay in data collection and reporting by the Centers for Disease Control and World Health Organization.

Despite their high mortality rates, heart disease and cancer have shown downward trends. The incidence of heart disease declined 2.8% from 2001 to 2002, while cancer declined 1.3% (National Center for Vital Statistics Reports, 2004). Although one would hope for a continual decline, the high prevalence of heart disease within our society is certain and will most likely remain for quite some time. Clearly, anything we can learn about the causes of this major killer will potentially extend many lives across age groups and genders.

THE MULTIFACTORIAL MODEL

Our particular interest in CHD here revolves around the long-standing speculation and evidence that caffeine consumption may be one of its causal or contributing factors (Lane, Pieper, Philips–Bute, Bryant, & Kuhn, 2002). Clinical observation suggested as early as the 1940s that CHD was not a function of any one or two simple factors. However, it was not until the 1960s and 1970s that randomized, controlled trials began the systematic effort to assess etiology. The major early—and continuing—investigation was the Framingham Heart Study (D. Smith, 2000), but many others have now been completed or are under way. By examining the factors derived from these studies, we will be better able to see just where caffeine might fit into the overall causal puzzle, if at all.

The classic etiological triad includes hypercholesterolemia, smoking, and hypertension (D. Smith, 2000), and the Framingham Study and others have added family history/genetics and diabetes mellitus (Singh, Wiegers, & Goldstein, 2001). However, a number of other factors have also been clearly implicated in recent scientific literature. Such factors include elevations in low-density lipoprotein, homocysteine, and C-reactive protein (Wilson, 2004). As we will see, some evidence suggests that caffeine may contribute to or interact with several of these and other factors.

FAMILY HISTORY AND GENETICS

Before the human genome was fully mapped, researchers had discovered that coronary heart disease and stroke run in families. Family history is a particularly strong factor when CHD occurs in younger people, but is also predictive in older age groups (Friedlander et al., 2001). In addition, behavior genetic research has demonstrated substantial heritability for cardiovascular diseases (Aoki et al., 2001; Katzmarzyk et al., 2000). For example, genetic and environmental influences on coronary heart disease were examined in the HERITAGE Family Study. The investigators assessed several CHD risk factors, including age, family history, LDL cholesterol, HDL cholesterol, blood pressure, diabetes, and smoking status. Based upon this information, a CHD risk index was created and familial heritability determined. Maximal heritability was 34% in Whites and 53% in Blacks (Katzmarzyk et al., 2000).

Further examinations of heritability have included molecular genetic studies using functional genomic methodology in an attempt to identify specific genes that may code for CHD. For example, high levels of fibrinogen have been found to predict future coronary heart disease. Fibrinogen is a large glycoprotein, which is a clotting factor that serves to activate thrombin and aggregate platelets. Variants of the h-fibrinogen gene subunit on 4q28 are associated with these elevated levels (Yang et al., 2005), though further research is needed to establish a direct causal link to CHD (G. Smith, Harbord, Milton, Ebrahim, & Sterne, 2005). Another genetic study focused on the involvement of the renin–angiotensin system (RAS) in premature CHD risk. Higher frequencies of the angiotensin-converting enzyme (ACE) and angiotensinogen (AGT) gene polymorphisms contributed to increased CHD risk, and the ACE genotype may thus be a risk factor (Sekuri et al., 2005).

A number of other specific genes also have been tentatively identified as contributing to CHD risk. They include the MEF2A, LTA, LGALS2, and ALOX5AP, all of which appear to be associated with myocardial infarction (Wang, 2005). Like CHD, the consumption and effects of caffeine have a hereditary component that may partially explain its role as a potential risk factor (Luciano, Kirk, Heath, & Martin, 2005).

DISEASES AND CONDITIONS

The genetic factors in CHD may be expressed through a variety of mechanisms, including those that underlie blood lipids, homocysteine, and C-reactive protein. Further complicating the causal model is the fact that these same mechanisms may also be subject to environmental and behavioral influences.

Blood Lipids

Among the major factors in this broad category is lipid status, and caffeine may be a factor in that status (see later discussion in this chapter and, for a more comprehensive review, chapter 7). Our understanding of the role of lipids in heart disease has evolved from the relatively simple idea that higher levels of total cholesterol are associated with CHD to an increasing understanding of the roles of various lipid components.

A steroid alcohol that regulates membrane fluidity, cholesterol comprises two major subtypes, low-density (LDL) and high-density (HDL) lipoproteins. High levels of LDL cholesterol and low levels of HDL cholesterol represent significant risk factors for CHD. Both types exhibit high heritability, but both can also be altered through behaviors and drugs (Wang & Paigen, 2005). At least four large clinical trials to date confirm that cholesterol is a factor in cardiovascular disease and that modifying its levels is an important aspect of primary prevention (Lloyd–Jones et al., 2001). A recent study involving data from several European countries confirms this finding by demonstrating that a single cholesterol measurement at baseline was a strong predictor of CHD-related death 35 years later (Menotti et al., 2005).

Although total cholesterol does predict CHD, the breakdown into LDL and HDL adds precision to that prediction, providing a better understanding of the mechanisms that underlie the role of cholesterol in CHD. Accordingly, high levels of LDL) are consistently associated with coronary heart disease (Slapikas, 2005). However, recent investigations suggest that low levels of HDL may be even more predictive of CHD mortality (Rosenson, 2005). HDL serves to break down LDL and prevent it from forming plaques on the walls of the coronary arteries. When inadequate HDL is present, LDL plaque formation increases, narrowing the arterial lumen and increasing probability of the complete blockage seen in a myocardial infarction (MI). The Helsinki Heart Study has shown that a 1-mg/dl increase in HDL can decrease the probability of a cardiac event by 2 to 3% (Young, Karas, & Kuvin, 2004).

Accordingly, some scientists now hypothesize that low HDL (below about 35 mg/dl) may be a significant independent predictor of CHD (McGovern, 2005). A genetic mechanism involved in hyperlipidemia that is specifically linked to LDL particle size and apolipoprotein B (apoB) has been proposed. Approximately 37% of variance of LDL particle size and 23% of the variance of the apoB can be explained by this genetic factor (Juo, Bredie, Kiemeney, Demacker, & Stalenhoef, 1998). Lipid and lipoprotein levels have also been attributed to APOE polymorphism E, as well as apolipoprotein B (Medina–Urrutia, Liria, Posadas–Romero, Cardoso–Saldaga, & Zamora–Gonzalez, 2004).

Plasma Homocysteine

An elevation in plasma homocysteine levels (hyperhomocysteinemia) is another substantial risk factor for cardiovascular disease, accounting for an estimated 10% of CHD risk (Fowler, 2005). Homocysteine is a sulfur-containing amino acid derived from methionine during its metabolism. Hyperhomocysteinemia promotes the development of thrombosis, atherosclerosis, and oxidative damage. As many as 10 to 20% of coronary heart disease cases are causally linked to homocysteine elevation (Rogers,

Sanchez–Saffon, Frol, & Diaz–Arrastia, 2003). A case-control study, for example, evaluated the relationship of homocysteine levels to 149 coronary events (74 deaths and 75 MIs) that occurred in women over a 13-year follow-up period and compared them with matched control subjects. Among women with heart disease at baseline, relative coronary risk, adjusted for other known factors, was 3.32 in the highest homocysteine quintile as compared to the lowest quintile (Knekt et al., 2001).

Elevated plasma homocysteine has also been linked to premature coronary artery disease (CAD) risk. In one investigation, three groups were studied: one with traditional risk factors, one with nontraditional risk factors, and a normal/control group. Enzyme-linked immunosorbent assay (ELISA) was used to estimate the homocysteine levels, and a significant association between premature CAD risk and elevated levels of homocysteine was found (Barghash, Barghash, El Dine, Elewa, & Hamdi, 2004). Other studies show that those with a history of myocardial infarction tend to have much higher homocysteine levels than controls (Boufidou et al., 2004).

As with cholesterol, genetic and environmental factors contribute to homocysteine levels. Numerous studies have reported significant heritability for homocysteine levels, and the recent AtheroGene study confirmed that homocysteine level is strongly influenced by genetic predisposition (Schnabel et al., 2005). At the molecular level, the genetic mutation C677T at the methylenetetrahydrofolate reductase (MTHFR) gene is associated with a substantially elevated risk of hyperhomocysteinemia and of developing CHD at an early age (Mager, Harell, Battler, Koren–Morag, & Shohat, 2005).

In addition to the genetic factor, hyperhomocysteinemia is associated with folate and vitamin B-12 deficiencies (Saibeni et al., 2005); the former is of less concern due to the folic acid fortification found in many foods today (Green & Miller, 2005). Vitamin B-6 and riboflavin are also involved in homocysteine metabolism and have been shown to decrease homocysteine levels (Strain, Pentieva, McNulty, Dowey, & Ward, 2004). Additionally, alcoholics tend to have elevated levels of homocysteine, with the highest levels seen in those with liver damage. Thus, methionine metabolism, a factor in liver deterioration, may play a role (Blasco et al., 2005). Some evidence suggests that components of coffee may affect homocysteine levels (Strandhagen & Thelle, 2003).

Inflammation: C-Reactive Protein and White Cell Count

Elevations in serum C-reactive protein (CRP) indicate the presence of inflammation and appear to be associated with an increased risk of coronary artery disease (Bello & Mosca, 2004; Luc et al., 2003). A recent 10-year prospective study showed that higher baseline levels of CRP were associated with elevated CHD risk, even in the absence of other cardiac risk factors (Cushman et al., 2005). Another study of 30,000 American women also demonstrated that CRP is an independent predictor of CHD incidence when all other known factors are controlled for (Ridker, Rifai, Rose, Buring, & Cook, 2002). Mackness and colleagues showed that higher levels of CRP and lower levels of paroxanase1, an anti-inflammatory agent, were present in individuals with CHD than in controls (Mackness, Hone, McElduff, & Mackness, 2005).

A second marker for inflammation, white blood cell count, may also be a useful predictor of CHD risk (Koren–Morag, Tanne, & Goldbourt, 2005). Additionally, a recent review of 32 investigations showed that exercise, which reduces cardiovascular risk (Courville, Lavie, & Milani, 2005; CDC, 2005; Frank et al., 2005), increases short-term but reduces long-term inflammation, further supporting the role of arterial inflammation in CHD (Kasapis & Thompson, 2005).

Plasma Catecholamines

Several amines that derive from tyrosine and contain dihydroxybenzene rings constitute the group of plasma catecholamines, including norepinephrine, epinephrine, and dopamine. Some investigators have reported higher levels of plasma catecholamines in CHD patients than in controls (Tjeerdsma et al., 2001). However, it thus far appears that these amines are probably not direct causal factors in CHD (Forslund et al., 2002). Rather, they may be associated indirectly through their role in autonomic dysfunction (Carney, Freedland, & Veith, 2005) and stress reactivity (Brunner et al., 2002) in metabolic syndrome. The latter is a condition characterized by three or more factors (such as hypertension, abdominal obesity, and high cholesterol) that are believed to lead to CHD and/or type 2 diabetes.

Thus, current research indicates that the plasma catecholamines are most likely a part of the pathway involved in the development of metabolic syndrome. Higher catecholamine levels lead to autonomic dysfunction and stress reactivity, which then give rise to hypertension, abdominal obesity, and other factors that collectively result in metabolic syndrome. The presence of metabolic syndrome then poses a general risk for CHD. Evidence suggests that caffeine increases catecholamine levels in a dose-dependent fashion (Papadelis et al., 2003).

Diabetes

Diabetes mellitus, a disorder of carbohydrate metabolism resulting from insufficient secretion or exploitation of insulin, is commonly regarded as a prime risk factor for CHD (Geronimo, Abarquez, Punzalan, & Cabral, 2005; Kengne, Amoah, & Mbanya, 2005). Type 1 diabetes (Dahl–Jorgensen, Larsen, & Hanssen, 2005; Skrivarhaug et al., 2005) and type 2 diabetes (Shai et al., 2005; Wannamethee, Shaper, Lennon, & Morris, 2005) have been linked to CHD and other cardiac events. Evidence indicates that a genetic predisposition combines with environmental factors to create the phenotype for diabetes (Roche, Phillips, & Gibney, 2005; Wolford & Vazarova de Courten, 2004). Currently, the proportion of variance attributable to genetics for type 1 and type 2 diabetes, respectively, is 40 to 50% (Kim & Polychronakos, 2005) and about 26% (Poulsen, Ohm–Kyvik, Vaag, & Beck–Nielsen, 1999).

The mechanism by which diabetes increases CHD risk is poorly understood. One theory is that diabetic patients have diminished sympathetic responses to exercise, including lower peak heart rates and smaller plasma epinephrine responses, both of which have been linked to an elevated risk of cardiovascular events (Endo et al., 2000). Other work has shown that increases in hemoglobin A may indicate increased risk for CHD (Selvin et al., 2005). A marker for long-term glycemic control, elevated hemoglobin A signals chronic hyperglycemia, which may be the culprit in the increased risk of CHD seen in diabetics (Selvin et al., 2005). Considerable further research is needed to assess the mechanisms underlying the relationship between diabetes and CHD. Some evidence suggests that coffee consumption may actually lower the risk for type 2 diabetes, although further work is needed to confirm this association (van Dam, Willett, Manson, & Hu, 2006).

Hypertension

A well-documented CHD risk factor, hypertension involves genetic and environmental factors (Aras, Sowers, & Arora, 2005). Research has demonstrated that 30 to 50% of the variance in hypertension is genetic, with such environmental and behavioral factors as obesity, stress, and lack of exercise completing the causal model (Marteau, Zajou, Siest, & Visvikis–Siest, 2005). The genetic component may be expressed in the reduction in endothelial progenitor cells that is associated with hypertension (Urbich & Dimmeler, 2005). In animal and in human trials, increasing the number of these cells appears to reduce atherosclerosis by promoting vascularization. The role of caffeine in hypertension is addressed briefly later in this chapter and more comprehensively in chapter 6.

Heart Rate and Arrhythmias

Absolute heart rate and cardiac arrhythmias have been suggested as risk factors. Lower peak heart rates during exercise (Endo et al., 2000), as well as high resting heart rates (Jouven et al., 2005) may be related to myocardial infarction. Similarly, arrhythmias are associated with acute cardiac events such as sudden cardiac death (Antezano & Hong, 2003; Buxton et al., 2003; de Sutter, Firsovaite, & Tavernier, 2002; Pacifico & Henry, 2003). The effects of caffeine on heart rate and rhythm are addressed briefly later in this chapter and more fully in chapter 4.

Smoking

Smoking is a major risk factor for CHD and cardiac death (Weisz et al., 2005). In fact, smokers have a 70% greater risk of death due to CHD than nonsmokers, and 30 to 40% of CHD deaths result from smoking (Kabat, 2003). Nicotine and carbon monoxide may be the chief pathogens in smoke, but tars may also be involved (Kabat). Moreover, the nitrogen oxides present in smoke are such powerful pathogens that CHD mortality is higher in neighborhoods where air pollution includes elevations in the levels of these chemicals (Maheswaran et al., 2005).

There is a strong dose-dependent relationship between smoking and CHD, and it appears that smoking may have synergistic interactions with hypertension and hyperlipidemia, thereby further increasing CHD risk (Rigotti & Pasternak, 1996). In addition, smoking has been shown to reduce the oxygen-carrying capacity of hemoglobin (Sansores, Pare, & Abboud, 1992), create higher blood levels of carbon monoxide (Gottlieb, 1992; McDonough & Moffitt, 1999), contribute to atherosclerosis (Ramos & Moorthy, 2005), stimulate platelet production and thereby clotting (Bell, 2004), and increase LDL cholesterol levels (Sharma et al., 2005).

The causal mechanisms underlying the smoking–CHD relationship have been at least partially described:

Smoking may interfere with arterial wall collagen metabolism, which weakens arteries and contributes to atherosclerosis (Raveendran et al., 2004).

Nicotine appears to alter the expression of endothelial genes that regulate vascular tone and thrombogenicity, which also increases the risk of atherosclerosis (Zhang, Day, & Ye, 2000).

Components of smoke may cause or exacerbate proinflammatory and procoagulatory responses (MacCallum, 2005) and may increase blood levels of homocysteine (Stein et al., 2002).

Smokers exhibit poor dietary habits. As compared to nonsmokers, smokers consume less vitamin C and vitamin E, fiber, and important nutrients, such as beta carotene, thereby increasing their levels of LDL cholesterol (Dallongeville, Marecaux, Fruchart, & Amouyel, 1998; Galan et al., 2005).

Caffeine is associated with smoking in a way that makes some caffeine studies more difficult to interpret, as we will see later in this chapter.

Obesity and Exercise

Obesity has a well-established relationship to CHD and is influenced by genetic as well as environmental factors (Liu, Xiao, Xiong, Recker, & Deng, 2005). Abdominal obesity, in particular, has been linked to higher plasma fibrinogen, a protein important in blood clotting, and other coagulatory abnormalities that are further linked to atherothrombosis (de Pergola & Pannacciulli, 2002). Additionally, left ventricular mass, which can be affected by obesity, is related to CHD (Post, Larson, Myers, Galderisi, & Levy, 1997). On the other hand, regular exercise is associated with improved cardiovascular function and reduced CHD risk (Wamhoff, Bowles, Dietz, Hu, & Sturek, 2002). In fact, some evidence suggests a dose–response relationship. However, the combination of frequent, intense exercise with a proper diet appears to provide the best cardiovascular outcomes (Al-Ajlan & Mehdi, 2005).

Interactions Among Factors

Although literature assessing the associations among the multiple risk factors is scant, there has been some speculation as to the nature of their interactions. Burns (2003), for example, has recently suggested that the presence of smoking as a risk factor is multiplicative when other risk factors are also present and there is little doubt that overall cardiovascular risk increases with the number of pathogenic factors present in a given individual. We will consider shortly just where caffeine may fit into the overall risk pattern and how it may interact with other factors.

BEHAVIORAL AND EMOTIONAL FACTORS IN CHD

CHD risk is tied not only to physiological factors, but also to emotions and behaviors. Although results relating to most such factors are less definitive than those for biological influences, they are nevertheless important.

Anger and Hostility

A recent comprehensive review of investigations examining the relationship of anger and hostility to CHD indicates a significant association between hostility scores on psychometric measures and CHD incidence and mortality (T. Smith, Glazer, Ruiz, & Gallo, 2004). The effect sizes in most of these studies are as large as those when using traditional risk factors, and the significant association remains even when physiological influences are controlled. The authors concluded that this relationship could occur as a result of psychophysiological reactivity to stressors, such as increases in blood pressure and reactive inflammatory responses. Another possibility is that hostility contributes indirectly through such mechanisms as reduced social support or a generally unhealthy lifestyle (such as poor diet and smoking) associated with hostility (T. Smith et al.).

Some studies, however, do not support the hostility–CHD relationship. One recent investigation showed that hostility scores in middle- to late-age adults do not predict cardiovascular mortality, perhaps suggesting that this relationship could diminish over time or involves a variety of other specific factors (Surtees, Wainwright, Luben, Day, & Khaw, 2005). Thus, the role of hostility remains unclear and further research is needed to provide clarification.

Stress

Another proposed cardiovascular risk factor is stress, which may contribute in two ways: (a) as a short-term factor that leads to an MI; and (b) as a long-term factor contributing to the gradual development of CHD over many years. First, myocardial infarction is associated with the occurrence of stressful life events in the year preceding the MI (Rafanelli et al., 2005). Tension and anxiety were also recently shown to be strong, independent factors in CHD incidence and mortality in men from the Framingham Offspring Study (Eaker, Sullivan, Kelly–Hayes, D'Agostino, & Benjamin, 2005). Stress indicators are also higher in people with metabolic syndrome, a precursor to CHD (Vitaliano et al., 2002). Activation of the sympathetic nervous system may thus be hypothesized as a cause of CHD and MI (Brunner et al., 2002). One recent theoretical model proposes that a type D personality, involving social avoidance and internalization of stress, results in higher cortisol levels and could contribute to CHD (Sher, 2005). Caffeine often interacts with stress to affect cardiovascular parameters (see later discussion).

Alcohol Consumption

In a recent review of literature concerning the role of alcohol consumption in CHD, Hill (2005) concludes that a J-shaped relationship exists between the two, with only moderate consumption being protective (Hill, 2005). Moderate consumption equals a maximum of approximately two drinks, or 25 g, of ethanol per day and does not appear to be related to the type of alcohol consumed. Previous research has also supported the idea that moderate levels of alcohol consumption, particularly 1 to 21 drinks per week, may specifically have an effect on sudden cardiac death in pre-existing CHD (de Vreede–Swagemakers et al., 1999).

Multiple mechanisms mediating the alcohol–CHD relationship have been proposed. They include increases in HDL levels, inhibition of platelet activation, decreased levels of fibrinogen, slightly decreased BP, increased antioxidant activity, and reduced general risk for diabetes. A study testing the effect of a single administration of wine per day found no change in cholesterol levels; however, it is quite possible that this dosage was too small to produce any noticeable changes (Ziegler et al., 2005).

THE ROLE OF CAFFEINE IN CORONARY HEART DISEASE

Caffeine is an alkaloid compound that acts as a CNS stimulant, resulting in increased autonomic arousal. The impact of caffeine consumption on coronary heart disease has been repeatedly assessed in numerous investigations and debated for several decades. However, a final resolution as to its causal or contributory role remains elusive. Here, we will review the relevant literature, past and recent, to arrive at informed conclusions as to the effects of caffeine on the cardiovascular system. It might be noted at the outset that earlier studies addressed the binary question of whether or not caffeine consumption is involved in CHD, while more recent work has focused instead on a more detailed analysis of the extent to which and the circumstances under which the drug may have cardiovascular effects.

A search of Medline from inception through 2005 yielded a total of 20,107 publications dealing with caffeine. Of these, 2,520 deal with the relationship of caffeine, coffee, or tea to heart function or CHD. Of these papers, the search was limited to those published in English that studied the effect of any caffeinated substance on myocardial infarction and/or coronary heart disease. These studies are summarized in Table 5.1.

RESEARCH HISTORY

Early Studies: 1960s and 1970s

Investigations that began in the 1960s indicated a likely relationship between caffeine or coffee use and CHD. A. Brown (1962) was the first to investigate the relationship. This initial investigation showed that control subjects, who had not suffered from a coronary thrombosis, were actually consuming more coffee than individuals who died due to coronary thrombosis. The following year, in a classic prospective study, Paul and colleagues (1963) found a strong association between coffee consumption and the development of CHD approximately 5 years later. They also reported a substantial correlation between smoking and caffeine use. However, they later reinterpreted the caffeine–CHD association as due primarily to the fact that these coffee drinkers smoked more than nondrinkers did (Paul, MacMillan, McKean, & Park, 1968; Paul, 1968).

Five studies addressing the relationship between coffee or caffeine and coronary heart disease were published during the 1970s, and only one of those reported a positive association. The Boston Collaborative Drug Surveillance Program (Vessey, 1972) compared myocardial infarction patients with controls hospitalized for other

TABLE 5.1
Role of Caffeinated Substances in Myocardial Infarction and Coronary Heart Disease

Country	Year	Caffeine source and presence of caffeine	Critical amount of caffeine	Brewing method	Study description	Outcome variable	Time to measure DV	Population	Total N	Main conclusion	Limitations	Interactions with other factors?	Ref.
England	1962	Coffee and tea, not specified	1 to 5 cups coffee daily; more than 10 cups tea daily	Not reported	Retrospective interviews of family of deceased individuals whose deaths were officially recorded as resulting from coronary thrombosis compared to living controls	Coronary thrombosis mortality	Not specified	Males and females aged 45 to 64 years	892	Coffee consumption associated with fewer deaths (control group); first study to document the role of caffeine in CHD			Brown
United States	1963	Coffee, not specified	0 to 200 cups per month	Not reported	Prospective study of a random sample	CHD incidence	5 years (average)	Male aged 40 to 55 years, free of CHD symptoms	1,989	Coffee consumption in the first year was associated with CHD development during the follow-up	Did not account for smoking; these conclusions rescinded in Paul et al., 1968	Correlated to smoking	Paul et al.

Country	Year	Substance	Amount		Study design	Outcome	Duration	Subjects	N	Results	Limitations	Correlated to	Reference
United States, Canada, Israel, New Zealand	1972	Coffee and tea, not specified	>5 cups per day	Not reported	Acute MI hospital patients each matched to four controls who were admitted for conditions other than MI	MI incidence	Not specified	Mostly male, White subjects with acute MI compared to controls with conditions other than MI	1,380	Acute MI patients drank more coffee than controls after controlling for smoking; drinking >5 cups/day doubles risk; no association between tea and MI	Did not use healthy controls; did not control for previous MI	Correlated to smoking	Vessey (Boston Collaborative Drug Surveillance Program)
United States	1974	Coffee, not specified	0 to >6 cups per day	Not reported	Prospective study of a random sample	CHD and MI incidence	12 years	Males and females aged 30 to 62 years, no CHD symptoms	5,209	No significant association between coffee consumption and CHD and MI	None outstanding		Dawber, Kannel, and Gordon (Framingham)
United States	1976	Coffee, caffeinated	Not reported	Not reported	Retrospective interviews of wives of deceased men whose deaths were officially recorded as resulting from CHD; case-control design	CHD mortality	3 months	White males aged 3 to 70 years, deceased	1,298	Risk ratios were similar between controls and CHD-death patients	Retrospective data		Hennekens et al.
Sweden	1977	Coffee, not specified	1 to 5 and 6+ cups per day	Not reported	Case-control prospective design	MI incidence	12 years (average)	Males aged 40 to 57 years	1,064	No significant relationship between coffee usage and MI	None outstanding	Associated with smoking and alcohol use	Wilhelmsen et al.

(continued)

TABLE 5.1 (Continued)
Role of Caffeinated Substances in Myocardial Infarction and Coronary Heart Disease

Country	Year	Caffeine source and presence of caffeine	Critical amount of caffeine	Brewing method	Study description	Outcome variable	Time to measure DV	Population	Total N	Main conclusion	Limitations	Interactions with other factors?	Ref.
United States	1977	Coffee, not specified	0 to >10 cups per day	Not reported	Prospective study of a random sample	CHD incidence	6 years	Japanese men in Hawaii	7,705	Association between coffee usage and CHD disappears when smoking is taken into account	Did not collect information regarding decaffeinated coffee use		Yano, Rhoads, and Kagan (Honolulu Heart Study)
United States	1980	Coffee, caffeinated	>5 cups per day	Not reported	MI patients compared to a control of non-MI emergency patients	MI incidence	Not specified	Females aged 30 to 49 years	1,467	No significant association between coffee use of >5 cups/day and MI when all other factors were controlled; greater coffee use associated with controls	None outstanding		Rosenberg et al.
United States	1981	Coffee, not specified	1 to >7 cups per day	Not reported	Prospective study of a random sample	IHD mortality	11.5 years (average)	Males aged 35 years and over with no history of IHD	16,911	No association between coffee consumption and IHD mortality	None outstanding	Interaction with smoking	Murray et al. (Lutheran Brotherhood Study)

Norway	1986	Coffee, not specified	0 to >7 cups per day	Not reported	Prospective study of a random sample	IHD mortality	11.5 years (average)	Mostly males, history of CHD not reported	16,555	No significant association between coffee use and IHD mortality	None outstanding	Jacobsen et al.
United States	1986	Coffee, not specified	>5 cups per day	Not reported	Prospective study of convenience sample	CHD incidence, CHD death, MI	25 years (average)	Male medical students, mostly White, ages 19 to 49, no CHD history at baseline	1,130	Heavy coffee drinkers three times as likely to develop CHD; when other risk factors are accounted for, this association decreases but continues to persist	Did not control for other important risk factors	LaCroix et al.
United States	1987	Coffee, caffeinated and decaffeinated	>6 cups per day	Not reported	Prospective study relating causes of death to coffee consumption	CHD mortality	19 years	White males aged 40 to 56 years at baseline	45,589	Elevated risk ratios for men consuming >6 cups coffee/day, even when other risk factors are controlled for	None outstanding	LeGrady et al. (Western Electric Power Study)
United States	1988	Caffeinated coffee, tea, and medications	0 to >4 cups per day	Not reported	Prospective study of a convenience sample	All cardiovascular mortality	4 years	Hypertensive males and females aged 30 to 69 years	10,064	No association between caffeine and cardiovascular mortality	Did not collect information regarding decaffeinated coffee/tea use	Correlated with smoking	Martin et al.

(continued)

TABLE 5.1 (Continued)
Role of Caffeinated Substances in Myocardial Infarction and Coronary Heart Disease

Country	Year	Caffeine source and presence of caffeine	Critical amount of caffeine	Brewing method	Study description	Outcome variable	Time to measure DV	Population	Total N	Main conclusion	Limitations	Interactions with other factors?	Ref.
United States	1988	Coffee, caffeinated and decaffeinated	>5 cups per day	Not reported	Case-control design of acute MI cases compared to controls admitted for conditions unrelated to caffeine	MI incidence	Not specified	Males under age 55 years, hospitalized with first nonfatal MI event	3,034	Drinking >5 cups caffeinated coffee/day can double MI risk; same with decaf, but not if decaf consumption of >5 cups had occurred for at least 5 years	Did not control for other important risk factors		Rosenberg et al.
United States	1989	Coffee, not specified	<3 cups per day	Not reported	Prospective study of a random sample	All CVD-related outcomes	20 years	Males and females aged 30 to 62 years, free of CHD symptoms	6,214	No association between coffee consumption and CVD occurrences	Did not assess decaffeinated coffee consumption	Correlated to smoking	Wilson et al. (Framingham Heart Study)
United States	1990	All sources of caffeine; decaffeinated tea and coffee	0 to >6 cups per day	Not reported	Two-year prospective study	MI and CHD mortality	2 years	Male health professionals, aged 40 to 75 years at baseline with no previous cardiovascular history	45,589	Caffeine consumption did not significantly affect relative-risk ratios	None outstanding		Grobbee et al.

Country	Year	Substance	Amount	Type	Study design	Outcome	Duration	Population	Sample	Results	Limitations	Correlations	Reference
Norway	1990	Coffee, not specified	0 to >9 cups per day	Not reported	Prospective study of a random sample	Coronary death	6.4 years (average)	Males and females aged 35 to 54 years without CVD symptoms, diabetes, or angina	38,564	Coffee consumption affects CHD mortality above and beyond cholesterol even when other risk factors are controlled for	Did not account for diet, behavioral factors		Tverdal et al.
Sweden	1991	Coffee, not specified	0 to >9 cups per day	Mostly filtered	Prospective study of a random sample	CHD mortality; nonfatal MI	7.1 years (average)	Men aged 51 to 59 years, free of MI symptoms	6765	No significant associations between coffee intake and CHD events	None outstanding	Correlated to smoking, cholesterol, alcohol, BP, and stress	Rosengren and Wilhelmsen
United States	1994	Coffee, caffeinated and decaffeinated	>5 cups per day	Not reported	Prospective study examining coffee consumption every 5 years and its relation to CHD	CHD incidence	28 to 44 years	White, male medical students	1,040	Elevated risk for >5 cups at baseline	None outstanding		Klag et al.
Denmark	1995	Coffee, caffeinated; tea, caffeinated	1 to >9 cups per day	Filtered	Prospective study of differences in coffee consumption between individuals with and without an IHD event	IHD incidence	21 years	Males, average age of 48 years at baseline	2,975	No significant association between IHD and coffee consumption, but significant inverse relationship in nonsmokers and very light smokers	None outstanding		Gyntelberg et al.

(continued)

TABLE 5.1 (Continued)
Role of Caffeinated Substances in Myocardial Infarction and Coronary Heart Disease

Country	Year	Caffeine source and presence of caffeine	Critical amount of caffeine	Brewing method	Study description	Outcome variable	Time to measure DV	Population	Total N	Main conclusion	Limitations	Interactions with other factors?	Ref.
United States	1995	Coffee, caffeinated and decaffeinated	>5 cups per day	Not reported	Case-controlled, retrospective design of MI patients	MI	Not specified	Females aged 45 to 69 years, mostly White	1,716	Relative risk for caffeinated coffee increases at >5 cups/day; for decaffeinated coffee, at >7 cups/day	Did not control for diet, behavioral factors		Palmer et al.
Norway	1995	Coffee, caffeinated	>9 cups per day	Boiled, filtered	Comparison of self-reported coronary events and coffee consumption	MI and angina pectoris	5 to 10 years	Males and females aged 40 to 54 years with no cardiovascular history at baseline	38,500	Relative risk ratios were higher for both DVs in those drinking >9 cups/day	Self-report of DVs; did not adequately control for cholesterol and other risk factors		Stensvold and Tverdal
Norway	1996	Coffee, caffeinated	>9 cups per day	Boiled, filtered	Six-year follow-up to 6-year prospective study	Coronary death	12 years (average)	Males and females aged 40 to 54 years with no cardiovascular history at baseline	38,500	Association reported in 1995 was weakened after accounting for cholesterol	Did not collect information regarding changes in brewing method		Stensvold, Tverdal, and Jacobsen

United States	1996	All sources of caffeine	>6 cups per day	Not reported	Ten-year prospective cohort study	CHD incidence	1 year	Female nurses, mostly white	85,747	Risk ratios were similar between women who consumed none and those who consumed >6 cups/day	None outstanding	Willett et al.
Scotland	1997	Coffee, caffeinated	0 to 5 cups per day	Instant	Follow-up study of individuals within a sample who died of CHD compared to survivors	CHD mortality	17 to 21 years	Males aged 35 to 64 years (at time 1)	5,766	No significant increase in risk of CHD due to coffee consumption	Did not assess recent caffeine/coffee consumption; did not specify criteria of controls	Hart and Davey–Smith
The Netherlands	1999	Coffee, caffeinated	>10 cups per day	Not reported	Regression model of information concerning risk factors collected retrospectively; case-controlled design	Sudden cardiac arrest	Not specified	Heterogenous group of CAD patients matched with sudden cardiac arrest CAD patients in The Netherlands	117	Heavy coffee drinkers who consumed >10 cups/day had more sudden cardiac arrests	Nonexperimental design introduced possible confounds	de Vreede–Swagemakers et al.
Scotland	1999	Coffee and tea, not specified	<3 cups per day	Not reported	Prospective study of a random sample	CHD incidence and coronary death	7.7 years (average)	Males and females aged 40 to 59 years	11,629	Coffee consumption predicted better cardiac health while tea appeared to be irrelevant	Did not account for confounding lifestyle factors of tea vs. coffee drinking	Woodward et al.

(continued)

TABLE 5.1 (Continued)
Role of Caffeinated Substances in Myocardial Infarction and Coronary Heart Disease

Country	Year	Caffeine source and presence of caffeine	Critical amount of caffeine	Brewing method	Study description	Outcome variable	Time to measure DV	Population	Total N	Main conclusion	Limitations	Interactions with other factors?	Ref.
Finland	2000	Coffee, not specified	>4 cups per day	Not reported	Prospective study of a random sample	CHD mortality and nonfatal MI	10 years	Random sample of males and females aged 30 to 59 years at baseline	20,179	CHD mortality followed J-shaped curve, whereas there was no association between MI and coffee drinking	Effect found only in men; small sample of women		Kleemola et al.
Japan	2000	Green tea, caffeinated	>2 cups per day	Not applicable	Cross-sectional, correlational design	Coronary obstruction/stenosis	1 year	Cardiac patients undergoing arteriogram, ages >30 years	167	Inverse relationship of green tea consumption and coronary stenosis in men but not women; mechanism unknown	Other dietary confounds		Sasazuki et al.
United States	2002	Tea, caffeinated	>14 cups per week	Not applicable	Prospective cohort study of a hospitalized sample	MI mortality	3.8 years (average)	Males and females hospitalized for nonfatal MI event	1,900	Increased tea consumption the year before MI event is associated with lower rates of MI death almost 4 years later	Did not assess decaffeinated tea consumption		Mukamal et al.

Country	Year	Substance	Amount	Brewing method	Study design	Outcome measure	Duration	Population	Sample size	Findings	Limitations		Reference
Saudi Arabia	2003	Black tea, caffeinated	>6 cups per day	Not applicable	Case-control study of CHD-diagnosed patients with control	CHD incidence	Not specified	Males and females aged 30 to 70 years	3,430	Tea drinkers consuming >6 cups/day had significantly lower risk of CHD even when other risk factors were controlled; dose-response relationship of CHD and tea	Decaffeinated tea not examined; biological mechanism still unclear		Hakim et al.
Greece	2003	Coffee, caffeinated	>4 cups per day or 600 ml/day	Instant, filtered, boiled	Quasi-experimental cardiac group compared to healthy control group	Cardiac risk odds ratio	1 year	Cardiac patients presenting with first symptoms of CHD (e.g., angina)	848	J-shaped effect of the odds ratio; variations by brewing method not reported	Selection and recall biases	None found	Panagiotakos et al.
Finland	2004	Coffee and tea, caffeinated	>800 ml per day	Boiled, filtered	Prospective study of a random sample	CHD mortality and acute MI	14 years	Males 42 to 60 years and free of CHD symptoms at baseline; no effect of brewing method	1,971	CHD incidence and acute MI followed a J- or U-shaped curve even when conventional factors were accounted for	No biological mechanism examined		Happonen et al.

illnesses. It was found that drinking more than five cups of coffee per day doubled the risk of an MI, even after smoking was controlled. However, this study found no association between tea consumption and myocardial infarction, suggesting that compounds in coffee other than the caffeine may have been responsible for the coffee–CHD association. The remaining studies in the 1970s, including the Honolulu Heart Study, reported no association at all or no association after smoking was controlled (see Table 5.1).

These studies represented important initial attempts to determine the association of caffeine and coffee with CHD. However, as in many bodies of research, early investigators were unable to anticipate the complexities of the question they were addressing fully; as a result, most studies did not have adequate controls in place to address important variables. Such potential confounds as smoking, a history of previous MIs, and consumption of caffeine from sources other than coffee were not uniformly measured. In addition, only one study determined whether the coffee or tea consumed was caffeinated or decaffeinated; brewing method, which may be an important factor, was specified in only one investigation.

Two More Decades of Research: 1980s and 1990s

The largest portion of CHD-related caffeine research was published in the 1980s and 1990s, with a total of 20 papers published in English. During this period, such potentially confounding variables as smoking and caffeination (decaffeinated vs. caffeinated coffee) were more frequently assessed, and Rosengren & Wilhelmsen (1991) became the first investigators to report differences among brewing methods. The majority of studies over the two decades in question employed prospective cohort designs, and a few studies added a case-control dimension. Results spanned the range of possibilities: Some studies reported a positive association between coffee or caffeine consumption and heart disease and others found no relationship; one reported that coffee drinking improves cardiovascular health.

Only seven studies—less than half the total in this period—reported positive findings. In one investigation, medical students were studied prospectively over an average of 25 years; those who drank five or more cups a day had the highest rate of CHD, and heavy coffee drinkers were almost three times more likely to develop the disease (LaCroix, Mead, Liang, Thomas, & Pearson, 1986). This risk decreased after adjustment for such CHD-related factors as number of cigarettes smoked, age, cholesterol level, and baseline coffee consumption. However, the risk persisted after controlling these factors, yielding a time-dependent model of average and most recent coffee consumption. The association between CHD and coffee intake was strongest when the time between the two was shortest—suggesting that recent coffee consumption may be a more potent predictor than past or average coffee consumption.

In line with the LaCroix (1986) study, six other studies reported a "critical" cutoff for caffeine intake such that consumption at or above that level greatly increased risk for CHD. Depending on the study, the threshold was found to be five or more cups per day (Klag et al., 1994; LaCroix et al., 1986; Palmer, Rosenberg, Rao, & Shapiro, 1995; Rosenberg, Palmer, Kelly, Kaufman, & Shapiro, 1988), more than six cups (LeGrady et al., 1987), and more than ten cups (deVreede–Swagemakers et al., 1999).

More recent research has addressed these discrepancies and, more generally, the dose–response relationship.

As Table 5.1 indicates, the remaining studies in the 1980s and 1990s found no association between caffeine and CHD. The Lutheran Brotherhood Study (Murray, Bjelke, Gibson, & Schuman, 1981), for instance, studied ischemic heart disease (IHD) mortality in over 16,000 males aged 35 and over with no prior history of IHD. These subjects were prospectively studied over an average period of 11.5 years. No significant associations were found between subgroups consuming anywhere from one to seven or more cups of coffee per day. The article did not, however, report whether the coffee studied was caffeinated or decaffeinated. Subsequent studies (e.g., Rosengren & Wilhelmsen, 1991; Stensvold, Tverdal, & Jacobsen, 1996) similarly demonstrated a lack of association between coffee or caffeine and heart disease after controlling for other risk factors. Reviewing much of this literature, Chou and Benowitz (1994) concluded that normal levels of coffee intake were not related to CHD.

One final study, published at the end of this two-decade period, showed that increased coffee consumption predicted better cardiac health (Woodward & Tunstall–Pedoe, 1999), though tea consumption had no effect. The authors pointed out that their results may have been confounded by lifestyle factors that were left unaccounted for. For example, it was found that coffee drinking was associated with youth, higher SES, and a more "cosmopolitan" lifestyle. When multiple potential confounding variables, including age and class, were controlled, the association for tea was removed and the association for coffee was greatly reduced. However, a mild protective effect of coffee drinking persisted, though only in the male subsample.

The studies of the 1980s and 1990s clearly reflect an improved knowledge of necessary controls. Nevertheless, the results of these investigations are widely discrepant: Seven studies show a positive relationship between coffee or caffeine consumption and heart disease, one shows a negative association, and thirteen show no relationship at all. Differences among samples may partially account for the discrepancies in results; however, it is likely that uncontrolled variables were primarily responsible. The LaCroix et al. (1986) study, for example, did not control for such factors as family history, diet, and demographic variables, and this is characteristic of many of the other studies (e.g., Klag et al., 1994; Palmer et al., 1995).

Therefore, it is still difficult to reach firm conclusions concerning the effect of caffeine on CHD. Indeed, the problem of confounding variables in caffeine research is limiting (Pirich, O'Grady, & Sinzinger, 1993). For example, one investigation showed that tea drinking is associated with preventative behaviors in relation to CHD, such as healthier diet and increased physical activity, whereas coffee drinking is associated with smoking, low levels of exercise, and fattier diets; these lifestyle indicators present powerful confounds (Schwarz, Bichoff, & Kunze, 1994). In fact, of the studies represented in Table 5.1, three did not control for diet (LaCroix et al., 1986; Palmer et al., 1995; Tverdal et al., 1990), two did not control for decaffeinated coffee/tea usage (Martin et al., 1988; Wilson, Garrison, Kannel, McGee, & Castelli, 1989), and one did not adequately control for cholesterol (Stensvold & Tverdal, 1995). Moreover, none of the studies explored personality or behavioral risk factors, such as stress and trait anger.

More Studies: 21st Century

Research conducted since 1999 has continued to exhibit increasing sophistication in identifying and controlling confounding variables and in specifying and operationalizing variables of interest. Additional strengths of this recent collection of research studies are greater inclusion of women and minorities, as well as a new focus on tea, especially green tea.

The majority of recent research on coffee intake, in particular, has demonstrated a J- or U-shaped relationship between the amount consumed and CHD incidence (Happonen, Voutilainen, & Salone, 2004; Kleemola, Jousilahti, Pietinen, Vartiainen, & Tuomilehto, 2000; Panagiotakos et al., 2003). Although the nuances of the curve can vary somewhat depending upon the study, the basic idea behind this finding is that moderate coffee intake may actually confer protective or beneficial effects where CHD is concerned.

By contrast, drinking no coffee or excessive amounts of coffee increases CHD-related risk. For instance, one study involving a large Finnish sample showed that those who did not drink coffee actually suffered from higher CHD mortality rates than their coffee-drinking cohorts. In men, the relationship between coffee drinking and CHD mortality was J-shaped, and no association existed between nonfatal MI risk and coffee consumption. In women, no relationship was found between coffee drinking and CHD mortality; however, the risk ratios for developing a nonfatal MI were higher in participants who did not drink coffee. In other words, when such CHD risk factors as cholesterol and smoking status were adjusted, nondrinkers actually appeared to have a higher risk of CHD mortality than drinkers.

This effect was found only in males, however, perhaps due to the small number of CHD cases in the female segment of the sample (Kleemola et al., 2000). Though the data were not presented graphically in this paper, the odds ratios indicate that CHD mortality risk follows a backward J-shaped curve; thus, individuals who drink zero to one cup of coffee per day are at highest risk (risk ratio = 1.88). The curve "dips" at one to three cups per day, signaling the potential protective benefit of drinking an average of two cups of coffee per day (risk ratio = 1.00). Finally, the risk ratios increase gradually from four cups per day onward; however, even at over seven cups, the risk ratio does not approach that of the zero-to-one cup per day group (risk ratio = 1.22). Detailed information concerning cup sizes, strength of coffee, and related issues is contained in chapter 2.

Similarly to the J-shaped curve, the U-shaped function between CHD and caffeine consumption implies that no or light consumption of coffee may be just as hazardous as drinking very large amounts. One recent investigation followed participants at 5 and 14 years and measured a variety of factors, including HDL and LDL cholesterol, blood pressure, smoking, diabetes, and income (Happonen et al., 2004). When these covariates were controlled for, the association between coffee drinking and CHD indicated a J- or perhaps U-shaped dose–response function. Based on calculations of average coffee intake, the researchers found that moderate coffee drinkers, who habitually consumed 376 to 813 ml of coffee per day, had lower risk ratios (1.00) when compared to individuals who drank no coffee (risk ratio = 1.12), light drinkers (1 to 375 ml per day; risk ratio = 1.24), or heavy drinkers (>813 ml per day; risk ratio = 1.43) up to 14 years later.

Although the risk ratios of the abstinent and light drinkers clearly approximate those of the heavy drinking group, heavy consumers of coffee still had the highest risk ratios for CHD events. Thus, the results of this study actually resemble those of the Kleemola (2000) study; the risk ratios are, in fact, quite similar, thus indicating a relationship better represented by a J-shaped curve. Furthermore, when smokers are examined as a separate group, the function is notably more "J-like" and steeper than the curve representing the nonsmokers.

Happonen and colleagues (2004) interpreted the curve they found in an interesting way. In Finland, where this study was conducted, coffee is a primary food source for antioxidants. Moderate coffee drinkers are thus reaping the protective effects of the antioxidants present in coffee by their regular, modest consumption. Abstinent and light drinkers, however, do not incur this benefit and, in fact, consume caffeine so intermittently that tolerance has not developed. Therefore, consuming coffee on an intermittent basis acts to make the consumer vulnerable to the negative effects of caffeine, such as high blood pressure, but does not offer any protective benefit, resulting in higher rates of CHD. Finally, heavy coffee drinkers consume large amounts of caffeine due to high tolerance and thus are more prone to its negative biochemical effects. The latter may outweigh any antioxidant activity to result in such chronic conditions as increased homocysteine levels that contribute to the development of CHD. This study did not offer a direct test of this hypothesis, but explanations such as this may help scientists understand the nuances of the J-shaped curve.

Studies such as these are clearer illustrations of the J- or U-shaped relationship between caffeine and CHD. Taken together, they suggest little or no harmful effect of moderate coffee consumption and that light or no coffee drinking may actually pose a modest risk for CHD. Furthermore, heavy coffee use appears to be more clearly associated with higher risk ratios. These studies collectively seem to indicate also that the increased risk for CHD and associated mortality in "heavy" drinkers begins at approximately four cups of coffee per day (about 600 ml).

POSSIBLE CAUSAL MECHANISMS

To the extent that coffee and caffeine contribute to development of coronary heart disease and cardiovascular morbidity and mortality, it is important to gain an understanding of the major causal mechanisms. Although we certainly do not yet have a definitive causal model, some of the likely mechanisms have been elucidated in recent research and theory development.

Caffeine, Heart Rate, and Blood Pressure

When excessive coffee drinking is found to be associated with CHD, caffeine is usually assumed to be the culprit (Lane et al., 2002). If so, what are the mechanisms through which caffeine impairs cardiovascular functioning? One of the most common lines of reasoning theorizes that caffeine activates stress reactivity systems, releasing epinephrine. As a result, blood pressure and heart rate are elevated, leading to the conclusion that long-term consumption of caffeine may cause hypertension, a well-established factor in CHD development.

To test the hypothesis that caffeine consumption would cause short-term blood pressure effects, one study employed a double-blind crossover design to compare members of a caffeine group, who received 500 mg of the drug, with those receiving placebo (Lane et al., 2002). Members of both groups were habitual coffee drinkers, consuming an average of two to seven cups per day. Ambulatory blood pressure and heart rate were measured during the waking hours for 1 day, and it was determined that the caffeine group had experienced significantly higher ambulatory blood pressure. These effects were especially pronounced during stressful situations over the test period and caused diastolic and heart rate elevations. It was concluded that caffeine does have at least an acute effect on heart rate and blood pressure, which may develop into hypertension in the long run.

Several other studies report similar results, with caffeine producing short-term increases in diastolic blood pressure (Berube–Parent, Pelletier, Dore, & Tremblay, 2005), systolic blood pressure (Farag et al., 2005; Roberts, de-Jonge–Levitan, Parker, & Greenway, 2005), and ambulatory blood pressure (Savoca et al., 2005). These results suggest that, at the very least, caffeine produces short-term blood pressure elevations. Although the theory is certainly a reasonable one, C. Brown and Benowitz (1989) found no effect of caffeine on heart rate or blood pressure over a 4-day dosing period, and some subsequent studies have found weak or inconsistent relationships between caffeine consumption and increases in heart rate, and blood pressure (e.g., Barry et al., 2005; Lewis et al., 1993).

Further analysis of this literature permits some refinement of the conclusions. First, some evidence suggests that caffeine causes an increase in systolic blood pressure during mental stress in nonhabitual coffee drinkers, whereas in habitual drinkers, cardiovascular responses are blunted when caffeine is introduced (Sudano et al., 2005). There is also evidence that blood pressure and heart rate changes are greater in caffeine consumers who have not developed tolerance (Farag et al., 2005). There also appear to be some differences in results between caffeine and coffee trials. For example, a recent meta-analysis of 16 clinical trials involving caffeine or coffee administration showed that caffeine did appear to increase blood pressure and pressor effects diminished when the coffee studies were examined alone. No effects on heart rate were found (Noordzij et al., 2005).

At this time, the literature does not unequivocally support the long-term impact of caffeine on blood pressure, but several studies have produced clear, direct evidence substantiating its acute effects. Indeed, the weight of this literature suggests that caffeine does affect blood pressure. If that result holds up in future research, blood pressure may be among the mechanisms through which caffeine can contribute to CHD. A much more extensive review of this literature can be found in chapter 6 and a more complete review of the heart rate literature in chapter 4.

Coffee, Cholesterol, and Brewing Method

If blood pressure may be one mechanism through which coffee relates to CHD, another may be its effects on blood lipids. The hypothesis that coffee may contribute to CHD by increasing LDL cholesterol has been proposed since the 1960s (e.g., A. Brown, 1962; Paul et al., 1963), but current evidence is mixed; some studies have found positive effects (Cheung, Gupta, & Ito, 2005; Happonen et al., 2004; Miyake et al., 1999) and others have found no relationship (Du et al., 2005; Sakamoto et al., 2005). The relevant literature is addressed in depth in chapter 7 in this volume. Therefore, our focus here is on the possible role of the boiling method of coffee preparation in the lipid effect.

Two diterpene lipids—cafestol and kahweol—present in coffee oil appear to increase cholesterol levels by as much as 32% in a dose-dependent fashion (Urgert & Katan, 1997). These compounds are typically removed from the final product in coffee-brewing methods that use filtering, but when a boiling method is used and the final coffee beverage is not passed through filter paper, these chemicals are not removed. Examples of boiled coffees with no filtration include French press/caffetiere, Turkish, Scandinavian, and Israeli "mud" coffees. The drip method, in particular, filters out the cafestol and kahweol. Brewing method may thus be one factor in the contradictory findings regarding the relationship between coffee and CHD.

Early studies, such as the one conducted by Bak and Grobbee (1989), showed that drinking boiled coffee for as little as 9 weeks could raise serum cholesterol levels by 10%. In a randomized clinical trial, subsequent researchers found that the hypercholesteremic element of coffee could be removed after boiling by filtering (van Dusseldorp, Katan, van Vliet, Demacker, & Stalenhoef, 1991). On the other hand, in a prospective study, regular consumers of filtered coffee abstained from coffee drinking for a 6-week period. Those who normally consumed four or more cups daily actually lowered their cholesterol levels by 0.28 mmol/L and homocysteine concentrations by 1.08 mmol/L on average, suggesting that filtering does not entirely eliminate the cholesterol effect (Strandhagen & Thelle, 2003).

A meta-analysis of 14 published studies on cholesterol and coffee showed that drinking six or more cups of boiled coffee per day can significantly raise total and LDL cholesterol. Levels rose minimally when filtered coffee was consumed. Moreover, similar effects were seen in drinkers of regular and decaffeinated coffee, making it likely that chemicals in the coffee other than caffeine are responsible for the increase in LDL cholesterol (Jee et al., 2001).

Overall, substantial, but mixed, evidence indicates that coffee, at least when boiled, affects cholesterol. However, considerable further research on the relationship between preparation method and cholesterol effects is clearly needed. One complicating factor is that some studies have not taken into account the possible role of the milk or cream that many drinkers add to coffee. In addition, as much as 85% of the variance in cholesterol level may be genetic. Thus, the effects of coffee, as well as milk products, must be viewed in light of this substantial heritability factor (Strandhagen et al., 2004).

Tea

Though coffee is the most widely consumed source of caffeine in the United States and is thus better represented in this literature, the study of tea and CHD proves illustrative. The increasing, widespread use of tea has prompted stand-alone tea research in recent years; the first study looking solely at CHD and tea was published in 2000. This small but growing literature on caffeinated tea finds that consumption may be protective against CHD (Hakim et al., 2003; Mukamal, Maclure, Muller, Sherwood, & Mittleman, 2002; Sasazuki et al., 2000). These three recent studies suggest that anywhere from two to fourteen cups of tea daily may buffer CHD development and protect against CHD-related mortality.

In one study, regular black tea (at a rate of five cups per day) was compared to decaffeinated placebo. Participants in both conditions received placebo with added caffeine, and participants' diets were controlled. Individuals in the black tea condition reaped the largest benefits in lowered cholesterol and LDL, followed by the placebo with added caffeine, and then finally the plain placebo. Thus, caffeine in tea may help to reduce cholesterol, a long-established risk factor in the development of CHD (Davies et al., 2003).

In a second investigation, the results were less clear. Short-term effects were independent of caffeine; results for vasodilation were similar in caffeinated and placebo groups. However, it is unclear whether long-term effects involve caffeine. Black tea may improve arterial flow and endothelial function, possibly due to the presence of polyphenols (Duffy et al., 2001). Therefore, tea does appear to have some beneficial effects as far as CHD is concerned, but because this literature is still in its early stages, further research is warranted. More extensive coverage of the tea literature appears in chapter 14.

CONCLUSIONS

For over 40 years now, the scientific literature has addressed what would seem to be a simple question: Does the consumption of coffee—or of caffeine more generally—contribute to cardiac morbidity and mortality? More specifically, does caffeine contribute to development of coronary heart disease, occurrence of myocardial infarctions, or both? Unfortunately, the answer has proven to be as elusive as it is complex. Substantial numbers of investigations have demonstrated statistically significant, positive relationships between coffee or caffeine consumption and CHD. However, many others have found no relationship at all, an inverse relationship, or a positive relationship that holds up whether the coffee is caffeinated or decaffeinated.

Much of the difficulty in interpreting the overall literature lies in the fact that the nature and extent of the variables examined and the controls employed vary markedly from study to study. Some investigators separate drinkers of caffeinated and decaffeinated coffee, while others do not. Some take into account the use of milk products in coffee, while others ignore this variable. Some assess and report preparation method, while others do not. Some take into account such other factors as smoking, alcohol consumption, and diet, while others choose not to collect data on these variables.

Although this variability in the literature precludes any firm and final conclusions, one variable that has been consistently assessed is the amount of coffee or caffeine consumed. Although there is some variability in the definition of "cup," most studies do at least report the number of cups consumed per day, providing a basis for reaching some tentative conclusions concerning the dose–response relationship. In addition, a few other conclusions are possible at this time.

THE CAFFEINE–CHD RELATIONSHIP

Although some variability in the literature remains, the overall relationship between caffeine consumption and CHD appears to follow a J-shaped curve, with moderate consumption producing the optimal cardiovascular outcomes. For coffee, optimal consumption ranges around 300 to 450 ml (two to three cups) per day. Consumption markedly above and below this amount is related to higher CHD incidence.

HEART RATE AND BLOOD PRESSURE

Caffeine does acutely raise blood pressure and, in some studies, heart rate, although some evidence indicates that these effects may dissipate as tolerance develops. Although chronically elevated blood pressure and heart rate are associated with development of CHD and occurrence of MIs, it has thus far been difficult to tie caffeine directly to the necessary chronic elevations. Thus, caffeine causes acute elevations, at least in blood pressure, but may or may not contribute to the chronic elevations associated with cardiovascular morbidity and mortality.

COFFEE AND CHOLESTEROL

Considerable evidence suggests that consuming coffee can increase levels of LDL cholesterol and that caffeine per se may not be responsible of this elevation. Instead, two diterpene lipids found in chemical analyses of coffee—cafestol and kahweol—appear to be the culprits. With ongoing coffee consumption, these lipids may raise LDL levels, thus contributing to the development of CHD and eventually to the occurrence of MIs.

BOILING AND FILTERING METHODS

Fairly consistent, though somewhat mixed, evidence suggests that coffee preparation method may influence long-term cardiovascular risk. In particular, it appears that coffee prepared by the boiling method is much more likely to increase CHD risk than that same coffee prepared by filtering. Theory and some evidence suggest that, again, the diterpene lipids underlie this difference. When coffee is boiled, these lipids remain in the product, but filtering largely removes them.

PROTECTIVE EFFECTS OF COFFEE

The fact that consuming relatively small amounts of coffee may reduce CHD risk suggests a protective effect. Preliminary evidence has been interpreted as suggesting that coffee may contain antioxidants that work to improve cardiovascular function. Considerable further work is needed to confirm this hypothesis, however.

PROTECTIVE EFFECTS OF TEA

Increasing evidence suggests that green tea and perhaps other teas may have beneficial effects in protecting against CHD. To some extent, these benefits may result from the caffeine found in tea. However, work to date suggests that the catechins in tea are more important.

FUTURE RESEARCH DIRECTIONS

As we have seen, a number of problems in the scientific literature on coffee and caffeine limit the generalizability of the empirical findings to date. First, caffeine is frequently equated with coffee to the point that other sources of caffeine, such as chocolate, medications, soft drinks, and tea, are not assessed. When risk-odds ratios were computed, it was found that when other such sources of caffeine are ignored in data collection, a 10-fold risk is not taken into account when coffee consumption alone is assessed (J. Brown, Krieger, Darlington, & Sloan (2001). Therefore, when assessing caffeine effects, it is important in future research to consider all major sources of caffeine, not just coffee.

A related concern is the paucity of research focusing primarily on tea, cola, and chocolate as sources of caffeine. Although this literature has certainly grown in the last 5 years, much more systematic research is needed to investigate the role of these sources of caffeine. A further advantage of studying caffeine intake from tea and cola is that they do not contain the other chemical compounds found in coffee, such as the diterpenes, thus making the differential role of caffeine across caffeinated substances easier to assess.

A further need is to better evaluate the causal mechanisms underlying caffeine- and coffee-related increases and decreases in CHD risk. Although the prospective paradigms characteristic of many past studies are certainly important, future research involving randomized designs should allow better exploration of etiology, leading to a more complete causal model. The available research to date is reviewed in chapter 4.

A final consideration in future studies is the establishment of more uniform assessments and controls. As we have seen, the research of the past 40 years has yielded in-depth information as to many of the variables that may contribute to the apparent caffeine–CHD relationship. At this point, investigators would do well to consider applying this knowledge systematically to future studies. For example, we now know that it is critical to assess whether coffee is caffeinated, whether milk products and sugar are added to coffee, and what preparation method is used.

We also need to assess caffeinated substances other than coffee (tea, chocolate, cola, etc.) that are consumed and in what quantities; ideally, there should be a full assessment of the presence of other known cardiovascular risk factors. These might include family history/genetics, smoking, alcohol consumption, diet, levels of HDL and LDL cholesterol, plasma homocysteine, C-reactive protein, plasma catechola- mines, diabetes, hypertension, obesity, exercise, level of chronic stress, anger/ hostility, and, perhaps, heart rate and arrhythmias. Assessing all of these variables may be impractical in some studies; however, our understanding of the roles of coffee and caffeine will increase considerably if investigations take into account as many of these important substances and risk factors as possible.

REFERENCES

Al-Ajlan, A. R., & Mehdi, S. R. (2005). Effects and a dose response relationship of physical activity to high-density lipoprotein cholesterol and body mass index among Saudis. *Saudi Medical Journal, 26*(7), 1107–1111.

American Heart Association. (2004). *Heart disease and stroke statistics.* (2005). Update. American Heart Association.

Antezano, E. S., & Hong, M. (2003). Sudden cardiac death. *Journal of Intensive Care Medicine, 18*(6), 313–329.

Aoki, S., Mukae, S., Itoh, S., Sato, R., Nishio, K., Ueda, H., Iwata, T., & Katagiri, T. (2001). Genetic background in patients with acute myocardial infarction. *Japanese Heart Journal, 42*, 15–28.

Aras, R., Sowers, J. R., & Arora, R. (2005). The proinflammatory and hypercoagulable state of diabetes mellitus. *Review of Cardiovascular Medicine, 6*(2), 84–97.

Bak, A. A., & Grobbee, D. E. (1989). The effect on serum cholesterol levels of coffee brewed by filtering or boiling. *The New England Journal of Medicine, 321,* 432–437.

Barghash, N. A., Barghash, A. A., El Dine, R., Elewa, S. M., & Hamdi, E. A. (2004). Role of plasma homocysteine and lipoprotein (a) in coronary artery disease. *British Journal of Biomedical Science, 61*, 78–83.

Barry, R. J., Rushby, J. A., Wallace, M. J., Clarke, A. R., Johnstone, S. J., & Zlojutro, I. (2005). Caffeine effects on resting-state arousal. *Clinical Neurophysiology, 116*(11), 2693–2700.

Bell, D. S. (2004). Advances in diabetes for the millennium: The heart and diabetes. *Medscape General Medicine, 22(6),* 7.

Bello, N., & Mosca, L. (2004). Epidemiology of coronary heart disease in women. *Progressive Cardiovascular Disease, 46*(4), 287–295.

Berube–Parent, S., Pelletier, C., Dore, J., & Tremblay, A. (2005). Effects of encapsulated green tea and Guarana extracts containing a mixture of epigallocatechin-3-gallate and caffeine on 24-h energy expenditure and fat oxidation in men. *British Journal of Nutrition, 94*(3), 432–436.

Blasco, C., Caballeria, J., Deulofeu, R., Lligona, A., Pares, A., Lluis, J. M., et al. (2005). Prevalence and mechanisms of hyperhomocysteinemia in chronic alcoholics. *Alcoholism—Clinical and Experimental Research, 29*, 1044–1048.

Boufidou, A. I., Karvounis, H. I., Makedou, K. G., Gourassas, J. T., Makedou, A. D., Adamidis, D. N., et al. (2004). Association between plasma homocysteine levels and coronary artery disease: A population-based study in northern Greece. *Current Medical Research and Opinion, 20*, 175–180.

Brown, A. (1962). Coronary thrombosis: An environmental study. *British Medical Journal, 5304*, 567–573.

Brown, C. P., & Benowitz, N. L. (1989). Caffeine and cigarette smoking: Behavioral, cardiovascular, and metabolic interactions. *Pharmacology Biochemistry and Behavior, 34*, 565–570.

Brown, J., Krieger, N., Darlington, G. A., & Sloan, M. (2001). Misclassification of exposure: Coffee as a surrogate for caffeine intake. *American Journal of Epidemiology, 153*(8), 815–820.

Brunner, E. J., Hemingway, H., Walker, B. R., Page, M., Clarke, P., Juneja, M., et al. (2002). Adrenocortical, autonomic, and inflammatory causes of the metabolic syndrome: Nested-case control study. *Circulation, 106*, 2650–2665.

Burns, D. M. (2003). Epidemiology of smoking-induced cardiovascular disease. *Progressive Cardiovascular Disease, 46*(1), 11–29.

Buxton, A. E., Ellison, K. E., Kirk, M. M., Frain, B., Koo, C., Gandhi, G., et al. (2003). Primary prevention of sudden cardiac death: Trials in patients with coronary artery disease. *Journal of Interventional Cardiac Electrophysiology, 9*(2), 203–206.

Carney, R. M., Freedland, K. E., & Veith, R. C. (2005). Depression, the autonomic nervous system, and coronary heart disease. *Psychosomatic Medicine, 67*(1), S29–S33.

Centers for Disease Control. (1999). *Achievements in Public Health 1900–1999: Control of Infectious Diseases. Morbidity and Mortality Weekly Report.* Retrieved November 16, 2005, from www.cdc.gov/od/oc/media/mmwrnews/n990730.htm#mmwr1.

Centers for Disease Control. (2005). Adult participation in recommended levels of physical—United States, 2001 and 2003. *Morbidity and Mortality Weekly Report, 54*(47), 1208–1212.

Cheung, R. J., Gupta, E. K., & Ito, M. K. (2005). Acute coffee ingestion does not affect LDL cholesterol level. *Annals of Pharmacotherapy, 39*(7–8), 1209–1213.

Chou, T. M., & Benowitz, N. L. (1994). Caffeine and coffee: Effects on health and cardiovascular disease. *Comparative Biochemistry & Physiology, 109C*, 173–189.

Courville, K. A., Lavie, C. J., & Milani, R. V. (2005). Lipid-lowering therapy for elderly patients at risk for coronary events and stroke. *American Heart Hospital Journal, 3*(4), 256–262.

Cushman, M., Arnold, A. M., Psaty, B. M., Manolio, T. A., Kuller, L. H., Burke, G. L., et al. (2005). C-reactive protein and the 10-year incidence of coronary heart disease in older men and women: The Cardiovascular Health Study. *Circulation, 112*, 25–31.

Dahl–Jorgensen, K., Larsen, J. R., & Hanssen, K. F. (2005). Atherosclerosis in childhood and adolescent type 1 diabetes: Early disease, early treatment? *Diabetologia, 48*(8), 1445–1253.

Dallongeville, J., Marecaux, N., Fruchart, J. C., & Amouyel, P. (1998). Cigarette smoking is associated with unhealthy patterns of nutrient intake: A meta-analysis. *Journal of Nutrition, 128*, 1450–1457.

Davies, M. J., Judd, J. T., Baer, D. J., Clevidence, B. A., Paul, D. R., Edwards, A. J., et al. (2003). *Journal of Nutrition, 133*, 3298S–3302S.

Dawber, T. R., Kannel, W. B., & Gordon, T. (1974). Coffee and cardiovascular disease: Observations from the Framingham study. *New England Journal of Medicine, 291*, 871–4.

de Pergola, G., & Pannacciulli. (2002). Coagulation and fibrinolysis abnormalities in obesity. *Journal of Endocrinology Investigation, 25*, 899–904.

de Sutter, J., Firsovaite, V., & Tavernier, R. (2002). Prevention of sudden death in patients with coronary artery disease: Do lipid-lowering drugs play a role? *Preventive Cardiology, 5*(4), 177–182.

de Vreede–Swagemakers, J. J., Gorgels, A. P. M., Weijenberg, M. P., Dubois–Arbouw, W. I., Golombeck, B., van Ree, J. W., et al. (1999). Risk indicators of out-of-hospital cardiac arrest in patients with coronary artery disease. *Journal of Clinical Epidemiology, 52*(7), 601–607.

Du, Y., Melchert, H. U., Knopf, H., Braemer–Hauth, M., Gerding, B., & Pabel, E. (2005). Association of serum caffeine concentrations with blood lipids in caffeine-drug users and nonusers—Results of German National Health Surveys from 1984 to 1999. *European Journal of Epidemiology, 20*(4), 311–316.

Duffy, S. J., Keaney, J. F., Holbrook, M., Gokce, N., Swerdloff, P. L., Frei, B., et al. (2001). Short- and long-term black tea consumption reverses endothelial dysfunction in patients with coronary artery disease. *Circulation, 104*, 151–156.

Eaker, E. D., Sullivan, L. M., Kelly–Hayes, M., D'Agostino, R. B., & Benjamin, E. J. (2005). Tension and anxiety in the prediction of the 10-year incidence of coronary heart disease, atrial fibrillation, and total mortality: The Framingham Offspring Study. *Psychosomatic Medicine, 67*, 692–696.

Endo, A., Kinugawa, T., Ogino, K., Kato, M., Hamada, T., Osaki, S., et al. (2000). Cardiac and plasma catecholamine responses to exercise in patients with type 2 diabetes: Prognostic implications for cardiac–cerebrovascular events. *American Journal of Medical Science, 320*(1), 24–30.

Farag, N. H., Vincent, A. S., Sung, B. H., Whitsett, T. L., Wilson, M. F., & Lovallo, W. R. (2005). *American Journal of Hypertension, 18*(5), 714–719.

Forslund, L., Björkander, I., Ericson, M., Held, C., Katan, T., Rehnqvist, N., et al. (2002). Prognostic implications of autonomic function assessed by analyses of catecholamines and heart rate variability in stable angina pectoris. *Heart, 87*, 415–422.

Fowler, B. (2005). Homocystein—An independent risk factor for cardiovascular and thrombotic diseases. *Therapeutische Umschau Revue Therapeutique, 62*, 641–646.

Frank, L. L., Sorensen, B. E., Yasui, Y., Tworoger, S. S., Schwartz, R. S., Ulrich, C. M., et al. (2005). Effects of exercise on metabolic risk variables in overweight postmenopausal women: A randomized clinical trial. *Obesity Research, 13*(3), 615–625.

Friedlander, Y., Arbogast, P., Schwartz, S. M., Marcovina, S. M., Austin, M. A., Rosendaal, F. R., et al. (2001). Family history as a risk factor for early onset myocardial infraction in young women. *Atherosclerosis, 156*, 201–207.

Galan, P., Viteri, F. E., Bertrais, S., Czernichow, S., Faure, H., Arnaud, J., et al. (2005). Serum concentrations of beta-carotene, vitamins C and E, zinc and selenium are influences by sex, age, diet, smoking status, alcohol consumption and corpulence in a general French adult population. *European Journal of Clinical Nutrition, 59*(10), 1181–1190.

Geronimo, F. R., Abarquez, R. F., Punzalan, F. E., & Cabral, E. I. (2005). Clustering of risk factors, metabolic syndrome, and coronary heart disease in hypertensive patients. *Asia Pacific Journal of Clinical Nutrition, 14*, S44.

Gottlieb, S. O. (1992). Cardiovascular benefits of smoking cessation. *Heart Disease & Stroke, 1*(4), 173–175.

Green, R., & Miller, J. W. (2005). Vitamin B12 deficiency is the dominant nutritional cause of hyperhomocysteinemia in a folic acid-fortified population. *Clinical Chemistry and Laboratory Medicine: CCLM/FESCC, 43*, 1048–1051.

Grobbee, D. E., Rimm, E. R., Giovannucci, E., Colditz, G., Stampfer, M. & Willett, W. (1990). Coffee, caffeine, and cardiovascular disease in men. *New England Journal of Medicine, 323*, 1026–1032.

Gyntelberg, F., Hein, H. O., Suadicani, P., & Sorensen, H. (1995). Coffee consumption and risk of ischaemic heart disease — a settled issue? *Journal of Internal Medicine, 237*, 55–61.

Hakim, I. A., Alsaif, M. A., Alduwaihy, M., Al-Rubeaan, K., Al-Nuaim, A. R., & Al-Attas, O. S. (2003). Tea consumption and the prevalence of coronary heart disease in Saudi adults: Results from a Saudi national study. *Preventive Medicine, 36*, 64–70.

Happonen, P., Voutilainen, S., & Salone, J. T. (2004). Coffee drinking is dose-dependently related to the risk of acute coronary events in middle-aged men. *Journal of Nutrition, 134*, 2381–2386.

Hart, C., & Davey-Smith, G. (1997). Coffee consumption and coronary heart disease mortality in Scottish men: A 21 year follow-up study. *Journal of Epidemiology & Community Health, 51*, 461–462.

Hennekens, C. H., Drolette, M. E., Jesse, M. J., Davies, J. E., & Hutchinson, G. B. (1976). Coffee drinking and death due to coronary heart disease. *New England Journal of Medicine, 294*, 633–636.

Hill, J. A. (2005). In vino veritas: Alcohol and heart disease. *American Journal of the Medical Sciences, 329*(3), 124–135.

Hoyert, D., Kung H., & Smith, B. (2005). Deaths: Preliminary data for 2003. *National Vital Statistics Reports, 53*, 1–48.

Jacobsen, B.K., Bjelki, E., Kvale, G., & Heuch, I. (1986). Coffee drinking, mortality, and cancer incidence: results from a Norwegian prospective study. *Journal of the National Cancer Institute, 76*, 823–831.

Jee, S. H., He, J., Appel, L. J., Whelton, P. K., Suh, I., & Klag, M. J. (2001). Coffee consumption and serum lipids: A meta-analysis of randomized controlled clinical trials. *American Journal of Epidemiology, 153*(4), 353–362.

Jemal, A., Murray, T., Ward, E., Samuels, A., Tiwari, R.C., Ghafoor, A., et al. (2005). Cancer statistics. *CA: A Cancer Journal for Clinicians, 55*, 10–30.

Jouven, X., Empana, J. P., Schwartz, P. J., Desnos, M., Courbon, D., & Ducimetiere, P. (2005). Heart-rate profile during exercise as a predictor of sudden death. *New England Journal of Medicine, 352*(19), 1951–1958.

Juo, S. H., Bredie, S. J., Kiemeney, L. A., Demacker, P. N., & Stalenhoef, A. F. (1998). A common genetic mechanism determines plasma apolipoprotein B levels and dense LDL subfraction distribution in familial combined hyperlipidemia. *American Journal of Human Genetics, 63*(2), 586–594.

Kabat, G. C. (2003). Fifty years' experience of reduced-tar cigarettes: What do we know about their effects? *Inhalation Toxicology, 15*, 1059–1102.

Kasapis, C., & Thompson, P. D. (2005). The effects of physical activity on serum C-reactive protein and inflammatory markers: A systematic review. *Journal of the American College of Cardiology, 45*, 1563–1569.

Katzmarzyk, P. T., Perusse, L., Rice, T., Gagnon, J., Skinner, J. S., Wilmore, J. H., et al. (2000). Familial resemblance for coronary heart disease risk: The HERITAGE Family Study. *Ethnicity & Disease, 10*, 138–147.

Kengne, A. P., Amoah, A. G., & Mbanya, J. C. (2005). Cardiovascular complications of diabetes mellitus in sub-Saharan Africa. *Circulation, 112*(23), 3592–3601.

Kim, M. S., & Polychronakos, C. (2005). Immunogenetics of type 1 diabetes. *Hormone Research, 64*, 180–188.

Klag, M. J., Mead, L. A., LaCroix, A. Z., Wang, N. Y., Coresh, J., Liang, K. Y., et al. (1994). Coffee intake and coronary heart disease. *Annals of Epidemiology, 4*(6), 425–433.

Kleemola, P., Jousilahti, P., Pietinen, P., Vartiainen, E., & Tuomilehto, J. (2000). Coffee consumption and the risk of coronary heart disease and death. *Archives of Internal Medicine, 160*, 3393–3400.

Knekt, P., Alfthan, G., Aromaa, A., Heliovaara, M., Marniemi, J., Rissanen, H., et al. (2001). Homocysteine and major coronary events: a prospective population study among women. *Journal of Internal Medicine, 249*, 461–465.

Koren–Morag, N., Tanne, D., & Goldbourt, U. (2005). White blood cell count and the incidence of ischemic stroke in coronary heart disease patients. *American Journal of Medicine, 18*, 1004–1009.

LaCroix, A. Z., Mead, L. A., Liang, K. L., Thomas, C. B., & Pearson, T. (1986). Coffee consumption and the incidence of coronary heart disease. *The New England Journal of Medicine, 315*(16), 977–982.

Lane, J. D., Pieper, C. F., Phillips–Bute, B. G., Bryant, J. E., & Kuhn, C. M. (2002). Caffeine affects cardiovascular and neuroendocrine activation at work and home. *Psychosomatic Medicine, 64*, 595–603.

LeGrady, D., Dyer, A. R., Shekelle, R. B., Stamler, J., Liu, K., Paul, O., et al. (1987). Coffee consumption and mortality in the Chicago Western Electric Company Study. *American Journal of Epidemiology, 126*(5), 803–812.

Lewis, C. E., Caan, B., Funkhouser, E., Hilner, J. E., Bragg, C., Dyer, A., et al. (1993). Inconsistent associations between caffeine-containing beverages with blood pressure and with lipoproteins. *American Journal of Epidemiology, 138*(7), 502–507.

Liu, Y. J., Xiao, P., Xiong, D. H., Recker, R. R., & Deng, H. W. (2005). Searching for obesity genes: Progress and prospects. *Drugs Today, 41*(5), 345–362.

Lloyd–Jones, D. M., Wilson, P. W., Larson, M. G., Leip, E., Beiser, A., D'Agostino, et al. (2003). Lifetime risk of coronary heart disease by cholesterol levels at selected ages. *Archives of Internal Medicine, 163,* 1966–1972.

Luc, G., Bard, J. M., Juhan–Vague, I., Ferrieres, J., Evans, A., Amouyel, P., et al. (2003). C-reactive protein, interleukin-6, and fibrinogen as predictors of coronary heart disease: The PRIME study. *Arteriosclerosis Thrombosis and Vascular Biology, 23,* 1255–1261.

Luciano, M., Kirk, L. M., Heath, A. C., & Martin, N. G. (2005). The genetics of tea and coffee drinking and preference for source of caffeine in a large community sample of Australian twins. *Addiction, 100,* 1510–1517.

MacCallum, P. K. (2005). Markers of hemostasis and systemic inflammation in heart disease and atherosclerosis in smokers. *Proceedings of the American Thoracic Society, 2,* 34–43.

Mackness, B., Hine, D., McElduff, P., & Mackness, M. (2006). High C-reactive protein and low paraoxonase1 in diabetes as risk factors for coronary heart disease. *Atherosclerosis, 182,* 396–401.

Mager, A., Harell, D., Battler, A., Koren–Morag, N., & Shohat, M. (2005). Family history, plasma homocysteine, and age at onset of symptoms of myocardial ischemia in patients with different methylenetetrahydrofolate reductase genotypes. *The American Journal of Cardiology, 95,* 1420–1424.

Maheswaran, R., Haining, R. P., Brindley, P., Law, J., Pearson, T., Fryers, P. R., et al. (2005). Outdoor air pollution, mortality, and hospital admissions from coronary heart disease in Sheffield, U.K.: A small-area level ecological study. *European Heart Journal, 26,* 2543–2549.

Marteau, J. B., Zaiou, M., Siest, G., & Visvikis–Siest, S. (2005). Genetic determinants of blood pressure regulation. *Journal of Hypertension, 23*(12), 2127–2143.

Martin, J. B., Annegers, J. F., Curb, J. D., Heyden, S., Howson, C., Lee, E. S., et al. (1988). Mortality patterns among hypertensives by reported level of caffeine consumption. *Preventive Medicine, 17*(3), 310–320.

McDonough, P., & Moffatt, R. J. (1999). Smoking-induced elevations in blood carboxyhaemoglobin levels. Effect on maximal oxygen uptake. *Sports Medicine, 27*(5), 275–283.

McGovern M. E. (2005). Taking aim at HDL-C. Raising levels to reduce cardiovascular risk. *Postgraduate Medicine, 117,* 29–39.

Medina–Urrutia, A., Liria, Y. K., Posadas–Romero, C., Cardoso–Saldaqa, G. C., & Zamora–Gonzalez, J. (2004). Apolipoprotein E polymorphism is related to plasma lipids and apolipoproteins in Mexican adolescents. *Human Biology: An International Record of Research, 76,* 605–614.

Menotti, A., Lanti, M., Kromhout, D., Kafatos, A., Nedeljkovic, S., & Nissinen, A. (2005). Short- and long-term association of a single serum cholesterol measurement in middle-aged men in prediction of fatal coronary and other cardiovascular events: A cross cultural comparison through Europe. *European Journal of Epidemiology, 20,* 597–604.

Miyake, Y., Kono, S., Nishiwaki, M., Hamada, H., Nishikawa, H., Koga, H., & Ogawa, S. (1999). Relationship of coffee consumption with serum lipids and lipoproteins in Japanese men. *Annals of Epidemiology, 9,* 121–126.

Mukamal, K. J., Maclure, M., Muller, J. E., Sherwood, J. B., & Mittleman, M. A. (2002). Tea consumption and mortality after acute myocardial infarction. *Circulation, 105,* 2476–2481.

Murray, S. S., Bjelke, E., Gibson, R. W., & Schuman, L. M. (1981). Coffee consumption and mortality from ischemic heart disease and other causes: Results from the Lutheran Brotherhood Study, 1966–1978. *American Journal of Epidemiology, 113*(6), 661–667.

Noordzij, M., Uiterwaal, C. S., Arends, L. R., Kok, F. J., Grobbee, D. E., & Geleijnse, J. M. (2005). Blood pressure response to chronic intake of coffee and caffeine: A meta-analysis of randomized controlled trials. *Journal of Hypertension, 23*(5), 921–928.

Pacifico, A., & Henry, P. D. (2003). Structural pathways and prevention of heart failure and sudden death. *Journal of Cardiovascular Electrophysiology, 14*(7), 764–775.

Palmer, J. R., Rosenberg, L., Rao, R. S., & Shapiro, S. (1995). Coffee consumption and myocardial infarction in women. *American Journal of Epidemiology, 141*(8), 724–731.

Panagiotakos, D. B., Pitsavos, C., Chrysohoou, C., Kokkinos, P., Toutouzas, P., & Stefanadis, C. (2003). The J-shaped effect of coffee consumption on the risk of developing acute coronary syndromes: The CARDIO2000 Case-Control Study. *Journal of Nutrition, 133*, 3228–3232.

Paul, O. (1968). Stimulants and coronaries. *Postgraduate Medicine, 44*(3), 196–199.

Paul, O., Lepper, M. H., Phelan, W. H., Supertuis, G. W., MacMillian, A., McKean, H., et al. (1963). A longitudinal study of coronary heart disease. *Circulation, 28*, 20–31.

Paul, O., MacMillian, A., McKean, H., & Park, H. (1968). Sucrose intake and coronary heart disease. *Lancet, 7577*(2), 1049–1051.

Pirich, C., O'Grady, J., & Sinzinger, H. (1993). Coffee, lipoproteins, and cardiovascular disease. *Wiener Klinische Wochenschrift, 105*(1), 3–6.

Post, W. S., Larson, M. G., Myers, R. H., Galderisi, M., & Levy, D. (1997). Heritability of left ventricular mass: The Framingham Heart Study. *Hypertension, 30*(5), 1025–1028.

Poulsen, P., Ohm–Kyvik, K., Vaag, A., & Beck–Nielsen, H. (1999). Heritability of type II (non-insulin dependent) diabetes mellitus and abnormal glucose tolerance—A population-based twin study. *Diabetologia, 24*(2), 139–145.

Rafanelli, C., Roncuzzi, R., Milaneschi, Y., Tomba, E., Colistro, M. C., Pancaldi, L. G., et al. (2005). Stressful life events, depression and demoralization as risk factors for acute coronary heart disease. *Psychotherapy and Psychosomatics, 74*, 179–184.

Ramos, K. S., & Moorthy, B. (2005). Bioactivation of polycyclic aromatic hydrocarbon carcinogens within the vascular wall: Implications for human atherogenesis. *Drug Metabolism Reviews, 37*(4), 595–610.

Raveendran, M., Senthil, D., Utama, B., Shen, Y., Dudley, D., Wang, J., et al. (2004). Cigarette suppresses the expression of P4Halpha and vascular collagen production. *Biochemical and Biophysical Research Communications, 323*(2), 592–598.

Ridker, P. M., Rifai, N., Rose, L., Buring, J. E., & Cook, N. R. (2002). Comparison of C-reactive protein and low-density lipoprotein cholesterol levels in the prediction of first cardiovascular events. *The New England Journal of Medicine, 347*(20), 1557–1565.

Rigotti, N. A., & Pasternak, R. C. (1996). Cigarette smoking and coronary heart disease: Risks and management. *Cardiology Clinics, 14*(1), 51–68.

Roberts, A. T., de Jonge–Levitan, L., Parker, C. C., & Greenway, F. (2005). The effect of an herbal supplement containing black tea and caffeine on metabolic parameters in humans. *Alternative Medicine Review, 10*(4), 421–325.

Roche, H. M., Phillips, C., & Gibney, M. J. (2005). The metabolic syndrome: The crossroads of diet and genetics. *Proceedings of the Nutrition Society, 64*(3), 371–377.

Rogers, J. D., Sanchez–Saffon, A., Frol, A. B., & Diaz–Arrastia, R. (2003). Elevated plasma homocysteine levels in patients treated with levodopa: Association with vascular disease. *Archives of Neurology, 60*, 59–64.

Rosenberg, L., Slone, D., Shapiro, S., Kaufman, D. W., Stolley, P. D., & Miettinen, O. S. (1980). Coffee drinking and myocardial infarction in young women. *American Journal of Epidemiology, 111*, 675–681.

Rosengren, A., & Wilhelmsen, L. (1991). Coffee, coronary heart disease and mortality in middle-aged Swedish men: Findings from the Primary Prevention Study. *Journal of Internal Medicine, 230*(1), 67–71.

Rosenson, R. S. (2005). Low HDL-C: A secondary target of dyslipidemia therapy. *American Journal of Medicine, 118*, 1067–1077.

Saibeni, S., Lecchi, A., Meucci, G., Cattaneo, M., Tagliabue, L., Rondonotti, E., Formenti, S., De Franchis, R., & Vecchi, M. (2005). Prevalence of hyperhomocysteinemia in adult gluten-sensitive enteropathy at diagnosis: Role of B12, folate, and genetics. *Clinical Gastroenterology & Hepatology, 6*, 574–580.

Sakamoto, W., Isomura, H., Fujie, K., Takahashi, K., Nakao, K., & Izumi, H. (2005). Relationship of coffee consumption with risk factors of atherosclerosis in rats. *Annals of Nutrition & Metabolism, 49*(3), 149–154.

Sansores, R. H., Pare, P. D., & Abboud, R. T. (1992). Acute effect of cigarette smoking on the carbon monoxide diffusing capacity of the lung. *American Review of Respiration Disorders, 146*(4), 951–958.

Sasazuki, S., Kodama, H., Yoshimasu, K., Liu, Y., Washio, M., Tanaka, K., et al. (2000). Relation between green tea consumption and the severity of coronary atherosclerosis among Japanese men and women. *Annals of Epidemiology, 10*, 401–408.

Savoca, M. R., MacKey, M. L., Evans, C. D., Wilson, M., Ludwig, D. A., & Harshfield, G. A. (2005). Association of ambulatory blood pressure and dietary caffeine in adolescents. *American Journal of Hypertension, 18*(1), 116–120.

Schnabel, R., Lackner, K. J., Rupprecht, H. J., Espinola–Klein, C., Torzewski, M., Lubos, E., et al. (2005). Glutathione peroxidase-1 and homocysteine for cardiovascular risk prediction: Results from the AtheroGene study. *Journal of the American College of Cardiology, 45*, 1631–1637.

Schwarz, P., Bichoff, H. P., & Kunze, M. (1994). Coffee, tea, and lifestyle. *Preventative Medicine, 23*, 377–384.

Sekuri, C., Cam, F. S., Ercan, E., Tengiz, I., Sagcan, A., Eser, E., et al. (2005). Renin–angiotensin system gene polymorphisms and premature coronary heart disease. *Journal of the Renin–Angiotensin Aldosterone System, 6*, 38–42.

Selvin, E., Coresh, J., Golden, S. H., Brancati, F. L., Folsom, A. R., & Steffes, M. W. (2005). Glycemic control and coronary heart disease risk in persons with and without diabetes: The Atherosclerosis Risk in Communities Study. *Archives of Internal Medicine, 165*, 1910–1916.

Shai, I., Schulze, M. B., Manson, J. E., Stampfer, M. J., Rifai, N., & Hu, F. B. (2005). A prospective study of lipoprotein (a) and risk of coronary heart disease among women with type 2 diabetes. *Diabetologia, 48*(12), 2691–2692.

Sharma, S. B., Dwivedi, S., Prabhu, K. M., Singh, G., Kumar, N., & Lal, M. K. (2005). Coronary risk variables in young asymptomatic smokers. *Indian Journal of Medical Research, 122*(3), 205–210.

Sher, L. (2005). Type D personality: The heart, stress, and cortisol. *Quarterly Journal of Medicine, 98*, 323–329.

Singh, R., Wiegers, S. E., & Goldstein, B. J. (2001). Impact of gender on diabetes mellitus and its associated cardiovascular risk factors. *Journal of Gender-Specific Medicine, 4*, 28–36.

Skrivarhaug, T., Bangstad, H. J., Stene, L. C., Sandvik, L., Hanssen, K. F., & Joner, G. (2005). Long-term mortality in a nationwide cohort of childhood-onset type 1 diabetic patients in Norway. *Diabetologia, 49*, 298–305.

Slapikas, R., Babarskiene, M. R., Slapikiene, B., Grybauskiene, R., Luksiene, D., & Linoniene, L. (2005). Prevalence of cardiovascular risk factors in coronary heart disease patients with different low-density lipoprotein phenotypes. *Medicina, 41*, 925–931.

Smith, D. (2000). Cardiovascular disease: A historic perspective. *Japanese Journal of Veterinary Research, 48*, 147–166.

Smith, G. D., Harbord, R., Milton, J., Ebrahim, S., & Sterne, J. A. (2005). Does elevated plasma fibrinogen increase the risk of coronary heart disease? Evidence from a meta-analysis of genetic association studies. *Arteriosclerosis, Thrombosis, & Vascular Biology, 25*, 2228–33.

Smith, T. W., Glazer, K., Ruiz, J. M., & Gallo, L. C. (2004). Hostility, anger, aggressiveness and coronary heart disease: An interpersonal perspective on personality, emotion, and health. *Journal of Personality, 72*(6), 1217–1270.

Stein, J. H., Bushara, M., Bushara, K., McBride, P. E., Jorenby, D. E., & Fiore, M. C. (2002). Smoking cessation, but not smoking reduction, reduces plasma homocysteine levels. *Clinical Cardiology, 25*, 23–26.

Stensvold, I., & Tverdal, A. (1995). The relationship of coffee consumption to various self-reported cardiovascular events in middle-aged Norwegian men and women. *Scandinavian Journal of Social Medicine, 23*(2), 103–109.

Stensvold, I., Tverdal, A., & Jacobsen, B. K. (1996). Cohort study of coffee intake and death from coronary heart disease over 12 years. *British Medical Journal, 312*, 544–545.

Strain, J. J., Pentieva, K., McNulty, H., Dowey, L., & Ward, M. (2004). B-vitamins, homocysteine metabolism and CVD. *Proceedings of the Nutrition Society, 63*, 597–603.

Strandhagen, E., & Thelle, D. S. (2003). Filtered coffee raises serum cholesterol: Results from a controlled study. *European Journal of Clinical Nutrition, 57*, 1164–1168.

Strandhagen, E., Zetterberg, H., Aires, N., Palmér, M., Rymo, L., Blennow, K., et al. (2004). The apolipoprotein E polymorphism and the cholesterol-raising effect of coffee. *Lipids in Health and Disease, 3*, 26.

Sudano, I., Spieker, L., Binggeli, C., Ruschitzka, F., Luscher, T. F., Noll, G., & Corti, R. (2005). Coffee blunts mental stress-induced blood pressure increase in habitual but not in nonhabitual coffee drinkers. *Hypertension, 46*(3), 521–526.

Surtees, P. G., Wainwright, N. W., Luben, R., Day, N. E., & Khaw, K. (2005). Prospective cohort study of hostility and the risk of cardiovascular disease mortality. *International Journal of Cardiology, 100*, 155–161.

Tjeerdsma, G., Szabo, B. M., van Wijk, L. M., Brouwer, J., Tio, R. A., Crijns, H. J., et al. (2001). Autonomic dysfunction in patients with mild heart failure and coronary artery disease and the effects of add-on beta-blockade. *European Journal of Heart Failure, 3*(1), 33–39.

Tverdal, A., Stensvold, I., Solvoll, K., Foss, O. P., Lund–Larsen, P., & Bjartveit, K. (1990). Coffee consumption and death from coronary heart disease in middle-aged Norwegian men and women. *British Medical Journal, 6724*(300), 566–569.

Urbich, C., & Dimmeler, S. (2005). Risk factors for coronary artery disease, circulating endothelial progenitor cells, and the role of HMG-CoA reductase inhibitors. *Kidney International, 67*(5), 1672–1676.

Urgert, R., & Katan, M. B. (1997). The cholesterol-raising factor from coffee beans. *Annual Review of Nutrition, 17*, 305–324.

van Dusseldorp, M., Katan, M. B., van Vliet, T., Demacker, P. N., & Stalenhoef, A. F. (1991). Cholesterol-raising factor from boiled coffee does not pass a paper filter. *Arteriosclerosis & Thrombosis, 11*(3), 586–593.

Vessey, M.P. (1972). Coffee drinking and acute myocardial infarction: Report from the Boston Collaborative Drug Surveillance Program. *Lancet, 7790*(20), 1278–1281.

Vitaliano, P. P., Scanlan, J. M., Zhang, J., Savage, M. V., Hirsch, I. B., & Siegler, I. C. (2002). A path model of chronic stress, the metabolic syndrome, and coronary heart disease. *Psychosomatic Medicine, 64*(3), 418–435.

Wamhoff, B. R., Bowles, D. K., Dietz, N. J., Hu, Q., & Sturek, M. (2002). Exercise training attenuates coronary smooth muscle phenotypic modulation and nuclear Ca2 signaling. *American Journal of Physiology—Heart and Circulatory Physiology, 283,* 2397–2410.

Wang, Q. (2005). Molecular genetics of coronary artery disease. *Current Opinion in Cardiology, 20,* 182–188.

Wang, X., & Paigen, B. (2005). Genetics of variation in HDL cholesterol in humans and mice. *Circulation Research, 96*(1), 27–42.

Wannamethee, S. G., Shaper, A. G., Lennon, L., & Morris, R. W. (2005). Metabolic syndrome vs. Framingham Risk Score for prediction of coronary heart disease, stroke, and type 2 diabetes mellitus. *Archives of Internal Medicine, 165*(22), 2644–2650.

Weisz, G., Cox, D. A., Garcia, E., Tcheng, J. E., Griffin, J. J., Guagliumi, G., et al. (2005). Impact of smoking status on outcomes of primary coronary intervention for acute myocardial infarction: The smoker's paradox revisited. *American Heart Journal, 150,* 358–364.

Wilhelmsen, L., Tibblin, G., Elmfeldt, D., Wedel, H., & Werko, L. (1977). Coffee consumption and coronary heart disease in middle-aged Swedish men. *Acra Med Scand., 201,* 547–552.

Willett, W. C., Stampfer, M. J., Manson, J. W., Colditz, G. A., Rosner, B. A. Speizer, F. E., et al. (1996). Coffee consumption and coronary heart disease in women. A ten-year follow-up. *JAMA, 275,* 458–462.

Wilson, P. W. (2004). Assessing coronary heart disease risk with traditional and novel risk factors. *Clinical Cardiology, 27,* III-7–III-11.

Wilson, P. W., Garrison, R. J., Kannel, W. B., McGee, D. L., & Castelli, W. P. (1989). Is coffee consumption a contributor to cardiovascular disease? Insights from the Framingham Study. *Archives of Internal Medicine, 149*(5), 1169–1172.

Wolford, J. K., & Vozarova de Courten, B. (2004). Genetic basis of type 2 diabetes mellitus: Implications for therapy. *Treatments in Endocrinology, 3(4),* 257–267.

Woodward, M., Moohan, M., & Tunstall-Pedoe, H. (1999). Self-reported smoking, cigarette yields and inhalation biochemistry related to the incidence of coronary heart disease: Results from the Scottish Heart Health Study. *Journal of Epidemiology Biostatistics, 4,* 285–295.

Woodward, M., & Tunstall–Pedoe, H. (1999). Coffee and tea consumption in the Scottish Heart Health Study follow up: Conflicting relations with coronary risk factors, coronary disease, and all-cause mortality. *Journal of Epidemiology & Community Health, 53,* 481–487.

Yang, X., Gao, Y., Zhou, J., Zhen, Y., Yang, Y., Wang, J., et al. (2005). Plasma homocysteine thiolactone adducts associated with risk of coronary heart disease. Electronic version. *Clinica Chimica ACTA.*

Yano, K., Rhoads, G. G., & Kagan, A. (1977). Coffee, alcohol and risk of coronary heart disease among Japanese men living in Hawaii. *New England Journal of Medicine, 297,* 405–409.

Young, C. E., Karas, R. H., & Kuvin, J. T. (2004). High-density lipoprotein cholesterol and coronary heart disease. *Cardiology in Review, 12,* 107–119.

Zhang, S., Day, I., & Ye, S. (2000). Nicotine induced changes in gene expression by human coronary artery endothelial cells. *Atherosclerosis, 154,* 277–283.

Ziegler, S., Kostner, K., Thallinger, C., Bur, A., Brunner, M., Woltz, M., et al. (2005). Wine ingestion has no effect on lipid peroxidation products. *Pharmacology, 75*(3), 152–156.

6 Blood Pressure Effects of Dietary Caffeine Are a Risk for Cardiovascular Disease

Jack E. James

CONTENTS

The aim of this chapter is to examine the effects of dietary caffeine on blood pressure and to consider the implications of those effects for cardiovascular disease. The focus on cardiovascular disease is well justified because the group of syndromes subsumed under that classification represents the major cause of death and disease in the developed countries of the world (Wilson & Culleton, 1998; van den Hoogen, Seidell, Menotti, & Kromhout, 2000; Wolf–Maier et al., 2003). For example, statistics published by the World Health Organization show that approximately half of all deaths in Europe are attributable to cardiovascular disease, with approximately half of these due specifically to coronary heart disease (http://data.euro.who.int/hfadb/profile/prfile.php?id=prf retrieved May 6, 2005). In the near future, cardiovascular disease will also be the major cause of mortality and morbidity throughout much of the developing world (Pearson, 1999; Rodgers, Lawes, & MacMahon, 2000; Rodgers & MacMahon, 1999).

Blood pressure was chosen as a focus for this review because it is the single most important predictor of cardiovascular disease (MacMahon, 2000; Prospective Studies Collaboration, 2002) and, compared to several other key indices of cardiovascular function, blood pressure is particularly responsive to dietary caffeine. Specifically, although elevated heart rate is a risk factor for cardiovascular disease (Palatini & Julius, 1999), extensive research shows that caffeine at dietary levels has little effect on heart rate (e.g., James, 1990; Lane & Williams, 1987; Smits, Temme, & Thien, 1993).

Similarly, there is little evidence of caffeine having consistent electrocardiographic effects (Ammar, Song, Kluger, & White, 2001), whether in persons with cardiac disease (Chelsky et al., 1990; Sutherland, McPherson, Renton, Spencer, & Montague, 1985) or those free from disease (Prineas, Jacobs, Crow, & Blackburn, 1980; Stamler, Goldman, Gomes, Matza, & Horowitz, 1992). Furthermore, although various coffee preparations have been found to elevate the cardiovascular risk factors of serum cholesterol and plasma homocysteine significantly (Ahola, Jauhiainen, & Aro, 1991; Christensen, Mosdol, Rettstol, & Thelle, 2001; De Roos et al., 2000; Fried et al., 1992; Urgert, van Vliet, Zock, & Katan, 2000), neither caffeine specifically nor caffeine beverages other than coffee have these effects.

Within the extensive literature concerning caffeine and blood pressure, particular attention has been given to the acute effects of a single dose of the drug. Dietary intake, however, mostly involves daily intermittent ingestion of caffeine; therefore, caution is needed when drawing conclusions from the many studies of acute effects. Although this chapter does not ignore studies of acute effects, it focuses on studies of chronic caffeine effects because these are likely to be more directly indicative of the effects of caffeine as ordinarily consumed.

WHY SHOULD WE BE CONCERNED ABOUT DIETARY CAFFEINE AS A POSSIBLE RISK FACTOR FOR CARDIOVASCULAR DISEASE?

Several facts have particular significance when considering dietary caffeine as a possible risk factor for cardiovascular disease. As indicated elsewhere in this book, population exposure to caffeine is high. More than 80% of the world's population consumes coffee, tea, or caffeine soft drinks daily, making the contemporary consumption of caffeine more prevalent than that of any other drug in history (James, 1997). Although caffeine is frequently ingested in food (e.g., chocolate) and not infrequently in medication (e.g., some compound analgesics), global consumption is overwhelmingly attributable to three beverages: coffee, tea, and caffeine soft drinks (including "energy" drinks).

Moreover, for the majority of consumers, exposure to caffeine is essentially life long (James, 1991). Typically, the first exposure occurs in the womb, a situation attributable to the fact that most pregnant women consume caffeine, which in turn crosses the placenta (Goldstein & Warren, 1962). Caffeine consumption is widespread during childhood and patterns of use tend to consolidate during adolescence and early adulthood. Subsequently, usage tends to stabilize, generally undergoing little change during the remainder of life (James, 1997).

The unparalleled prevalence of caffeine exposure introduces significant multiplying factors that should be taken into account when assessing the impact of the drug on population health. That is, because caffeine use is widespread and essentially life long, even relatively small effects at the level of the individual may have a substantial cumulative impact on the population as a whole. An additional multiplying factor is introduced in the context of cardiovascular disease because it too (as mentioned earlier) has high prevalence. The causes of cardiovascular disease, which are complex and multifactorial, include behavior and lifestyle variables (Wilson & Culleton, 1998), with dietary caffeine possibly one such variable.

When a variable is under consideration as a possible risk factor for disease, it is important to consider the question of biological plausibility, which in the present context means taking account of the mechanisms responsible for the effects of caffeine. Although multiple specific mechanisms may be involved, a strong consensus is that antagonism of endogenous adenosine is the main mechanism responsible for many of the actions of caffeine (e.g., Dunwiddie & Masino, 2001).

Adenosine is a neuromodulator that acts upon specific cell-surface receptors distributed throughout the body, including the central nervous system and the cardiovascular system. Having a similar molecular structure to adenosine, caffeine occupies adenosine receptor sites, thereby antagonizing the normal physiological actions of adenosine. The fact that adenosine has an important role in the regulation of cardiovascular function provides biological plausibility to the hypothesis that caffeine is a cardiovascular risk factor. Thus, taking account of these various facts about caffeine (i.e., high prevalence of use, life-long exposure for most consumers, high prevalence of cardiovascular disease, and high plausibility regarding suspected biological mechanisms of action), interest in dietary caffeine as a possible cause of cardiovascular disease is well justified.

ACUTE EFFECTS OF CAFFEINE ON BLOOD PRESSURE

It has been shown conclusively that caffeine can elevate blood pressure in the range of 5 to 15 mg Hg systolic and 5 to 10 mg Hg diastolic across a wide age range, with effects lasting for up to several hours in healthy men and women (see James, 1997 and 2004, for a discussion). In addition, caffeine-induced pressor effects have been reported for persons with hypertension (e.g., Hartley et al., 2000; Shepard, al'Absi, Whitsett, Passey, & Lovallo, 2000), are additive to the effects of cigarette smoking (Freestone, Yeo, & Ramsay, 1995; James & Richardson, 1991; Smits et al., 1993), and have generally been found to be at least additive (e.g., France & Ditto, 1992; Greenberg & Shapiro, 1987; James, 1990, 1994a; Lane & Williams, 1987) and possibly synergistic (e.g., al'Absi et al., 1998; Lane et al., 2002) to the effects of psychological stress.

Furthermore, recent studies show that caffeine produces acute increases in aortic stiffness and enhances wave reflection, both of which contribute to increased blood pressure as well as being independent risk factors for cardiovascular disease. These effects have been observed in persons who are normotensive (Karatzis et al., 2005; Mahmud & Feely, 2001; Vlachopoulos, Hirata, & O'Rourke, 2003) as well as those being treated for hypertension (Vlachopoulos, Hirata, Stefanadis, Toutouzas, &

O'Rourke, 2003), and appear to be synergistic to similarly adverse effects of smoking (Vlachopoulos et al., 2004). An important recent finding is that caffeine and coffee appear to have more pronounced effects on aortic blood pressure than brachial blood pressure, leading to the suggestion that caffeine-induced pressor effects may generally have been underestimated (Karatzis et al., 2005; Mahmud & Feely, 2001; Waring, Goudsmit, Marwick, Webb, & Maxwell, 2005).

The large number and diversity of relevant studies provide unassailable evidence of adverse acute effects of caffeine on cardiovascular function, especially blood pressure. As such, the available evidence provides a reasonable basis for concern about dietary caffeine as a factor in development of cardiovascular disease. In turn, such concern suggests possible grounds for the formulation of primary prevention appeals to consumers to avoid caffeine in the interests of cardiovascular health. Until recently, however, concern and action have been largely absent, and the main reasons for this appear to be twofold: (a) confusion regarding the epidemiology of caffeine and cardiovascular disease; and (b) the belief that habitual caffeine use leads to the development of tolerance to the cardiovascular effects of the drug.

Epidemiology of Caffeine and Cardiovascular Disease

More than 100 large epidemiological studies in more than a dozen countries have reported data on the relationship between dietary caffeine and cardiovascular function, morbidity, and/or mortality (James, 2004). One feature of this large literature is the many inconsistencies in the reported findings, a fact that has inclined some commentators and reviewers towards dismissing concerns about caffeine. In addition, caffeine has been cursorily dismissed as a cause for concern in a number of reviews that have been partial (i.e., have been selective in their choice of studies to review), while omitting to state clearly the criteria used for including or excluding studies (e.g., Chou & Benowitz, 1994; Fredholm, Battig, Holmen, Nehli, & Zyartau, 1999; Stavric, 1992). The conclusions reached by those reviews do not represent relevant epidemiological knowledge and do not withstand scrutiny.

When all relevant studies are considered, critical reviews have found that the majority of studies implicate dietary caffeine as a possible cardiovascular risk factor (James, 1991, 1997, 2004). Moreover, caffeine has also been implicated in meta-analytic reviews of relevant studies selected as satisfying carefully defined methodological criteria (Greenland, 1993; Jee, He, Whelton, Suh, & King, 1999; Kawachi, Colditz, & Stone, 1994). An earlier meta-analysis, which reported no caffeine–disease association (Myers & Basinski, 1992), was shown by Greenland to have been "improperly conducted and interpreted" (p. 372).

The assumption that clear consistency should have emerged in the epidemiological findings if caffeine were having substantive effects on the population fails to take account of the many methodological shortcomings in the epidemiological studies published to date. In particular, there are grounds for concluding that the many "null" reports (i.e., nonsignificant associations) in the epidemiological literature on caffeine and cardiovascular disease reflect a high rate of type II error (i.e., failure to observe a real effect when one exists).

A major shortcoming of many studies is poor measurement of the key "exposure" variable, namely, caffeine consumption. Although this shortcoming has long been the subject of criticism (e.g., Gilbert, 1976; James, 1991; Schreiber et al., 1988), relatively little improvement or innovation has occurred over the past three decades to try to overcome the problem. For example, although dietary caffeine levels can be measured reliably using detailed self-report protocols (James et al., 1988), most studies provide no data concerning the reliability of measurements employed and many provide few details of the measurements used (e.g., a researcher may state simply that "coffee was recorded" without supplying any further details).

Moreover, although at least half of the relevant epidemiological studies conducted to date collected blood samples (mostly for the purpose of measuring serum lipid levels), none has taken the obvious next step of measuring systemic levels of caffeine or its metabolites. As such, advantage has not been taken of the fact that good estimates of dietary caffeine levels can be obtained by analyzing plasma and saliva caffeine or paraxanthine (the major metabolite in humans) using HPLC (e.g., James et al., 1988; Lelo, Miners, Robson, & Birkett, 1986a) or enzyme immunoassay techniques (James & Gregg, 2004a). The inadequate methods frequently used to date are likely to have produced largely undifferentiated (i.e., random) measurement error; therefore, the effect in many epidemiological studies will have been to underestimate the true association between caffeine and cardiovascular disease. Thus, although overall epidemiological findings suggest that dietary caffeine has a modest detrimental effect on cardiovascular health, actual effects may be larger, considering the generally imprecise methods that have been employed.

Confounding in Epidemiological Research

A frequent erroneous observation about the epidemiology of caffeine and cardiovascular health is that much of the research has ignored the influence of confounders. This "confounder myth" (James, 1997) asserts that reports of significant positive correlations between caffeine consumption and cardiovascular disease are the result of failure to control confounders, especially cigarette smoking. As well as being a cardiovascular risk factor, smoking has been found to be positively correlated with caffeine use (e.g., Klesges, Ray, & Klesges, 1994; Patton et al., 1995; Ungemack, 1994). The myth, however, arises from the fact that, for the past three decades, epidemiological studies of caffeine have routinely controlled for cigarette smoking. Excepting one or two earlier studies, virtually all of the literature reporting a positive correlation between caffeine consumption and cardiovascular disease has included controls for the influence of cigarette smoking.

Of course, in the context of population studies, there is always a risk of unanticipated influence of an as yet unidentified confounder. However, the level of such risk is probably lower in epidemiological studies of dietary caffeine and health than in many other areas because the list of potential confounders controlled for in caffeine studies (including those that reported positive findings) is very long and includes (James, 1991):

age
gender
cigarette smoking
alcohol consumption

body mass index
dietary factors
serum cholesterol
blood pressure
medical history
use of oral contraceptives
family history of heart disease
physical activity
personality
region of residence
education level
religion

Moreover, Schreiber et al. (1988) specifically examined associations between a wide range of potential confounders and coffee/caffeine consumption; they found that smoking accounted for approximately 13% of the variation in coffee/caffeine use and that none of the remaining variables explained more than 1% of the variation. Indeed, rather than being inadequately controlled for confounder effects, there has probably been a tendency toward overadjustment for confounders in epidemiological studies of caffeine (e.g., LaCroix, Mead, Liang, Homas, & Pearson, 1987; Rosenberg, Palmer, Kelly, Kaufman, & Shapiro, 1988). In particular, findings have frequently been adjusted for blood pressure and cholesterol, which may be caffeine- and coffee-related causal pathways in their own rights. Thus, as with measurement error, the likely affect of overadjustment for confounder effects would be to underestimate the actual strength of the association between caffeine consumption and cardiovascular disease (i.e., increased risk of Type II error).

Epidemiology of Caffeine and Blood Pressure

As part of the much larger body of epidemiological research on caffeine and cardiovascular disease, 18 population studies have been specifically concerned with caffeine and blood pressure (James, 2004). Of these, five reported no association between dietary caffeine and BP, six reported a significant positive association for systolic and/or diastolic pressure, and seven reported an inverse association for systolic or diastolic pressure. It is unlikely, however, that this pattern of results represents the true state of affairs because the populations studied were similar in demographics and socioeconomics.

Moreover, this inconsistency in findings from epidemiological research contrasts the largely consistent pattern of pressor effects reported in experimental studies of chronic caffeine use (discussed later), further undermining confidence in the methodological adequacy of epidemiological attempts to characterize the effects of dietary caffeine. A particular concern is that epidemiological studies have generally ignored the plasma caffeine concentration time course and concomitant pattern of effects on blood pressure. The general pattern is shown in Figure 6.1, which is a schematic representation of the estimated 24-hour plasma caffeine concentration time course, assuming an elimination half-life of 5 hours

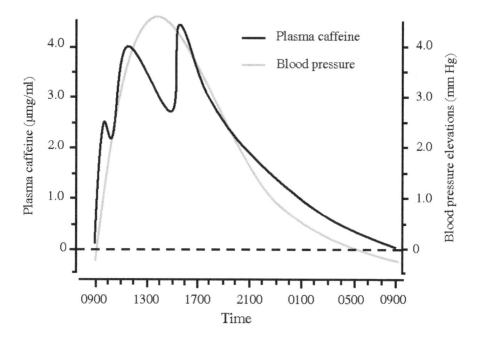

FIGURE 6.1 Schematic representation of estimated 24-hour plasma caffeine concentration time course and associated caffeine-induced elevations in blood pressure. Estimated plasma caffeine concentration assumes an elimination half-life of 5 hours and ingestion of one cup of coffee in the morning, midmorning, and midafternoon. Associated increases in blood pressure were estimated on the basis of experimental studies involving ambulatory blood pressure monitoring (see text).

and ingestion of the approximate equivalent of one cup of coffee in the morning, midmorning, and midafternoon.

Figure 6.1 helps to show that the strength and even the sign of the correlation between dietary caffeine and blood pressure level depend on the timing of blood pressure measurement relative to when caffeine was last ingested (James, 2004). Using 24-hour ambulatory monitoring, James (1994b) found that overnight absti-nence produced transient modest *decreases* in blood pressure. Thus, taking a cross-section of the population, recent caffeine consumption is likely to have a pressor effect (positive association), whereas brief caffeine abstinence (10 to 12 hours) may have no effect, and longer periods of abstinence (12 to 24 hours) may decrease BP modestly (inverse association due to withdrawal).

In view of this analysis, a noteworthy feature of several of the studies in which dietary caffeine was said to have been protective (i.e., inverse association between intake and blood pressure) is that participants were asked to fast before being examined (James, 2004). Specifically, participants in five of the seven studies were reported to have fasted, while one reported nonfasting and one omitted to report whether participants fasted or not. Thus, in the majority of the studies involved, caffeine consumers' blood pressure readings were likely to have been spuriously lower than "normal" for themselves and potentially lower also than their nonconsuming counterparts'.

Although interpreting the findings of epidemiological studies of caffeine and blood pressure depends crucially on knowing when blood pressure was measured relative to when individual participants ingested caffeine, with one exception (Shirlow, Berry, & Stokes, 1988), none of the relevant studies provides that level of detail. In the one exception, an overall analysis revealed no association between caffeine consumption and blood pressure level after adjustment for age, body mass, cigarette smoking, alcohol consumption, serum cholesterol, and family history of hypertension (Shirlow et al., 1988).

Closer examination, however, revealed that participants who had consumed caffeine during the 3 hours prior to measurement had significantly elevated blood pressure compared with participants consuming no caffeine for the same period. Importantly, because the increases in blood pressure associated with recent ingestion of caffeine were independent of average daily intake (a measure of habitual use), the results also confirm experimental findings that habitual caffeine consumption does not lead to complete tolerance to the pressor action of the drug.

CAFFEINE TOLERANCE

Development of Hemodynamic Tolerance

Turning to the second of the two main reasons mentioned previously for the relative absence of concern and action regarding the high prevalence of dietary caffeine, there is a belief that the proven acute effects of caffeine on blood pressure are not generalizable to dietary caffeine because habitual use leads to development of hemodynamic tolerance. However, a search of the literature yields little support for this long-standing belief. The most often (and often the only) cited source for the claim of hemodynamic tolerance is Robertson, Wade, Workman, Woosley & Oates (1981), which is widely misquoted as having demonstrated complete hemodynamic tolerance to dietary caffeine.

The many methodological shortcomings of the Robertson et al. study have been considered in some detail previously (James, 1991, pp. 112–113). In summary, participants ingested caffeine three times daily over several days, and blood pressure levels on those days were compared to precaffeine baseline readings. One problem relates to the fact that changes in blood pressure level were determined by calculating daily averages of readings taken before and after caffeine ingestion—a procedure that would have reduced and possibly concealed evidence of sustained blood pressure elevations. Given that caffeine is frequently consumed separately from meals, the procedure of administering caffeine with meals may have been unwise because this would have slowed the rate of absorption of the drug and thereby may have dampened effects. Indeed, evidence of such an effect is to be found in the unusually long mean elimination half-life, which the authors estimated to have been 10 hours, compared to the more generally accepted estimate of 5 hours (Pfeifer & Notari, 1988).

Also, as suggested by Lane and Williams (1985), the relatively high doses of caffeine (750 mg per day) used in the Robertson et al. (1981) study may have encouraged development of tolerance to an extent not observed with more typical dietary doses (300 to 400 mg per day). Specifically, it is possible that the time between doses was not long enough to deplete plasma caffeine levels to a point at which subjects would be responsive to subsequent ingestion of the drug. Furthermore, although Robertson et al. state that baseline blood pressure levels "appeared stable," the results they present show that there had been a progressive reduction in blood pressure during the baseline period. This, in turn, could have had the effect of diminishing and possibly concealing sustained pressor effects and erroneously suggesting the development of caffeine tolerance.

Finally, the sample size of nine participants for the crucial comparisons was small, with the resulting statistical power possibly too low to detect a caffeine-induced pressor effect reliably. Indeed, this study shared the feature of small sample size with a number of subsequent studies (in which the number of participants ranged from five to eight) that also claimed to have demonstrated hemodynamic tolerance (Casiglia et al., 1992; Debrah, Haigh, Sherwin, Murphy, & Kerr, 1995; Haigh et al., 1993). Overall, then, the strength of the belief that hemodynamic tolerance develops in the context of dietary caffeine is not matched by the extent and quality of the evidence. On the contrary, substantial experimental evidence (summarized next) indicates that consumers do not develop complete tolerance to the hemodynamic effects of dietary caffeine.

Chronic Effects of Dietary Caffeine on Blood Pressure

As stated earlier, scores of studies have demonstrated that caffeine ingestion induces acute elevations in blood pressure, a fact that provides a common-sense basis for skepticism regarding claims that habitual use leads to complete caffeine tolerance. Acknowledging that the majority of people are habitual consumers of caffeine, it follows that the majority of participants in studies of caffeine-induced hemodynamic reactivity will also have been habitual consumers of the drug. As consumers, participants in such studies will generally have a pattern of caffeine consumption characterized by intermittent ingestion of caffeine during the day, with fewer portions consumed later in the day, followed by overnight abstinence.

Typically, participants in laboratory studies are required to abstain from caffeine overnight prior to submitting for laboratory testing. Thus, the question arises: Why, given that ordinary consumers after overnight abstinence show increased blood pressure in response to caffeine ingested in a laboratory, would these same consumers show no such response (due to tolerance) in the natural setting? As might be expected even from this simple line of reasoning, the relevant empirical evidence, direct and indirect, indicates that the inclusion of moderate levels of caffeine in the diet does *not* lead to immunity against the pressor effects of the drug.

Before the last decade, little direct examination of the chronic hemodynamic effects of dietary caffeine had been conducted. Among the first studies to undertake such an examination, modest sustained decreases in blood pressure were reported when caffeine beverages were removed from the diet (Bak & Grobee, 1990) or replaced by decaffeinated alternatives (van Dusseldorp, Smits, Thien, & Katan, 1989). Similar results were reported in a number of subsequent studies in which ambulatory monitoring was used to measure blood pressure level for extended time periods (Green & Suls, 1996; James, 1994b; Jeong & Dimsdale, 1990; Lane et al., 2002; Rakic, Burke, & Beilin, 1999; Superko et al., 1994). Although not all such studies reported persistent caffeine-induced elevations in blood pressure, it is noteworthy that studies failing to observe persistent effects generally shared a methodological feature: Blood pressure readings were averaged across relatively long epochs (Eggertsen, Andreasson, Hedner, Karlsberg, & Hansson, 1993; MacDonald et al., 1991; Myers & Reeves, 1991).

Because the hemodynamic effects of caffeine usually peak within about 1 hour postingestion and are substantially diminished within about 3 hours, significant pressor effects were probably obscured in those studies. In contrast, the 24-hour ambulatory blood pressure records reported by James (1994b) were averaged across 2-hour epochs, and these records correlated well with systemic caffeine levels. Compared to caffeine abstinence, caffeine-induced chronic increases in blood pressure peaked at 5 to 6 mm Hg; increases of 2 to 4 mm Hg persisted for several hours of the day. Notwithstanding the persistent increases in blood pressure observed, the study also found evidence of caffeine tolerance. However, the level of tolerance was partial, not complete. Compared to abstinence, habitual caffeine consumption diminished peak pressor effects by only 25% (James, 1994b).

It is known that blood pressure responses of similar magnitude may be accompanied by different patterns of change in cardiac output (CO) and total peripheral resistance (TPR), and these differences in hemodynamic profile may be implicated in cardiovascular pathology (Gregg, Matyas, & James, 2002). Speculation has existed as to whether caffeine-induced pressor effects are due to cardiac stimulation of contractility leading to increased CO or vasoconstriction leading to increased TPR. Findings generally suggest that the blood pressure elevating effect of caffeine is due primarily to increased vascular resistance (Coney & Marshall, 1998; Fuller, Maxwell, Conradson, Dixon, & Barnes, 1987; Hartley, Lovallo, Whitsett, Sung, & Wilson, 2001; James & Gregg, 2004a; Smits, Boekema, de Aberu, Thien, & van't Laar, 1987).

Because greater risk has been attached to hemodynamic reactivity in which vascular, rather than myocardial, responses predominate (Julius, 1988), available evidence adds to concerns regarding the possible implications of dietary caffeine for cardiovascular health. In the study by James and Gregg (2004a), sleep loss was also found to have a vascular effect on hemodynamic profile, which in turn was found to be additive to the vascular effects of caffeine. As such, current evidence suggests the possibility of combined adverse effects of caffeine and sleep loss on cardiovascular health; this may be of particular importance in light of the antisoporific action of caffeine and the frequent (sometimes recommended) use of caffeine when sleep cycles are disrupted.

As well as direct empirical evidence of sustained elevations in blood pressure due to dietary caffeine, an array of indirect evidence converges upon the same conclusion. For example, an examination of the large body of individual studies of caffeine-induced elevations in blood pressure shows that participants in those studies represent the entire spectrum of consumers, ranging from essential nonusers to high consumers (James, 1997). Nevertheless, when results of different studies are compared, there is no obvious systematic difference in reactivity as a function of reported dietary caffeine levels. This result is contrary to the tolerance hypothesis, which would predict greater reactivity in the context of low compared to high habitual caffeine intake.

Moreover, in a number of studies in which habitual levels of caffeine consumption were examined directly, no difference in caffeine reactivity was found between consumers of high and low amounts (James, 1990; Lane, Adcock, Williams, & Kuhn, 1990). In fact, rather than being a function of caffeine-consumer status, the magnitude of caffeine-induced pressor effects has been found to be proportional to plasma caffeine concentration at the time at which the drug is ingested, irrespective of prior history of use (e.g., Shirlow et al., 1988; Smits, Thien, & van't Laar, 1985a). That is, for an individual on any day, second and later cups of a caffeine beverage produce less hemodynamic reactivity than the initial cup (Goldstein, Shapiro, Hui, & Yu, 1990; Lane & Manus, 1989; Ratliff–Crain, O'Keefe, & Baum, 1989), but overall reactivity varies little between persons who consume caffeine regularly and those who do not (Smits, Thien, & van't Laar, 1985b).

It can be seen from Figure 6.1 that plasma caffeine concentration is typically highest in the late afternoon and lowest on awakening in the morning (Denaro, Brown, Jacob, & Benowitz, 1991; Lelo et al., 1986a). Overnight abstinence of 10 to 14 hours is a characteristic of dietary intake for the majority of consumers and leads essentially to complete depletion of systemic caffeine by early morning (Lelo, Miners, Robson, & Birkett, 1986b; Pfeifer & Notari, 1988; Shi, Benowitz, Denaro, & Sheiner, 1993). The most plausible interpretation of the available evidence is that the depleted levels, in turn, render the consumer sensitive to the hemodynamic effects of the drug when re-exposure next occurs (typically, shortly after awakening) (Denaro et al.; Shi et al., 1993; Smits et al., 1985b). Hence, as Figure 6.1 illustrates, for any day, caffeine-induced elevations in blood pressure are most pronounced following initial ingestion, with subsequent intake resulting in modest additional increases.

The cumulative effect of typical dietary levels is for blood pressure to be elevated modestly throughout most of the waking hours. The declines in plasma caffeine concentration levels that occur overnight are accompanied by declines in blood pressure level (James, 1994b). On awakening the following day, plasma caffeine concentration levels are depleted to near zero, apparently resensitizing the consumer to the hemodynamic effects of the drug.

In a recent meta-analysis of blood pressure response to chronic intake of caffeine and coffee, Noordzij et al. (2005) concluded that the pressor effect of coffee may be substantially less pronounced than that of caffeine. They selected randomized controlled trials in which coffee (containing caffeine) had been consumed, or caffeine in tablet or capsule form had been ingested, for 7 consecutive days or more. Blood pressure elevations were found to be two to three times larger for caffeine than for coffee, despite equal average doses of caffeine. In light of the diminished effect of coffee, the authors concluded that the impact of coffee consumption on population blood pressure may be inconsequential for cardiovascular health. They speculated as to why caffeine in coffee may not have the adverse effects on blood pressure suggested by effects observed when caffeine alone is ingested.

Among their speculations, the authors mention possible differences in the bioavailability of caffeine in coffee versus tablet form, a possible protective effect of constituents in coffee other than caffeine, and "side effects" of coffee (but not caffeine), including physical or mental relaxation. However, apart from the fact that none of these speculations is directly supported by the evidence of the study, there are reasons to question the central finding reported by Noordzij et al. (2005).

To begin, the large body of epidemiological research conducted to date has been exclusively concerned with caffeine as consumed in beverages, mostly coffee. As mentioned before, the overall finding of that research is that caffeine (i.e., coffee consumption) is associated with increased risk of cardiovascular disease. Similarly, epidemiological studies involving the more specific outcome variable of blood pressure have also been concerned with caffeine as consumed in beverages, again mostly coffee. Although that body of research has yielded inconsistent findings, it provides little support for the main finding reported Noordzij et al. (2005) that caffeine, but not coffee, chronically elevates blood pressure. Indeed, aspects of the Noordzij et al. study give cause for doubting the reliability and generality of their main finding.

As a meta-analysis, it was based on a small sample of studies: 11 trials in the coffee consumption group of studies and only 5 trials in the caffeine group. Moreover, the definition used to distinguish between coffee and caffeine studies is open to question. Specifically, studies in which the active treatment consisted of "caffeine tablets, either as the sole treatment or combined with decaffeinated coffee" (Noordzij et al., 2005, p. 922) were classified as caffeine trials. This operational definition is inconsistent with the study's objective of differentiating between trials in which caffeine alone was administered versus coffee because caffeine "combined with decaffeinated coffee" is functionally equivalent to "coffee." It appears that this definition may have resulted in one of the caffeine trials being misclassified, the effect of which would be to reduce the number of those trials to four.

Furthermore, whereas all the caffeine trials were classified as having been double blind, only one of the coffee trials was classified as such. Thus, differences in the conduct of the two trial groups suggest that reported differences in the effects of coffee and caffeine are as likely to be an artifact due to methodological confounding as any of the explanations offered by Noordzij et al. (2005).

Dietary Caffeine and Population Blood Pressure Levels

If, as this review indicates, dietary caffeine contributes to statistically significant elevations in blood pressure, it should be noted that such increases are modest in absolute terms, amounting to possibly 2 to 4 mm Hg for most waking hours of the day. The question that then needs to be considered is whether such increases are likely to have an appreciable effect on population cardiovascular mortality and morbidity. It is sometimes presumed that increases of such magnitude are not meaningful, on the grounds that blood pressure level is inherently variable. However, it should be remembered that the effects of caffeine are at least additive, and possibly synergistic, to blood pressure increases due to a variety of other factors (e.g., smoking, hypertension, stress). In this sense, caffeine represents a preventable additional burden on the cardiovascular system.

However, whether the influence of caffeine should be regarded as a burden on the cardiovascular system is sometimes questioned on the grounds that modest elevations in blood pressure may possibly be health enhancing. Specifically, it is pointed out that the modest elevations in blood pressure that underlie moderate physical exertion enhance rather than harm cardiovascular conditioning, health, and longevity (e.g., Booth, Gordon, Carlson, & Hamilton, 2000; Kohl, 2001).

The comparison with caffeine, however, is spurious. The blood pressure increases associated with physical exercise are metabolically appropriate. That is, the increased cardiac output and/or increased total peripheral resistance that accompany exercise-induced increases in blood pressure ensure that appropriate levels of oxygen and other nutrients carried in blood are transported to sites of increased demand in the body. The blood pressure increases that accompany ingestion of caffeine are not appropriate because they do not involve a commensurate increase in metabolic demand. It is precisely these metabolically inappropriate increases in blood pressure that are generally believed to contribute to the pathogenic processes that result in cardiovascular disease (e.g., Guyton, 1987).

The clearest insight into the contribution of blood pressure increases to cardiovascular disease is provided by population statistics of the relationship between blood pressure level and cardiovascular mortality and morbidity. The association between the population distribution of blood pressure and cardiovascular disease is primarily linear, so any contribution by caffeine to population blood pressure level may be expected to contribute to the overall incidence of cardiovascular mortality and morbidity (MacMahon et al., 1990; Rodgers et al., 2000; van den Hoogen et al., 2000). It is important to remember that exposure to caffeine is generally long (essentially life long for consumers), the prevalence of exposure is high (more than 80% in most countries), and the incidence of cardiovascular disease is high throughout the world. Although reduced blood pressure associated with reductions in dietary caffeine may be expected to be modest in absolute terms, even modest absolute changes in population levels of blood pressure translate to significant changes in the population burden of cardiovascular death and disease.

For example, it has been estimated that a downward shift of 2 to 3 mm Hg in the population distribution of blood pressure would produce life-saving benefits equal to the cumulative benefits achieved by antihypertensive treatment (Rodgers & MacMahon, 1999; Rose, 1981). It has also been estimated that population-wide reductions of 2 mm Hg could avert 5% of deaths from coronary heart disease and 15% of stroke deaths (Rodgers et al., 2000; Rodgers & MacMahon).

More specifically, James (1997) estimated that if caffeine consumption had the effect of elevating average population blood pressure by 2 to 4 mm Hg—a reasonable inference considering the relevant experimental data (e.g., James, 1994b; Jeong & Dimsdale, 1990; Lane et al., 2002; Superko et al., 1994)—extrapolation based on epidemiological blood pressure data (MacMahon et al., 1990) suggests that population-wide cessation of caffeine use could lead to a reduction of 9 to 14% of premature deaths from coronary heart disease and 17 to 24% of premature deaths from stroke. Were caffeine removed from the diet in populations where coffee specifically is widely consumed, additional benefits would be achieved due to the adverse impact of that beverage on serum cholesterol and homocysteine.

The conclusion that moderate caffeine consumption poses a risk to cardiovascular health is likely to come as something of a surprise to many consumers.

However, some may see consolation in the belief that there are benefits to offset the risk. In particular, it is widely believed that oral ingestion of the drug enhances performance and mood. It is also a common perception that caffeine has the potential to restore performance and mood adversely affected by lack or loss of sleep, as frequently experienced by shift workers and long-distance drivers (e.g., haulers).

However, the empirical evidence said to confirm the enhancing and restorative effects of caffeine has been questioned (James, 1994c), and there is now extensive evidence against such claims (e.g., Heatherley, Hancock, & Rogers, 2005; Heatherley, Hayward, Seers, & Rogers, 2005; James, 1998; James & Gregg, 2004b; James, Gregg, Kane, & Harte, 2005; Rogers et al., 2005). Appropriately controlled studies consistently show that caffeine has no significant net enhancing effects for performance or mood when consumers are rested, and no net restorative effects when performance and mood have been degraded by sleep restriction. Indeed, those studies show that the effects of caffeine on performance and mood are almost wholly attributable to reversal of adverse withdrawal effects associated with brief (e.g., overnight) abstinence from the drug (see James & Rogers, 2005, for a review of the evidence).

INDUSTRY INFLUENCES ON RESEARCH

The available experimental evidence and, to a lesser extent, the epidemiological evidence support the conclusion that caffeine is a likely cardiovascular disease risk factor. Notwithstanding the importance of the implications of this conclusion for population health, there is little organized effort to inform the public and to advise them in ways consistent with the magnitude of the threat. Indeed, it is evident from a close examination of the caffeine literature that this is a field of enquiry marred by a considerable amount of misinformation and misrepresentation.

There are probably many reasons for this. For example, almost by definition, most of the people engaged in caffeine research are caffeine consumers, and this could foster reticence about acknowledging the full implications of the empirical findings. More importantly, it is necessary to confront the reality that the academic pursuit of research on caffeine is linked in many ways to the trade in caffeine products. Each of the main sources of caffeine (namely, coffee, tea, and soft drinks) is a multinational, multibillion-dollar enterprise. These industries have sought to lessen the impact of scientific findings adverse to their commercial interests (James, 1994d, 2002).

A variety of methods have been employed by industry over the past two decades to influence public opinion about caffeine and caffeine products. Such attempts include dissemination of selective information and directed funding for caffeine research (James, 1994d). From 1962 to 1982, the average number of cups of coffee consumed per day in the United States declined 39% (Masterson, 1983), and it is evident from caffeine-industry publications that manufacturers attributed much of that decline to increased public awareness of scientific concern about possible caffeine-induced harmful effects (James, 1994c). Around 1990, the downward trend was arrested and thereafter a reversal was evidenced by substantially increased sales of coffee and tea.

Manufacturers of caffeine products appear to have been in no doubt about the reason for the improved commercial outlook for caffeine products. Industry representatives congratulated themselves on the success of their campaign to counter scientific findings adverse to their interests (Heuman, 1994; Richards, 1994). In this regard, actions by the caffeine industry to protect its commercial interests and similar activities by the tobacco industry appear to have parallels.

In particular, it is noteworthy that the International Life Sciences Institute (ILSI), a major body representing the interests of the caffeine industry, has been reported as having assisted the tobacco industry to counter World Health Organization (WHO) efforts to promote tobacco controls. A WHO Committee of Experts on Tobacco Industry Documents recently reported that for many years tobacco companies have operated with the "purpose of subverting the efforts of WHO to address tobacco issues [and that the] attempted subversion has been elaborate, well financed, sophisticated and usually invisible" (Zeltner, Kessler, Martiny, & Randera, 2000, p. 18).

Subsequently, the Tobacco-Free Initiative (TFI), a WHO project, identified ILSI as one such group, and that "outing" has been debated in a major medical journal (MacDonald, 2001; Murphy, 2001). Moreover, ILSI has recently been the subject of editorial comment for its reticence in declaring a possible conflict of interest regarding its involvement in a publication concerned with health issues related to alcohol consumption (Edwards & Savva, 2001). Furthermore, ILSI is directly involved in EU research into "food safety" (James, 2002).

Taken together, these examples of industry intervention in research serve as a warning to the research community. It is important that ways are found for ensuring exposure of possible conflicts of interest when they are not freely declared. When possible conflicts do exist (whether or not declared), ways must be found to safeguard against resulting threats to scientific integrity (James, 2002). The importance and urgency of steps by the scientific community to counter such threats is highlighted by empirical evidence of bias attributable to general industry involvement in biomedical research. For example, in a study of the association between funding source and conclusions in randomized drug trials, Als-Nielsen, Chen, Gluud, & Kjaergard (2003) found that after adjustment for study characteristics, industry-sponsored trials were five times more likely to yield conclusions favorable to industry's commercial interests than trials funded by nonprofit organizations.

CONCLUSION

It is evident that claims that dietary caffeine is of little importance to cardiovascular health are ill founded. Broadly, such claims reflect confusion concerning the epidemiological evidence relating dietary caffeine to cardiovascular disease and the belief that habitual caffeine use leads to development of tolerance to the cardiovascular effects of the drug. Although marred by persistent methodological shortcomings, the overall epidemiological evidence implicates dietary caffeine in the development of cardiovascular disease.

In addition, there is strong direct and indirect experimental evidence that blood pressure remains reactive to caffeine even when it is habitually consumed. Overall, study of the relationship between blood pressure and cardiovascular mortality and morbidity in populations leads to the conclusion that the blood pressure elevating effects of dietary caffeine represent a significant cardiovascular risk factor.

REFERENCES

Ahola, I., Jauhiainen, M., & Aro, A. (1991). The hypocholestrolemic factor in boiled coffee is retained by a paper filter. *Journal of Internal Medicine, 230,* 293–297.

al'Absi, M., Lovallo, W. R., McKey, B., Sung, B. H., Whitsett, T. L., & Wilson, M. F. (1998). Hypothalamic-pituitary-adrenocortical responses to psychological stress and caffeine in men at high and low risk for hypertension. *Psychosomatic Medicine, 60,* 521–527.

Als-Nielsen, B., Chen, W., Gluud, C., & Kjaergard, L. L. (2003). Association of funding and conclusions in randomized drug trials: a reflection of treatment effect or adverse events? *JAMA, 290,* 921–928.

Ammar, R., Song, J. C., Kluger, J., & White, C. M. (2001). Evaluation of electrocardiographic and hemodynamic effects of caffeine with acute dosing in healthy volunteers. *Pharmacotherapy, 21,* 437–442.

Bak, A. A., & Grobbee, D. E. (1990). A randomized study on coffee and blood pressure. *Journal of Human Hypertension, 4,* 259–264.

Booth, F. W., Gordon, S. E., Carlson, C. J., & Hamilton, M. T. (2000). Waging war on modern chronic diseases: Primary prevention through exercise biology. *Journal of Applied Physiology, 88,* 774–787.

Casiglia, E., Paleari, C. D., Petucco, S., Bongiovi, S., Colangeli, G., Baccilieri, M. S., Pavan, L., Pernice, M., & Pessina, A. C. (1992). Haemodynamic effects of coffee and purified caffeine in normal volunteers: A placebo-controlled clinical study. *Journal of Human Hypertension, 6,* 95–99.

Chelsky, L. B., Cutler, J. E., Griffith, K., Kron, H., McClelland, J. H., & McAnulty, J. H. (1990). Caffeine and ventricular arrhythmias. An electrophysiological approach. *JAMA, 264,* 2236–2240.

Chou, T. M., & Benowitz, N. L. (1994). Caffeine and coffee: effects on health and cardiovascular disease. *Comparative Biochemistry & Physiology: Pharmacology, Toxicology, Endocrinology, 109,* 173–189.

Christensen, B., Mosdol, A., Rettstol, L., & Thelle, D. S. (2001). Abstention from filtered coffee reduces the concentrations of plasma homocysteine and serum cholesterol— A randomized controlled trial. *American Journal of Clinical Nutrition, 74,* 302–307.

Coney, A. M., & Marshall, J. M. (1998). Role of adenosine and its receptors in the vasodilation induced in the cerbral cortex of the rat by systemic hypoxia. *Journal of Physiology, 509,* 507–518.

De Roos, B., Van Tol, A., Urgert, R., Scheek, L. M., Van Gent, T., Buytenhek, R., Princen, H. M., & Katan, M. B. (2000). Consumption of French-press coffee raises cholesteryl ester transfer protein activity levels before LDL cholesterol in normolipidaemic subjects. *Journal of Internal Medicine, 248,* 211–216.

Debrah, K., Haigh, R., Sherwin, R., Murphy, J., & Kerr, D. (1995). Effect of acute and chronic caffeine use on the cerebrovascular, cardiovascular and hormonal responses to orthostasis in healthy volunteers. *Clinical Science, 89,* 475–480.

Denaro, C. P., Brown, C. R., Jacob, P. I., & Benowitz, N. L. (1991). Effects of caffeine with repeated dosing. *European Journal of Clinical Pharmacology, 40,* 273–278.

Dunwiddie, T. V., & Masino, S. A. (2001). The role and regulation of adenosine in the central nervous system. *Annual Review of Neuroscience, 24,* 31–55.

Edwards, G., & Savva, S. (2001). ILSI Europe, the drinks industry, and a conflict of interest undeclared. *Addiction, 96,* 197–202.

Eggertsen, R., Andreasson, A., Hedner, T., Karlberg, B. E., & Hansson, L. (1993). Effect of coffee on ambulatory blood pressure in patients with treated hypertension. *Journal of Internal Medicine, 233,* 351–355.

France, C., & Ditto, B. (1992). Cardiovascular responses to the combination of caffeine and mental arithmetic, cold pressor, and static exercise stressors. *Psychophysiology, 29,* 272–282.

Fredholm, B. B., Bättig, K., Holmén, J., Nehli, A., & Zvartau, E. E. (1999). Actions of caffeine in the brain with special reference to factors that contribute to its widespread use. *Pharmacological Reviews, 51,* 83–133.

Freestone, S., Yeo, W. W., & Ramsay, L. E. (1995). Effect of coffee and cigarette smoking on the blood pressure of patients with accelerated (malignant) hypertension. *Journal of Human Hypertension, 9,* 89–91.

Fried, R. E., Levine, D. M., Kwiterovich, P. O., Diamond, E. L., Wilder, L. B., Moy, T. F., & Pearson, T. A. (1992). The effect of filtered-coffee consumption on plasma lipid levels. Results of a randomized clinical trial. *JAMA, 267,* 811–815.

Fuller, R. W., Maxwell, D. L., Conradson, T-B. G., Dixon, C. M. S., & Barnes, P. J. (1987). Circulatory and respiratory effects of infused adenosine in conscious man. *British Journal of Pharmacology, 24,* 309–317.

Gilbert, R. M. (1976). *Caffeine as a drug of abuse.* New York: John Wiley & Sons.

Goldstein, A., & Warren, R. (1962). Passage of caffeine into human gonadal and fetal tissue. *Biochemical Pharmacology, 11,* 166–168.

Goldstein, I. B., Shapiro, D., Hui, K. K., & Yu, J. L. (1990). Blood pressure response to the "second cup of coffee." *Psychosomatic Medicine, 52,* 337–345.

Green, P. J., & Suls, J. (1996). The effects of caffeine on ambulatory blood pressure, heart rate, and mood in coffee drinkers. *Journal of Behavioral Medicine, 19,* 111–128.

Greenberg, W., & Shapiro, D. (1987). The effects of caffeine and stress on blood pressure in individuals with and without a family history of hypertension. *Psychophysiology, 24,* 151–156.

Greenland, S. (1993). A meta-analysis of coffee, myocardial infarction, and coronary death. *Epidemiology, 4,* 366–374.

Gregg, M. E., Matyas, T. A., & James, J. E., (2002). A new model of individual differences in hemodynamic profile and blood pressure reactivity. *Psychophysiology, 39,* 64–72.

Guyton, A. (1987) *Human physiology and mechanisms of disease,* 4th ed. Philadelphia, PA: W. B. Saunders.

Haigh, R. A., Harper, G. D., Fotherby, M., Hurd, J., Macdonald, I. A., & Potter, J. F. (1993). Duration of caffeine abstention influences the acute blood pressure responses to caffeine in elderly normotensives. *European Journal of Clinical Pharmacology, 44,* 549–553.

Hartley, T. R., Lovallo, W. R., Whitsett, T. L., Sung, B. H., & Wilson, M. F. (2001). Caffeine and stress: Implications for risk, assessment, and management of hypertension. *Journal of Clinical Hypertension, 3,* 354–361.

Hartley, T. R., Sung, B. H., Pincomb, G. A., Whitsett, T. L., Wilson, M. F., & Lovallo, W. R. (2000). Hypertension risk status and effect of caffeine on blood pressure. *Hypertension, 36,* 1337–1341.

Heatherley, S. V., Hancock, K. M. F., & Rogers, R. J. (2005). Psychostimulant and other effects of caffeine in 9- to 11-year-old children. *Journal of Child Psychology and Psychiatry, 167,* 54–62.

Heatherley, S. V., Hayward, R. C. , Seers, H. E., & Rogers, P. J. (2005) Cognitive and psychomotor performance, mood, and pressor effects of caffeine after 4, 6 and 8 h caffeine abstinence. *Psychopharmacology, 178,* 461–470

Heuman, J. (1994). A look back on 1993. *Tea and Coffee Trade Journal, 166,* 5–7.

James, J. E. (1990). The influence of user status and anxious disposition on the hypertensive effects of caffeine. *International Journal of Psychophysiology, 10,* 171–179.

James, J. E. (1991). *Caffeine and health*. London: Academic Press.

James, J. E. (1994a). Psychophysiological effects of habitual caffeine consumption. *International Journal of Behavioral Medicine, 1*, 247–263.

James, J. E. (1994b). Chronic effects of habitual caffeine consumption on laboratory and ambulatory blood pressure levels. *Journal of Cardiovascular Research, 1*, 159–164.

James J. E. (1994c). Does caffeine enhance or merely restore degraded psychomotor performance? *Neuropsychobiology, 30*, 124–125.

James, J. E. (1994d). Caffeine, health and commercial interests. *Addiction, 89*, 1595–1599.

James, J. E. (1997). Caffeine and blood pressure: Habitual use is a preventable cardiovascular risk factor. *Lancet, 349*, 279–281.

James, J. E. (1998). Acute and chronic effects of caffeine on performance, mood, headache, and sleep. *Neuropsychobiology, 38*, 32–41.

James, J. E. (2002). "Third party" threats to research integrity in public-private partnerships. *Addiction, 97*, 1251–1255.

James, J. E. (2004). A critical review of dietary caffeine and blood pressure: A relationship that should be taken more seriously. *Psychosomatic Medicine, 66*, 63–71.

James, J. E., & Gregg, M. E. (2004a). Hemodynamic effects of dietary caffeine, sleep restriction, and laboratory stress. *Psychophysiology, 41*, 914–923.

James, J. E., & Gregg, M. E. (2004b). Effects of dietary caffeine on mood when rested and sleep restricted. *Human Psychopharmacology: Clinical & Experimental, 19*, 333–341.

James, J. E., Gregg, M. E., Kane, M., & Harte, F. (2005). Dietary caffeine, performance and mood: Enhancing and restorative effects after controlling for withdrawal relief. *Neuropsychobiology, 52*, 1–10.

James, J. E., Paull, I., Cameron–Traub, E., Miners, J. O., Lelo, A., & Birkett, D. J. (1988). Biochemical validation of self-reported caffeine consumption during caffeine fading. *Journal of Behavioral Medicine, 11*, 15–30.

James, J. E., & Richardson, M. (1991). Pressor effects of caffeine and cigarette smoking. *British Journal of Clinical Psychology, 30*, 276–278.

James, J. E., & Rogers, P. J. (2005). Effects of caffeine on performance and mood: Withdrawal reversal is the most plausible explanation. *Psychopharmacology, 182*, 1–8.

Jee, S. H., He, J., Whelton, P. K., Suh, I. & King, J. (1999). The effect of chronic coffee drinking on blood pressure: A meta-analysis of controlled clinical trials. *Hypertension, 33*, 647–652.

Jeong, D., & Dimsdale, J. E. (1990). The effects of caffeine on blood pressure in the work environment. *American Journal of Hypertension, 3*, 749–753.

Julius, S. (1988). The blood pressure seeking properties of the central nervous system. *Journal of Hypertension, 6*, 177–185.

Karatzis, E., Papaioannou, T. G., Aznaouridis, K., Karatzi, K., Stamatelopoulos, K., Zampelas, A., et al. (2005). Acute effects of caffeine on blood pressure and wave reflections in healthy subjects: Should we consider monitoring central blood pressure? *International Journal of Cardiology, 98*, 425–430.

Kawachi, I., Colditz, G. A., & Stone, C. B. (1994). Does coffee drinking increase the risk of coronary heart disease? Results from a meta-analysis. *British Heart Journal, 72*, 269–275.

Klesges, R. C., Ray, J. W., & Klesges, L. M. (1994). Caffeinated coffee and tea intake and its relationship to cigarette smoking: An analysis of the Second National Health and Nutrition Examination Survey. *Journal of Substance Abuse, 6*, 407–418.

Kohl, H. W., III. (2001). Physical activity and cardiovascular disease: Evidence for a dose response. *Medicine & Science in Sports & Exercise, 33*, S472–483.

LaCroix, A. Z., Mead, L. A., Liang, K. Y., Thomas, C. B., & Pearson, T. A. (1987). Coffee consumption and coronary heart disease. *New England Journal of Medicine, 316,* 947.

Lane, J. D., Adcock, R. A., Williams, R. B., & Kuhn, C. M. (1990). Caffeine effects on cardiovascular and neuroendocrine responses to acute psychosocial stress and their relationship to level of habitual caffeine consumption. *Psychosomatic Medicine, 52,* 320–336.

Lane, J. D., & Manus, D. C. (1989). Persistent cardiovascular effects with repeated caffeine administration. *Psychosomatic Medicine, 51,* 373–380.

Lane, J. D., Pieper, C. F., Phillips–Bute, B. G., Bryant, J. E., & Kuhn, C. M. (2002). Caffeine affects cardiovascular and neuroendocrine activation at work and home. *Psychosomatic Medicine, 64,* 323–331.

Lane, J. D., & Williams, R. B., Jr. (1985). Caffeine affects cardiovascular responses to stress. *Psychophysiology, 22,* 648–655.

Lane, J. D., & Williams, R. B. (1987). Cardiovascular effects of caffeine and stress in regular coffee drinkers. *Psychophysiology, 24,* 157–164.

Lelo, A., Miners, J. O., Robson, R., & Birkett, D. J. (1986a). Assessment of caffeine exposure: Caffeine content of beverages, caffeine intake, and plasma concentrations of methylxanthines. *Clinical Pharmacology and Therapeutics, 39,* 54–59.

Lelo, A., Miners, J. O., Robson, R. A., & Birkett, D. J. (1986b). Quantitative assessment of caffeine partial clearances in man. *British Journal of Clinical Pharmacology, 22,* 183–186.

MacDonald, R. (2001) WHO says tobacco industry "used" institute to undermine its policies. *British Medical Journal, 322,* 576.

MacDonald, T. M., Sharpe, K., Fowler, G., Lyons, D., Freestone, S., Lovell, H. G., Webster, J., & Petrie, J. C. (1991). Caffeine restriction: Effect of mild hypertension. *British Medical Journal, 303,* 1235–1238.

MacMahon, S. (2000). Blood pressure and the risk of cardiovascular disease. *New England Journal of Medicine, 342,* 50–52.

MacMahon, S., Peto, R., Cutler, J., Collins, R., Sorlie, P., Neaton, J., Abbott, R., Godwin, J., Dyer, A., & Stamler, J. (1990). Blood pressure, stroke, and coronary heart disease. Part 1. Prolonged differences in blood pressure: Prospective observational studies corrected for the regression dilution bias. *Lancet, 335,* 765–774.

Mahmud, A., & Feely, J. (2001). Acute effect of caffeine on arterial stiffness and aortic pressure waveform. *Hypertension, 38,* 227–231.

Masterson, J. (1983). Trends in coffee consumption. *Tea and Coffee Trade Journal,* March, 24–25.

Murphy, P. (2001). ILSI responds to March 10 *BMJ* article. *British Medical Journal, 322,* 576.

Myers, M. G., & Basinski, A. (1992). Coffee and coronary heart disease. *Archives of Internal Medicine, 152,* 1767–1772.

Myers, M. G., & Reeves, R. A. (1991). The effect of caffeine on daytime ambulatory blood pressure. *American Journal of Hypertension, 4,* 427–431.

Noordzij, M., Uiterwaal, C. S., Arends, L. R., Kok, F. J., Grobbee, D. E., & Geleijnse, J. M. (2005). Blood pressure response to chronic intake of coffee and caffeine: A meta-analysis of randomized controlled trials. *Journal of Hypertension, 23,* 921–928.

Palatini, P., & Julius, S. (1999). Relevance of heart rate as a risk factor in hypertension. *Current Hypertension Reports, 1,* 219–224.

Patton, G. C., Hibbert, M., Rosier, M. J., Carlin, J. B., Caust, J., & Bowes, G. (1995). Patterns of common drug use in teenagers. *Australian Journal of Public Health, 19,* 393–399.

Pearson, T. A. (1999). Cardiovascular disease in developing countries: Myths, realities, and opportunities. *Cardiovascular Drugs and Therapy, 13,* 95–104.

Pfeifer, R. W., & Notari, R. E. (1988). Predicting caffeine plasma concentrations resulting from consumption of food or beverages: A simple method and its origin. *Drug Intelligence and Clinical Pharmacy, 22,* 953–959.

Prineas, R. J., Jacobs, D. R., Crow, R. S., & Blackburn, H. (1980). Coffee, tea, and VPB. *Journal of Chronic Diseases, 33,* 67–72.

Prospective Studies Collaboration. (2002). Age-specific relevance of usual blood pressure to vascular mortality: A meta-analysis of individual data for one million adults in 61 prospective studies. *Lancet, 360,* 1903–1913.

Rakic, V., Burke, V., & Beilin, L. J. (1999). Effects of coffee on ambulatory blood pressure in older men and women: A randomized controlled trial. *Hypertension, 33,* 869–873.

Ratliff–Crain, J., O'Keefe, M. K., & Baum, A. (1989). Cardiovascular reactivity, mood, and task performance in deprived and nondeprived coffee drinkers. *Health Psychology, 8,* 427–447.

Richards, G. (1994). Tea in 1993. *Tea and Coffee Trade Journal, 166,* 42–50.

Robertson, D., Wade, D., Workman, R., Woosley, R. L., & Oates, J. A. (1981). Tolerance to the humoral and hemodynamic effects of caffeine in man. *Journal of Clinical Investigation, 67,* 1111–1117.

Rodgers, A., Lawes, C., & MacMahon, S. (2000). Reducing the global burden of blood pressure-related cardiovascular disease. *Journal of Hypertension, 18,* S3–S6.

Rodgers, A., & MacMahon, S. (1999). Blood pressure and the global burden of cardiovascular disease. *Clinical & Experimental Hypertension, 21,* 543-552.

Rogers, P. J., Heatherley, S. V., Hayward, R. C., Seers, H. E., Hill, J., & Kane, M. (2005). Effects of caffeine and caffeine withdrawal on mood and cognitive performance degraded by sleep restriction. *Psychopharmacology, 179,* 742–752.

Rose, J. (1981). Strategy of prevention: Lessons from cardiovascular disease. *British Medical Journal, 282,* 1847–1851.

Rosenberg, L., Palmer, J. R., Kelly, J. P., Kaufman, D. W., & Shapiro, S. (1988). Coffee drinking and nonfatal myocardial infarction in men under 55 years of age. *American Journal of Epidemiology, 128,* 570–578.

Schreiber, G. B., Robins, M., Maffeo, C. E., Masters, M. N., Bond, A. P., & Morganstein, D. (1988). Confounders contributing to the reported associations of coffee or caffeine with disease. *Preventive Medicine, 17,* 295–309.

Shepard, J. D., al'Absi, M., Whitsett, T. L., Passey, R. B., & Lovallo, W. R. (2000). Additive pressor effects of caffeine and stress in male medical students at risk for hypertension. *American Journal of Hypertension, 13,* 475–781.

Shi, J., Benowitz, N. L., Denaro, C. P., & Sheiner, L. B. (1993). Pharmacokinetic–pharmacodynamic modeling of caffeine: tolerance to pressor effects. *Clinical Pharmacology and Therapeutics, 53,* 6–14.

Shirlow. M. J., Berry, G., & Stokes, G. (1988). Caffeine consumption and blood pressure: An epidemiologic study. *International Journal of Epidemiology, 17,* 90–97.

Smits. P., Boekema, P., de Abreu, R., Thien, T., & van't Laar, A. (1987). Evidence for an antagonism between caffeine and adenosine in the human cardiovascular system. *Journal of Cardiovascular Pharmacology, 10,* 136–143.

Smits, P., Temme, L., & Thien, T. (1993). The cardiovascular interaction between caffeine and nicotine in humans. *Clinical Pharmacology and Therapeutics, 54,* 194–204.

Smits, P., Thien, T., & van't Laar, A. (1985a). The cardiovascular effects of regular and decaffeinated coffee. *British Journal of Clinical Pharmacology, 19,* 852–854.

Smits, P., Thien, T., & van't Laar, A. (1985b). Circulatory effects of coffee in relation to the pharmacokinetics of caffeine. *American Journal of Cardiology, 56,* 958–963.

Stamler, J. S., Goldman, M. E., Gomes, J., Matza, D., & Horowitz, S. F. (1992). The effect of stress and fatigue on cardiac rhythm in medical inters. *Journal of Electrocardiology*, *25*, 333–338.

Stavric, B. (1992). An update on research with coffee/caffeine (1989–1990). *Food Chemistry and Toxicology*, *30*, 533–555.

Superko, H. R., Myll, J., DiRicco, C., Williams, P. T., Bortz, W. M., & Wood, P. D. (1994). Effects of cessation of caffeinated-coffee consumption on ambulatory and resting blood pressure in men. *American Journal of Cardiology*, *73*, 780–784.

Sutherland, D. J., McPherson, D. D., Renton, K. W., Spencer, C. A., & Montague, T. J. (1985). The effect of caffeine on cardiac rate, rhythm, and ventricular repolarization. *Chest*, *87*, 319–324.

Ungemack, J. A. (1994). Patterns of personal health practice: men and women in the United States. *American Journal of Preventive Medicine*, *10*, 38–44.

Urgert, R., van Vliet, T., Zock, P. L., & Katan, M. B. (2000). Heavy coffee consumption and plasma homocysteine: a randomized controlled trial in healthy volunteers. *American Journal of Clinical Nutrition*, *72*, 1107–1110.

van den Hoogen, P. C., Seidell, J. C., Menotti, A., & Kromhout, D. (2000). Blood pressure and long-term coronary heart disease mortality in the Seven Countries study: Implications for clinical practice and public health. *European Heart Journal*, *21*, 1639–1642.

van Dusseldorp, M., Smits, P., Thien, T., & Katan, M. B. (1989). Effect of decaffeinated versus regular coffee on blood pressure. A 12-week, double-blind trial. *Hypertension*, *14*, 563–569.

Vlachopoulos, C., Hirata, K., & O'Rourke, M. F. (2003). Effect of caffeine on aortic elastic properties and wave reflection. *Journal of Hypertension*, *21*, 563–570.

Vlachopoulos, C., Hirata, K., Stefanadis, C., Toutouzas, P., & O'Rourke, M. F. (2003). Caffeine increases aortic stiffness in hypertensive patients. *American Journal of Hypertension*, *16*, 63–66.

Vlachopoulos, C., Kosmopoulou, F., Panagiotakos, D., Ioakeimidis, N., Alexopoulos, N., Pitsavos, C., et al. (2004). Smoking and caffeine have a synergistic detrimental effect on aortic stiffness and wave reflections. *Journal of the American College of Cardiology*, *44*, 1911–1917.

Waring, W. S., Goudsmit, J., Marwick, J., Webb, D. J., & Maxwell, S. R. (2003). Acute caffeine intake influences central more than peripheral blood pressure in young adults. *American Journal of Hypertension*, *16*, 919–924.

Wilson, P. W. & Culleton, B. F. (1998). Epidemiology of cardiovascular disease in the United States. *American Journal of Kidney Disease*, *32*, S56–S65.

Wolf–Maier K, Cooper, R. S., Banegas, J. R., Giampaoli, S., Hense, H. -W., Joffres, M., et al. (2003). Hypertension prevalence and blood pressure levels in six European countries, Canada, and the United States. *JAMA*, *289*, 2363–2369.

Zeltner, T., Kessler, D. A., Martiny, A., & Randera, F. (2000) *Tobacco company strategies to undermine tobacco control activities at the World Health Organization*. Geneva, World Health Organization.

7 Effects of Coffee and Caffeine Consumption on Serum Lipids and Lipoproteins

Ming Wei and Harvey A. Schwertner

CONTENTS

Coffee and beverages with caffeine represent one of the world's leading commodities. Over half of the adults in the United States and Europe consume coffee regularly and many people in the world are lifetime consumers of tea and caffeine-containing colas (Arnesen, Forde, & Thelle, 1984; Thelle, 1991, 1995; Thelle, Heyden, & Fodor, 1987; Thompson, 1994; Urgert, Kosmeijer–Schuil, & Katan, 1996; Urgert et al., 1997; van Dusseldorp & Katan, 1990; Wei, Macera, Horning, & Blair, 1995). Because of the large percentage of adults consuming coffee and caffeine, any adverse or beneficial effect of coffee or caffeine consumption would be of public interest. In this review, we present the major epidemiological and clinical trials that have examined the association between coffee or caffeine consumption and serum lipid and lipoprotein concentrations. In addition, we discuss the various *in vitro* and *in vivo* studies to identify the mechanisms by which coffee might increase serum lipid and lipoprotein concentrations.

EPIDEMIOLOGICAL STUDIES OF THE RELATIONSHIP BETWEEN COFFEE INTAKE AND SERUM LIPID AND LIPOPROTEIN CONCENTRATIONS

Numerous epidemiological studies have been published to assess the association between coffee and caffeine consumption and serum lipids (Table 7.1). Several epidemiological studies have examined the influence of tea and cola with caffeine on serum lipids and lipoproteins; however, most of them did not find an association between tea and cola consumption and cholesterol concentrations (Carson, Cauley, & Caggiula, 1993; Curb, Reed, Kautz, & Yano, 1986; Davis, Curb, Borhani, Prineas, & Molteni, 1988; Green & Harari, 1992; Haffner et al., 1985; Kark, Friedlander, Kaufmann, & Stein, 1985; Klatsky, Petitti, Armstrong, & Friedman, 1985; Wei et al., 1995). Other studies have focused almost exclusively on the relationship between coffee consumption and lipids, especially serum cholesterol. The majority of epidemiological studies were cross-sectional studies, but one was a prospective study (Wei et al.). Most of the studies described in this review have come from English language journals.

About 32 epidemiological studies have reported an association between coffee intake and serum cholesterol concentrations (Table 7.1). The strongest experimental evidence has come from several Scandinavian countries, which have the highest coffee consumption worldwide. In a study in Norway involving 7,213 women and 7,368 men between the ages of 20 and 54 years, coffee consumption was positively associated with the levels of total cholesterol and triglycerides (Thelle, Arnesen, & Forde, 1983). This association was found in men and in women. Coffee intake also was found to be inversely associated with the levels of HDL cholesterol in women.

The coffee–cholesterol relationship remained strong and statistically significant after adjustment for age, body mass index, physical activity, cigarette smoking, and alcohol consumption. After adjustment for all covariates, the mean total cholesterol level was 5.56 mmol/L (215 mg/dl) for men drinking less than one cup of coffee a day compared to 6.23 mmol/L (241mg/dl) for those consuming more than nine cups per day. The corresponding figures for women were 5.32 mmol/L (206 mg/dl) and 5.92 mmol/L (218 mg/dl).

The Cardiovascular Disease Risk Factor Study in Oppland, in southern Norway, was the largest epidemiological study of the effects of coffee on serum cholesterol concentrations. This study was one to take into account possible confounding variables from dietary sources. The study consisted of 11,912 men and 12,328 women between 35 and 49 years of age (Solvoll, Selmer, Loken, Foss, & Trygg, 1989). A positive relationship between coffee consumption and serum cholesterol was found for men and women. The relationship between coffee consumption and serum cholesterol levels remained statistically significant after adjusting for the potentially confounding dietary variables.

Haffner et al. (1985) performed studies to determine whether coffee and other caffeinated beverages might have an effect on serum lipids and lipoproteins. Their study included 1,228 women and 923 men, 25 to 64 years of age. The study confirmed the positive relationship between coffee consumption and total cholesterol and LDL cholesterol in males and females. This association persisted after adjustment for age, ethnicity, obesity, cigarette smoking, and alcohol consumption. In this study, tea or cola consumption was not found to have an effect on serum lipid concentrations.

TABLE 7.1
Epidemiological Studies of Coffee on Serum Lipids and Lipoprotein Concentrations

Author	Study subjects	Results—negative association between coffee intake and lipids
Dawber (1974)	1,992 men	Coffee intake was not associated with total cholesterol.
Philips (1981)	2,455 men and women	Coffee intake was not associated with total cholesterol.
Kovar (1983)	5,098 men and women	Coffee intake was not associated with total cholesterol.
Shekelle (1983)	1,900 men	Coffee intake was not associated with total cholesterol.
Hofman (1983)	4,323 men and women	Coffee intake was not associated with total cholesterol.
Folsom (1984)	632 men and women	Coffee intake was not associated with total cholesterol.
Donahue (1987)	472 young men and women	Coffee intake was unrelated to total cholesterol, LDL cholesterol, HDL cholesterol, or apoproteins AI, AII, or B.
Salonen (1987)	9,347 persons	High coffee consumption was associated with decreased HDL cholesterol levels in smokers but increased levels in nonsmokers.
Schwarz (1990)	1,203 men and women	Coffee intake was not associated with total cholesterol.
D'Avanzo (1993)	642 men and women	Although there was a dose–response association between coffee intake and serum cholesterol among coffee drinkers, cholesterol levels were higher in noncoffee drinkers than in moderate coffee drinkers.
Carson (1993)	1,035 elderly women	Adjustment for potential confounders yielded no significant associations between caffeine from coffee, tea, and cola and any of the lipid fractions.
Carson (1994)	541 premenopausal women	Coffee intake had no effect on lipids, except a negative association was found between coffee intake and triglycerides.
Lancaster (1994)	1,074 adults	Coffee intake was not associated with total cholesterol.
Du (2005)	814 caffeine-drug users and 623 nonusers	Coffee intake was not associated with total cholesterol and LDL cholesterol, but associated with triglycerides.

(*continued*)

TABLE 7.1 (Continued)
Epidemiological Studies of Coffee on Serum Lipids and Lipoprotein Concentrations

Author	Study subjects	Results—positive association between coffee intake and lipids
Bjelke (1974)	444 men	Coffee consumption was positively associated with total cholesterol.
Sacks (1975)	116 women and men	Coffee intake was positively associated with total cholesterol among smokers.
Nichols (1976)	3,395 women and men	Coffee intake was positively associated with total cholesterol in women.
Heyden (1979)	361 men and women	Smoking and coffee drinking interact in affecting LDL and total cholesterol, but coffee drinking alone did not appear to affect blood lipids.
Thelle (1983)	14,581 men and women	Coffee consumption was positively associated with total cholesterol and triglycerides, and inversely associated with HDL cholesterol.
Arab (1983)	770 men and women	Coffee intake was associated with total cholesterol in young but not in the elderly. No association was found between coffee consumption and triglyceride, apolipoprotein A and B, and HDL cholesterol.
Shirlow (1984)	4,757 men and women	Caffeine intake was positively associated with total cholesterol in women irrespective of the source of caffeine. No association was found in men.
Mathias (1985)	701 women and men	Coffee intake was positively associated with total cholesterol and LDL cholesterol in women but not in men. Decaffeinated coffee had no effect on lipids in either sex.
Kark (1985)	1,596 men and women	Caffeine intake was associated with total cholesterol and LDL cholesterol. Tea had no effect.
Klatsky (1985)	47,611 men and women	Caffeine intake was associated with total cholesterol and LDL cholesterol. Tea had no effect.
Haffner (1985)	2,151 men and women	Coffee intake was positively associated with total cholesterol. Tea and cola had no effect.
Williams (1985)	77 men	Coffee intake was positively associated with total cholesterol, LDL cholesterol and aprolipoprotein B.
Green (1986)	658 men	Coffee intake was positively associated with total cholesterol and LDL cholesterol.
Curb (1986)	5,858 men	Coffee intake was positively associated with total cholesterol. Tea and cola had no effect.
Tuomilehto (1987)	8,979 men and women	Serum cholesterol was higher in coffee drinkers than in noncoffee drinkers. No association was found between HDL cholesterol and coffee intake.
Pietinen (1988)	18,070 men and women	Coffee intake was positively associated with total cholesterol, but not HDL cholesterol.
Davis (1988)	9,034 men and women	Coffee intake was positively associated with cholesterol. Tea, cola, and decaffeinated coffee had no effect.
Stensvold (1989)	29,027 men and women	Coffee intake was positively associated with total cholesterol, most strongly for boiled coffee.

TABLE 7.1 (Continued)
Epidemiological Studies of Coffee on Serum Lipids and Lipoprotein Concentrations

Author	Study subjects	Results—positive association between coffee intake and lipid
Solvoll (1989)	24,240 men and women	Coffee intake was positively associated with total cholesterol.
Pietinen (1990)	5,704 men and women	Serum cholesterol was higher in coffee drinkers than in noncoffee drinkers. Consumers of boiled coffee had the highest cholesterol levels. A weak association between filtered coffee and cholesterol was found in women.
Lindahl (1991)	1,625 men and women	Consumers of boiled coffee had higher serum cholesterol levels than consumers of filtered coffee.
Salvaggio (1991)	8,983 men and women	Coffee intake was positively associated with total cholesterol and LDL cholesterol, even though the coffee drunk was mainly filtered and nonboiled.
Hostmark (1992)	165 middle-aged men	Coffee intake was positively associated with total cholesterol and LDL cholesterol.
Green (1992)	5,369 men and women	Coffee intake was positively associated with total cholesterol and LDL cholesterol. Tea had no effect.
Jossa (1993)	900 men	Coffee intake was positively associated with total cholesterol in smokers, but not in nonsmokers.
Berndt (1993)	1,879 men and women	Coffee intake was positively associated with total cholesterol and LDL cholesterol and inversely associated with triglycerides.
Mensink (1993)	6,822 men and women	Coffee intake was positively associated with total cholesterol among smokers and life-long abstainers but not in the group of ex-smokers.
El Shabrawy Ali (1993)	252 men and women	Serum cholesterol was higher in coffee drinkers than in noncoffee drinkers.
Ruzi–Lapuente (1995)	609 women	Coffee intake was positively associated with total cholesterol.
Wei (1995)	2,109 nonsmoking women and men	Dose response was found between increased coffee consumption and increased total cholesterol. Tea, cola, and decaffeinated coffee had no effect.
Jansen (1995)	319 men	Coffee intake was positively associated with total cholesterol.
Urgert (1996)	309 men and women	Chronic consumers of boiled coffee have higher levels of lipoprotein (a) concentrations than filtered coffee drinkers.
Miyake (1999)	4,587 men	Instant coffee intake was positively associated with LDL cholesterol and inversely associated with triglycerides. Brewed coffee had no effect.

The effect of coffee consumption on serum cholesterol levels was determined in a group of 9,043 hypertensive men and women participating in the Hypertension Detection and Follow-Up Program (Davis et al., 1988). The relationship between coffee consumption and serum cholesterol levels was examined along with potentially confounding variables including age, race, sex, diuretic status, diastolic blood pressure, cigarette smoking, relative weight, physical activity, stress, and education level. When these variables were included in the multiple regression equations, the positive association between coffee consumption and serum cholesterol level remained statistically significant. As in the other studies, tea, cola, or decaffeinated coffee consumption was not found to be associated with cholesterol levels.

In a prospective epidemiological study of the effects of coffee consumption on serum cholesterol concentrations, Wei et al. (1995) examined 2,109 healthy non-smokers, 25 to 65 years of age, who attended two clinic visits at a preventive medical center between 1987 and 1991 (mean interval between visits: 16.7 months). After adjusting for age and other potential confounders, each cup of coffee was found to increase serum total cholesterol by about 2 mg/dl (0.052 mmol/L). This dose response was found for individuals who decreased their regular coffee consumption, those who continued to consume the same amount of coffee, and those who increased their consumption of coffee.

The same trend was observed for individuals who quit drinking regular coffee, who never drank coffee, and who first started to drink coffee. Cholesterol concentrations did not change in individuals who continued to consume the same quantity of regular coffee. The change in cholesterol level was not found to be related to consumption of decaffeinated coffee, regular tea, decaffeinated tea, or cola.

Most of the epidemiological studies have shown that coffee increases serum cholesterol concentrations. However, in a few studies coffee consumption did not have an effect on serum lipid and lipoprotein concentrations. Coffee intake, for example, was not found to increase serum cholesterol concentrations in 5,098 women and men participating in the U.S. National Health and Nutrition Survey (Kovar & Feinleib, 1983). Also, no association was found between coffee intake and serum cholesterol levels in 1,990 men participating in a Chicago study (Shekelle & Paul, 1983). In this study, serum cholesterol concentrations were slightly higher for the heavy coffee drinkers (6.58 mmol/L; 254.4 mg/dl) than for the light coffee users (6.37 mmol/L; 246.6 mg/dl); however, the differences were not found to be statistically significant.

Carson, Caggiula, Meilahn, Matthews, and Kuller (1994) studied 541 randomly selected premenopausal women, 42 to 50 years of age. The correlation between coffee consumption and blood lipids as well as the multiple regression analyses controlling for menopausal status at follow-up was not found to be significant for any of the blood lipids studied except for the triglycerides. The triglyceride concentrations were found to be inversely related to coffee consumption at follow-up. The lack of an association between coffee and serum cholesterol also has been reported in several other studies (Carson et al, 1993; Dawber, Kannel, & Gordon, 1974; Donahue, Orchard, Stein, & Kuller, 1987; Du et al., 1998; Folsom, 1984; Hofman & Klein, 1983; Lancaster, Muir, & Silagy, 1994; Phillips, Havel, & Kane, 1981; Schwarz, Bischof, & Kunze, 1990).

Effects of Different Coffee Brewing Methods on Serum Cholesterol Concentrations in Epidemiological Studies

A number of studies have been performed to determine whether different coffee brewing methods have an effect on serum cholesterol concentrations (Lindahl, Johansson, Huhtasaari, Hallmans, & Asplund, 1991; Pietinen, Aro, Tuomilehto, Uusitalo, & Korhonen, 1990; Stensvold, Tverdal, & Foss, 1989; Urgert, Weusten–van der Wouw, et al., 1996). In most of the studies, consumption of boiled coffee was found to result in higher serum cholesterol concentrations than consumption of filtered coffee or instant coffee.

Significant increases in serum cholesterol concentrations were found in a Norwegian cross-sectional study of 14,168 men and 14,859 women who consumed boiled or filtered coffee (Stensvold et al., 1989). The serum cholesterol concentrations increased linearly with increasing coffee consumption, but most strongly with boiled coffee. After controlling for other potential confounders, boiled coffee was found to increase serum cholesterol levels by 8% in men and 10% in women. When filtered coffee was consumed, the coffee–cholesterol dose relationship remained significant only for women.

The effects of boiled and filtered coffee on blood cholesterol concentrations were also studied in an epidemiological study of 5,704 men and women in Finland (Pietinen et al., 1990). The mean serum cholesterol values of those consuming boiled coffee were found to be significantly higher than for those drinking filtered coffee for both sexes after adjusting for age, body mass index, smoking, serum gamma-glutamyltransferase, index of saturated fat intake, and physical activity.

The cholesterol concentrations obtained with boiled and filtered coffee were 6.37 versus 6.02 mmol/L (246.3 vs. 232.8 mg/dl), respectively, for men and 6.22 versus 5.84 mmol/L (240.5 vs. 225.8 mg/dl) for women (both significant at $p < 0.001$). A significant dose-dependent effect was observed between boiled coffee intake and serum cholesterol concentrations in men and in women. When filtered coffee was consumed, a weak coffee dose–cholesterol association was found for women but not for men.

Lindahl et al. (1991) examined the effects of boiled and filtered coffee on serum cholesterol in a population-based study of 1,625 middle-aged subjects. Approximately 50% of the participants drank boiled coffee and 50% drank filtered coffee. Consumption of boiled coffee resulted in significantly higher serum cholesterol levels than consumption of filtered coffee did. Linear multiple regression analysis performed with serum cholesterol as the dependent variable found boiled coffee to be an important independent determinant of cholesterol levels.

Urgert, Weusten–van der Wouw, et al. (1996) determined the effects of boiled coffee and filtered coffee on serum lipoprotein(a) concentrations. The cross-sectional study was performed on 309 healthy Norwegians, 40 to 42 years of age. The median lipoprotein(a) concentration was 13.0 mg/dl (10th and 90th percentiles: 2.5 and 75.0 mg/dl, respectively) for individuals consuming boiled coffee and 7.9 mg/dl (10th and 90th percentiles: 1.9 and 62.5 mg/dl, respectively) for individuals consuming filtered coffee. The mean lipoprotein(a) concentrations were 25.8 and 19.6 mg/dl, respectively. The results of the study indicate that individuals who chronically consume unfiltered, boiled coffee have higher serum lipoprotein(a) concentrations than individuals who consume filtered coffee.

The results indicate that coffee prepared by boiling is more likely to increase concentrations of cholesterols. Several studies, however, have shown that consumption of filtered and instant coffee also increases serum cholesterol concentrations. In a study conducted in northern Italy, where filtered coffee is mainly consumed, Salvaggio, Periti, Miano, Quaglia, and Marzorati (1991) investigated the possible association between coffee consumption and serum cholesterol levels in 8,983 subjects aged 18 to 65 years. A positive relationship was found between coffee intake and cholesterol concentrations.

The differences in serum cholesterol concentrations between coffee users and nonusers were 6.1 mg/dl for consumers of one to three cups/day (3.4 mg/dl after adjustment for age, body mass index, alcohol and cigarette consumption, and physical activity), 9.9 mg/dl for those drinking four to five cups/day (5.8 mg/dl after adjustment), and 14.8 mg/dl for those drinking more than five cups/day (9.6 mg/dl after adjustment). This relationship remained substantially unchanged when nonsmokers and smokers were analyzed separately and after adjusting for other potential confounders (Salvaggio et al., 1991).

A weak but significant association between filtered coffee intake and cholesterol concentrations was found in women in a study by Pietinen et al. (1990). In a 1999 study of 4,587 Japanese men 48 to 56 years of age, instant coffee consumption was found to be positively associated with serum LDL cholesterol levels and inversely associated with serum triglyceride levels. After adjustment for body mass index, smoking, alcohol use, and green tea consumption, each cup of instant coffee consumed per day was associated with an increase in LDL cholesterol levels of 0.82 mg/dl (Miyake et al., 1999). These associations remained significant after additional adjustments were made for selected foods and beverages known to increase serum lipids and lipoproteins.

To date, about 47 epidemiological studies have been published on the relationship between coffee consumption and serum cholesterol concentrations (Table 7.1). The majority of the studies have shown that serum cholesterol levels increase linearly with increase in coffee consumption. In addition, the studies show that drinking boiled coffee results in a higher cholesterol concentration than does drinking filtered or instant coffee. It is important to recognize that almost all of the studies were cross-sectional studies and that bias and confounders might have had an influence on the results of the epidemiological studies. For example, most coffee drinkers add cream or milk to their coffee. As a result, the association between coffee intake and serum cholesterol might be influenced by these additives (Thelle et al., 1983).

Another potential confounder is the possible difference in dietary patterns and dietary intake of individuals who consumed more coffee versus those who consumed less coffee or did not consume coffee. Differences in the dietary patterns of persons who consumed high amounts of coffee versus those who consumed low amounts of coffee have been found (Jacobsen & Thelle, 1987a, b; Puccio, McPhillipos, Barrett-Connor, & Ganiats, 1990). Several studies have shown that heavy coffee drinkers have a clustering of atherogenic behaviors (Aro, Pietinem, Uusitalo, & Tuomilehto, 1989; Brown & Benowitz, 1989; Haffner et al., 1985; Jacobsen & Thelle; Puccio et al.).

For example, heavy coffee drinkers had a higher consumption of butter or margarine, and hard margarine, as well as a higher consumption of eggs, dietary saturated fats, and cholesterol. In addition, coffee drinkers were more likely to smoke and less likely to exercise than were the noncoffee drinkers (Solvoll et al., 1989). However, in this large study of 24,000 men and women, only 20% of the variation in the association between coffee consumption and cholesterol concentration could be explained by dietary and lifestyle variables (Solvoll et al.).

Several other studies have also shown that dietary and lifestyle variables do not have a major effect on the coffee–cholesterol relationship (Davis et al 1988; Thelle et al., 1987; Tuomilehto et al., 1987). In a prospective study, the association between regular coffee intake and total cholesterol remained unchanged after adjustment for many potential confounders such as body mass index, alcohol consumption, physical activity index, consumption of meal, beef, pork, cheese, fried food, desserts, snacks, eggs, butter, hot dogs, fruit, vegetables, fish, poultry, and milk (Wei et al., 1995). It should be noted that there was no association between the consumption of tea and cola containing caffeine and cholesterol concentrations despite the association between coffee intake and cholesterol (Table 7.1). Likewise, caffeine intake per se was not found to be associated with changes in serum cholesterol concentrations.

CLINICAL TRIALS OF THE EFFECTS OF COFFEE ON LIPIDS AND LIPOPROTIENS

The relationship between coffee and serum lipid levels has been examined in 21 published clinical trials (Table 7.2). The clinical trials have an advantage over epidemiological studies in that the amount of coffee consumed is more precisely known and that potential confounder variables are controlled.

A significant coffee–cholesterol relationship was found in some (Ahola, Jauhiainen, & Aro, 1991; Aro, Teirila, & Greg, 1990; Aro, Tuomilrhto, Kostiainen, Utusitalo, & Pietinen, 1987; Bak & Grobbee, 1989; Burr et al., 1995; Christensen, Mosdol, Retterstol, Landaas, & Thelle, 2001; de Roos et al., 2000; Forde, Knutsen, Arnesen, & Thelle, 1985; Fried et al., 1992; Strandhagen & Thelle, 2003; Urget, Meyboom, et al., 1996; van Dusseldorp, Katan, van Vliet, Demacker, & Stalenhoef, 1991) but not all (Aro, Kostiainen, Huttnen, Seppala, & Vapaatalop, 1985; Bak & Grobbee, 1991; Burr, Gallacher, Butland, Bolton, & Downs, 1989; D'Amicis et al., 1996; Rosmarin, Applegate, & Somes, 1990; Sanguigni, Gallu, Ruffini, & Strano, 1995; Superko, Bortz, Williams, Albers, & Wood, 1991; van Dusseldorp, Katan, & Demacker, 1990; Wahrburg, Martin, Schulte, Walek, & Assmann, 1994) of the clinical trials. The factors responsible for the lack of agreement are not known, but could be due in part to the relatively small number of study subjects and to the variability in the brewing methods used in the studies.

The effects of coffee, tea, and caffeine intake on serum lipoproteins and thromboxane production were determined in 12 healthy, normolipidemic volunteers, 33 to 45 years of age (Aro et al., 1985). Each individual consumed eight cups of instant coffee, instant tea, or rosehip "tea" daily, during three successive periods of 3 weeks

TABLE 7.2
Effects of Coffee on Serum Lipid and Lipoprotein Concentrations in Clinical Trials

Author	Subjects	Design	Cups/ day	Intervention	Results
Aro (1985)	12 subjects	Crossover	8	Instant coffee or tea	No significant differences in the total cholesterol, LDL cholesterol, and triglyceride were observed between study periods.
Burr (1989)	54 subjects	Crossover	5	Coffee, decaffeinated coffee, or no coffee for 4 weeks	Decrease in HDL cholesterol and apolipoprotein A and increase in total cholesterol and apolipoprotein B with coffee intake, but none of these were statistically significant.
Rosmarin (1990)	21 healthy men	Crossover	3.6	Filtered coffee or no coffee for 4 weeks	No effect of coffee consumption on serum total cholesterol, HDL cholesterol, LDL cholesterol, or apolipoprotein B.
van Dusseldorp (1990)	45 healthy subjects	Crossover	5	Regular coffee or decaffeinated coffee for 6 weeks	Replacement of regular coffee by decaffeinated coffee has no effect on serum cholesterol and lipoproteins.
Bak (1991)	69 young, healthy subjects	Parallel	4–6	Filtered decaffeinated, caffeine, and placebo pills for 9 weeks	Abstinence from caffeine for a period of 9 weeks has no effect on serum lipids.
Superko (1991)	181 men	Parallel	4	Caffeinated coffee, decaffeinated coffee or no coffee for 8 weeks	Change from caffeinated to decaffeinated coffee increased LDL cholesterol, whereas change to no coffee showed no change.
Wahrburg (1994)	119 healthy subjects	Parallel	5–6.7	Caffeinated or decaffeinated coffee for 6 weeks	Switch from regular to decaffeinated coffee had no cholesterol-elevating effects, irrespective of the type of coffee.

TABLE 7.2 (Continued)
Effects of Coffee on Serum Lipid and Lipoprotein Concentrations in Clinical Trials

Author	Subjects	Design	Cups/ day	Intervention	Results
Sanguigni (1995)	49 men and women	Crossover	5	Caffeinated and decaffeinated coffee for 10 weeks	There was no evidence that the Italian method of brewing coffee affects serum lipoproteins.
D'Amicis (1996)	84 normo-lipidemic young men	Parallel	3	A 6-week break from espresso, mocha, and no coffee/tea intake	Coffee brewed in the Italian way does not alter blood levels of total cholesterol, HDL cholesterol, or LDL cholesterol.
Forde (1985)	33 men with hyperchol-esterolemia	Parallel	7	Boiled or filter coffee for 10 weeks	Cholesterol concentrations rose in subjects returning to boiled coffee but remained the same in those returning to filter coffee.
Aro (1987)	42 hyperchol-esterolemic subjects	Crossover	8	Boiled coffee, filtered coffee, and tea for 4 weeks	Boiled coffee increased the concentration of LDL cholesterol.
Bak (1989)	107 normo-lipidemic subjects	Parallel	6	Boiled coffee, filtered coffee, or no coffee for 9 weeks	Total and LDL cholesterol levels increased in boiled coffee group. No significant difference in cholesterol levels between filtered-coffee and no-coffee groups.
Aro (1990)	41 healthy subjects	Crossover	5.7	Boiled coffee and filtered coffee for 4 weeks	A dose-dependent increase on serum total and LDL cholesterol and apoprotein B concentrations with boiled coffee.
van Dusseldorp (1991)	64 healthy subjects	Parallel	6	Boiled coffee, filtered coffee, or no coffee for 79 days	Paper filters retain the lipid present in boiled coffee and in that way remove the hypercholesterolemic factor.

(continued)

TABLE 7.2 (Continued)
Effects of Coffee on Serum Lipid and Lipoprotein Concentrations in Clinical Trials

Author	Subjects	Design	Cups/day	Intervention	Results
Ahola (1991)	20 healthy subjects	Crossover	6–10	Boiled coffee or filtered coffee for 4 weeks	Serum total cholesterol, LDL cholesterol, triglyceride, and apoprotein B concentrations were significantly higher during boiled-coffee periods.
Fried (1992)	100 healthy men	Parallel	2.4–4.8	Caffeinated coffee, decaffeinated coffee, or no coffee for 8 weeks	Consumption of filtered, caffeinated coffee leads to an increase in total cholesterol and LDL and HDL cholesterol.
Burr (1995)	261 healthy subjects	Crossover	5	Instant coffee or no coffee for 6 weeks	Consumption of instant coffee leads to an increase in total cholesterol and apolipoprotein B.
Urgert (1996)	46 healthy men and women	Parallel	6	French-press or filtered coffee for 24 weeks	French-press coffee raised LDL cholesterol by 9 mg/dl (0.26 mmol/L) relative to filtered coffee.
de Roos (2000)	46 healthy normolipidemic subjects	Parallel	6	French-press or filtered coffee for 24 weeks	The increase in activity levels of cholesteryl ester transfer protein clearly preceded the increase in LDL cholesterol.
Christensen (2001)	191 filtered coffee drinkers	Parallel	0–≥4	Three groups (0, 1–3, ≥4) of filtered coffee for 6 week	Abstention from coffee for 6 weeks was associated with a decrease in the total cholesterol of 0.28 mmol/L.
Strandhagen (2003)	121 healthy, non-smoking men and women	Crossover	4	3-week placebo, 4-week coffee	Four cups of filtered coffee/day during 4 weeks raised total serum cholesterol by 0.15 to 0.25 mmol/L.

each. In these studies, instant coffee, instant tea, and rosehip tea did not increase the total serum cholesterol, serum lipoprotein (VLDL, LDL, HDL2, HDL3) cholesterol, or the triglyceride concentrations.

Rosmarin et al. (1990) conducted a randomized cross-over clinical trial involving 21 healthy white men who consumed an average of 3.6 cups of coffee a day for 28 days. In this study, coffee consumption did not have an effect on serum total cholesterol, HDL cholesterol, LDL cholesterol, or apolipoprotein B concentrations. Diet, creamer use, and cigarette use as well as group assignment and time factors were controlled in this study.

D'Amicis et al. (1996) performed studies to determine whether giving up Italian coffee might reduce blood cholesterol levels. They randomly assigned 84 young men to three different regimens of coffee consumption: espresso, mocha, and no coffee, but tea. The average daily consumption of espresso and mocha coffee was 3.1 and 2.8 cups per day, respectively. Total cholesterol, HDL cholesterol, LDL cholesterol, and triglycerides were measured eight times during the study. Dietary pattern, alcohol consumption, smoking habits, drug use, and anthropometric data were also taken into consideration. The changes observed in serum cholesterol concentration between baseline and intervention were not found to be statistically different in all the groups studied.

In some clinical trials, coffee consumption has been found to be associated significantly with increases in serum lipids and lipoproteins. For example, Forde et al. (1985) conducted a 10-week trial to assess the effects of coffee consumption and coffee brewing methods on serum cholesterol concentrations. Thirty-three men with hypercholesterolemia were randomly assigned to continue with their usual coffee intake; to stop drinking coffee altogether; or to stop drinking coffee for 5 weeks. After this period of time, the subjects started drinking boiled or filtered coffee. Cholesterol concentrations fell significantly in all subjects abstaining for the first 5 weeks compared to subjects who continued to consume coffee. Cholesterol concentrations continued to fall in those abstaining for 10 weeks.

The cholesterol concentrations rose again in subjects who returned to drinking boiled coffee, but remained the same in those who returned to drinking filtered coffee. Forde et al. (1985) concluded that abstention from heavy coffee drinking is an efficient way to reduce serum cholesterol concentrations in men with hypercholesterolemia.

A number of clinical trials have been performed to compare the effects of boiled and filtered coffee on cholesterol concentrations. The clinical trials indicate that boiled or unfiltered coffee and the coffee diterpene levels in the coffee have a significant effect on serum lipid and lipoprotein concentrations. Aro et al. (1990) evaluated the effects of boiled coffee and filtered coffee on serum lipoproteins in 41 healthy subjects whose serum cholesterol concentrations were less than 7 mmol/L (270.6 mg/dl). The subjects consumed, in random order, boiled coffee and filtered coffee for 4-week periods in a crossover design. The individual daily consumption ranged from 2 to 14 cups (mean 5.7 cups per day) and was similar during both study periods.

Serum total cholesterol, LDL cholesterol, and apolipoprotein B concentrations were higher ($P < 0.001$) and the HDL cholesterol concentrations were lower ($P < 0.05$) with consumption of boiled coffee than with consumption of filtered coffee.

Body weight, apoprotein A-I, and triglycerides remained unchanged. In the 16 subjects who consumed less than five cups of coffee per day, the differences in serum total cholesterol concentration of individuals consuming boiled coffee and filtered coffee periods were nonsignificant (P = 0.16). The differences in serum total cholesterol and LDL cholesterol concentrations between the periods were found to be linearly correlated with the amount of coffee consumed daily ($r = 0.52$, P < 0.001 and $r = 0.33$, P < 0.05, respectively). Other clinical trials have shown that drinking boiled coffee results in higher cholesterol concentrations than does drinking filtered or instant coffee (Ahola et al., 1991; Aro et al., 1987; de Roos et al., 2000; Urget, Meyboom, et al., 1996; van Dusseldorp et al., 1991).

The influence of coffee and caffeine consumption on hemostatic factors was studied in some randomized trials. In one study, 69 subjects received four to six tablets containing 75 mg caffeine or the same amount of placebo tablets, while using decaffeinated coffee (Bak & Grobbee, 1991). Caffeine intake from any other source was not allowed. Although boiled coffee intake raised serum LDL cholesterol, coffee consumption did not have an effect on fibrinogen concentration, clotting factor VII activity, factor VIII antigen level, or on protein C or protein S levels. Likewise, caffeine consumption did not alter the fibrinogen concentrations or the factor VII activities.

Urgert et al. (1997) experimentally studied the influence of coffee on lipoprotein(a) levels in healthy, normolipidemic volunteers in four randomized controlled trials. In 22 subjects who drank five to six cups of strong French-press coffee per day, the median fall in lipoprotein(a) relative to 24 subjects who drank filtered coffee was 1.5 mg/dl after 2 months (P = 0.03), and 0.5 mg/dl after 6 months (P > 0.05). In another study involving two separate trials, coffee oil doses equivalent to 10 to 20 cups of unfiltered coffee reduced lipoprotein(a) levels up to 5.5 mg/dl (P < 0.05). A purified mixture of cafestol and kahweol, as well as cafestol alone, was also found to be effective in reducing Lp(a) levels. Averaged over the four trials, each 10 mg/day of cafestol (plus kahweol), which is the amount present in two to three cups of French-press coffee, significantly decreased Lp(a) levels by 0.5 mg/dl after 4 weeks or 4% from baseline.

Significant associations between filtered-coffee or instant-coffee consumption and serum cholesterol concentrations were found in four clinical trials (Burr et al., 1995; Christensen et al., 2001; Fried et al., 1992; Strandhagen & Thelle, 2003). Fried et al. (1992) conducted a randomized controlled trial with filtered coffee with an 8-week washout period followed by an 8-week intervention period. One hundred healthy men were randomly assigned to drink 720 ml/day of caffeinated coffee, 360 ml/day of caffeinated coffee, or 720 ml/day of decaffeinated coffee or no coffee.

Men who consumed 720 ml/day of caffeinated coffee had increases in plasma total cholesterol (0.24 mmol/L [9.28 mg/dl], P = 0.001), LDL cholesterol (0.17 mmol/L [6.5 mg/dl], P = 0.04), and HDL cholesterol (0.08 mmol/L [3.1 mg/dl], P = 0.03). No significant changes in the plasma lipid and lipoprotein levels occurred in the groups receiving less coffee (360 ml/day) or in the groups receiving decaffeinated coffee or no coffee. Compared with the group that drank no coffee, the group that drank 720 ml/day of caffeinated coffee had increases in total cholesterol of 0.25 mmol/L (9.6 mg/dl; P = 0.02) after adjustment for changes in diet.

In a crossover clinical trial with a relatively large sample size of 261 healthy volunteers, subjects were given five cups of instant coffee or no coffee per day for

6 weeks. During the period of instant-coffee consumption, serum cholesterol concentrations increased by 0.12 mmol/L (4.6 mg/dl) (Burr et al., 1995). A total of 121 healthy, nonsmoking men and women aged 29 to 65 years were included in a controlled study with four consecutive trial periods (Strandhagen & Thelle, 2003).

The first and third periods were 3 weeks of total coffee abstention. The second and fourth periods consisted of 4 weeks with the subjects consuming 600 ml filter-brewed coffee/day. The two coffee abstention periods were associated with a decline in serum cholesterol of 0.22 mmol/L (8.5 mg/dl) (95% CI −0.31, −0.13) and 0.36 mmol/L (13.9 mg/dl) (95% CI −0.46, −0.26), respectively. The authors concluded that a volume of 600 ml (about four cups) of filtered coffee/day during 4 weeks raised total serum cholesterol between 0.15 and 0.25 mmol/L.

In summary, the effect of coffee consumption on cholesterol levels has been studied in about 21 clinical trials. The results from these studies were inconsistent, although more than half of the clinical trials found an effect of coffee on lipid levels, especially those with large sample sizes (Table 7.2). Experiments involving different brewing methods suggest that a major part of the cholesterol-increasing effect can be explained by the method used to brew the coffee. Boiled coffee, for example, was more likely to increase cholesterol levels than filtered coffee.

However, some studies had design problems in that not all of them accounted for the brewing method or the amount of coffee consumed. The inconsistent effect of coffee on serum cholesterol also may be attributable, in part, to the small sample size used in many of the studies, the mild effect that filtered-coffee consumption has on serum cholesterol levels, and the large variance in lipid profiles (Wei et al., 1995).

In a meta-analysis of clinical trials and a large prospective study, each cup of coffee consumed per day was found to be associated with about a 0.052 mmol/L (2 mg/dl) increase in total cholesterol (Jee et al., 2001; Wei et al., 1995). Assuming this is the true effect of a cup of coffee on cholesterol with a standard deviation of 20%, the corresponding sample size for detecting a significant coffee–cholesterol effect with intake of six cups of coffee per day at 80% power would be over 100 subjects in each comparison group, respectively. Unfortunately, only a few of the clinical trials had a sample size greater than 100 subjects in each group (Table 7.2).

Therefore, from a statistical point, it is not surprising that an association was found in some clinic trials but not in others, especially if instant coffee and filtered coffee were used in the clinical trials with small sample sizes. However, four large clinical trials with a sample size of over 100 subjects for instant coffee and filtered coffee all demonstrated the effect of coffee consumption on cholesterol levels (Burr et al., 1995; Christensen et al., 2001; Fried et al., 1992; Strandhagen & Thelle, 2003).

POSSIBLE MECHANISMS—EFFECTS OF COFFEE AND COFFEE CONSTITUENTS ON LIPID AND LIPOPROTEIN METABOLISM

A number of clinical studies have shown that two diterpenes in coffee—cafestol and kahweol—can cause an increase in serum lipid and lipoprotein concentrations (Table 7.3). Several studies have shown that these compounds are in higher concentrations in

TABLE 7.3
Effects of Coffee Oil on Serum Lipid and Lipoprotein Concentrations in Randomized Clinical Trials

Author	Subjects	Design	Intervention	Results
Weusten–Van der Wouw (1994)	15 subjects	Parallel	Pure cafestol and kahweol for 4 to 6 weeks	Coffee oil containing cafestol and kahweol raised serum cholesterol.
Urgert (1995)	15 subjects	Parallel and crossover	Coffee grounds containing cafestol and kahweol	Coffee grounds containing cafestol and kahweol raised serum cholesterol.
Heckers (1994)	10 subjects	Parallel	Pure cafestol and kahweol for 5 weeks	Coffee oil containing cafestol and kahweol raised serum cholesterol.
van Rooij (1995)	36 men and women	Parallel	Arabica coffee oil, Robusta coffee for 6 weeks	Arabica coffee oil elevated serum total cholesterol by 1.1 mmol/L, but Robusta coffee did not.
Mensink (1995)	11 subjects	Crossover	Arabica and Robusta coffee oil or placebo oil	Arabica and Robusta coffee oils elevated serum cholesterol levels.
Urgert (1997)	10 healthy men	Crossover	Cafestol and cafestol + kahweol for 4 weeks	The effect of cafestol on serum lipid concentrations was much larger than the additional effect of kahweol.
Urgert (1997)	46 healthy normolipidemic subjects	Parallel	Coffee, coffee oil, and pure diterpenes for 4 to 24 weeks	Each 10 mg/d of cafestol plus kahweol decreased Lp(a) levels by 0.5 mg/dl or 4% from baseline values after 4 weeks.
van Tol (1997)	10 healthy men	Crossover	Cafestol and kahweol for 4 weeks	Cafestol raised the activity of cholesterylester transfer protein by 18% and activity of phospholipid transfer protein by 21%.
Boekschoten (2003)	32 healthy men	Crossover	3-week placebo, 5-week coffee oil, then 3-week wash out, 3-week placebo, 5-week coffee oil	Coffee oil containing cafestol raised total cholesterol, LDL cholesterol, and triglycerides.

boiled coffee than in filtered coffee (Gross, Jaccaud, & Huggett, 1997; Ratnayake, Hollywood, O'Grady, & Stavric, 1993; Ruiz del Castillo, Herraiz, & Blanch, 1999; Urgert & Katan, 1996, 1997).

Gross et al. (1997) developed a simple and sensitive reverse-phase HPLC method using solid-phase extraction for the analysis of cafestol and kahweol in coffee brews. They found that Scandinavian-style boiled coffee and Turkish-style coffee contained the highest amounts, equivalent to 7.2 and 5.3 mg cafestol per cup and 7.2 and 5.4 mg kahweol per cup, respectively. By contrast, instant and drip-filtered coffee brews contained negligible amounts of these diterpenes, and espresso coffee contained intermediate amounts, about 1 mg cafestol and 1 mg kahweol per cup.

Zock, Katan, Merkus, van Dusseldorp, and Harryvan (1990) first reported that consumption of coffee oil from boiled coffee increases LDL cholesterol concentrations. Ten volunteers consumed coffee oil from boiled coffee for 6 weeks. Serum cholesterol rose in every subject. The mean rise was 0.74 mmol/L (28.6 mg/dl) after 3 weeks. The increase was mainly due to LDL cholesterol, but triglyceride concentrations also increased. The lipid levels returned to baseline when the coffee oil intake was stopped. Recently, the effects of coffee oil on serum lipid response were measured twice in 32 healthy volunteers in two separate 5-week periods (Boekschoten, Engberink, Katan, & Schouten, 2003). Total cholesterol levels increased by 24% in period 1 and 18% in period 2, LDL cholesterol by 29 and 20% in periods 1 and 2, and triglycerides by 66 and 58% in periods 1 and 2.

Weusten–Van der Wouw et al. (1994) examined the effect of purified coffee oils containing cafestol and kahweol on serum cholesterol in 15 volunteers. The serum cholesterol concentrations of subjects who ingested nontriglyceride coffee oil (85 mg of cafestol and 103 mg of kahweol per day) were found to be about 1.2 mmol/L (46 mg/dl) higher than those of the control group. In contrast, coffee oil stripped of cafestol and kahweol had no effect on serum cholesterol levels. These findings provide an explanation for the hypercholesterolemic effect previously observed with coffee oil.

In a randomized, double-blind crossover study, Urgert, Essed, and colleagues (1997) gave 10 healthy male volunteers pure cafestol (61 to 64 mg/day) or a mixture of cafestol (60 mg/d) and kahweol (48 to 54 mg/day) for 28 days. Cafestol raised the total serum cholesterol concentration by 0.79 mmol/L (31 mg/dl), LDL cholesterol by 0.57 mmol/L (22 mg/dl), and triglycerides by 0.65 mmol/L (58 mg/dl). A mixture of cafestol plus kahweol increased total cholesterol by an additional 0.23 mmol/L (9.0 mg/dl), LDL cholesterol by 0.23 mmol/L (9 mg/dl), and triglycerides by 0.09 mmol/L (8 mg/dl) (all $P > 0.05$).

Thus, the effect of cafestol on serum lipid concentrations was much larger than that of kahweol and the hyperlipidemic potential of unfiltered coffee appears to depend mainly on its cafestol content. The effects of purified coffee oils containing cafestol and kahweol on serum cholesterol concentrations were confirmed in a number of other studies (Table 7.3).

The mechanism by which coffee diterpenes influence lipoprotein metabolism is largely unknown (de Roos & Katan, 1999). Only a few *in vitro* studies have been published on this topic. Halvorsen, Ranheim, Nenseter, Huggett, and Drevon (1998) studied the effects of pure cafestol on cholesterol metabolism in human skin fibroblasts (HSF). The uptake of [125I]-labeled tyramine cellobiose-labeled LDL was decreased by about 50% (P < 0.05) after an 18-hour preincubation time with cafestol (20 µg/ml) compared to the control cells. The specific binding of radiolabeled LDL was reduced by 54% (P < 0.05) after preincubation for 18 hours with cafestol. Cafestol also reduced the number of LDL receptors as determined by a protein-normalized Scatchard plot analysis.

Furthermore, they transfected HSF cells with a promoter region for the LDL receptor gene linked to a reporter gene, chloramphenicol acetyl transferase (CAT). No change was seen in the CAT activity after incubation with cafestol (20 µg/ml). Moreover, cafestol caused a 2.3-fold (P < 0.05) higher incorporation of radiolabeled [14C] oleic acid into cholesteryl esters after 24-hour incubation, suggesting an increase in acyl-CoA:cholesterol acyl transferase activity. In addition, cafestol (20 µg/ml) reduced the incorporation of [14C] acetate into cholesterol by about 40% (P < 0.05) after 24 hours of preincubation. The *in vitro* results suggest that cafestol intake may increase plasma cholesterol concentrations via the downregulation of LDL receptors by post-transcriptional mechanisms.

Post, de Wit, and Princen (1997) studied the effects of cafestol and a mixture of cafestol, kahweol, and isokahweol (5 w/w) (Jacobsen & Thelle, 1987b; Jansen et al., 1995) on bile acid synthesis and on cholesterol 7-alpha-hydroxylase and sterol 27-hydroxylase activities in cultured rat hepatocytes. Dose-dependent decreases in bile acid mass production, cholesterol 7 alpha-hydroxylase activities, and sterol 27-hydroxylase activities were found when 20 µg/ml of cafestol was given. Maximal reductions of bile acid mass production, cholesterol 7 alpha-hydroxylase activities, and sterol 27-hydroxylase activities were –91, –79, and –49%, respectively. The mixture of cafestol, kahweol, and isokahweol was less potent in suppression of bile acid synthesis and cholesterol 7-alpha-hydroxylase activity. LDL-receptor, HMG-CoA reductase, and HMG-CoA synthase mRNAs were also significantly decreased by cafestol (–18, –20, and –43%, respectively).

The authors concluded that cafestol suppresses bile acid synthesis by downregulation of cholesterol 7-alpha-hydroxylase and, to a lesser extent, sterol 27-hydroxylase in cultured rat hepatocytes, whereas kahweol and isokahweol are less active. The results suggest that suppression of bile acid synthesis may provide an explanation for increases in cholesterol seen with cafestol intake in humans.

Several clinical studies have been performed to determine whether coffee diterpenes have an effect on lipid transfer proteins and lipid metabolism. van Tol et al. (1997) examined the effect of coffee diterpenes on serum lipid transfer proteins and on lecithin:cholesterol acyltransferase activities in a randomized, double-blind cross-over study with 10 healthy male volunteers. Cafestol (61 to 64 mg/day) or a mixture of cafestol (60 mg/day) and kahweol (48 to 54 mg/day) was given for 28 days.

Cafestol was found to increase the activity of cholesteryl ester transfer protein by 18% and the phospholipid transfer protein by 21% (both P < 0.001). Kahweol did not produce a significant additional effect over that achieved with cafestol. Cafestol plus kahweol, however, reduced lecithin:cholesterol acyltransferase activity by 11% (P = 0.02). The results of the studies indicate that the diterpene-induced increases in cholesterol may be related to increases in phospholipid transfer proteins and to inhibition of lecithin:cholesterol acyltransferase (LCAT) activity.

The long-term effects of unfiltered coffee consumption on the activity levels of cholesteryl ester transfer protein (CETP), phospholipid transfer protein (PLTP), and LCAT have been studied by de Roos et al. (2000). Forty-six healthy normolipidemic subjects consumed 0.9 L of unfiltered French-press or filtered coffee for 24 weeks. Fasting blood samples were obtained after 0, 2, 12, and 24 weeks of intervention and after 12 weeks of follow-up. The consumption of French-press coffee significantly increased CETP activity by 12% after 2 weeks, by 18% after 12 weeks, and by 9% after 24 weeks. PLTP activity was significantly increased by 10% after 12 and 24 weeks. LCAT activity was significantly decreased by 6% after 12 weeks and by 7% after 24 weeks.

The increase in CETP clearly preceded the increase in LDL cholesterol concentration, but not the increase in triglyceride concentrations. However, consumption of French-press coffee caused a persistent rise in CETP activity, whereas the rise in serum triglycerides was transient. The conclusions were that consumption of cafestol and kahweol causes a long-term increase in CETP as well as PLTP activity and that the increase in CETP activity may contribute to the rise in LDL cholesterol.

The diterpenes do not appear to account for all of the cholesterol increases associated with coffee oil consumption. For example, al-Kanhal (1997) conducted a study to identify the cholesterol-raising factors in coffee oil free of the two well-known diterpenes, cafestol and kahweol. This researcher found that female rats fed coffee oil for 4 weeks showed significantly higher levels of plasma cholesterol ($P < 0.01$) and triglycerides ($P < 0.01$). These results provide some evidence that cafestol and kahweol diterpene alcohols may not be the only cholesterol-raising factors in coffee oil. However, the results need to be confirmed in humans.

CONCLUSIONS

The majority of cross-sectional and prospective epidemiological studies found an association between regular coffee consumption and total cholesterol. However, in a few studies coffee intake was not associated with an increase in serum cholesterol concentrations. Consumption of decaffeinated coffee, tea, and cola did not result in increased cholesterol concentrations. Also, HDL cholesterol levels were not found to be related to any kind of coffee or caffeine consumption.

In the majority of clinical trials, boiled coffee raised total cholesterol and LDL cholesterol concentrations. The effect of coffee on cholesterol metabolism appears to be due largely to two diterpenes: cafestol and kahweol. These diterpenes have been shown to be present in much higher concentrations in unfiltered and boiled coffee than in instant or filtered coffee. These findings are consistent with the weak associations found between instant coffee and filtered coffee consumption and cholesterol concentrations and the weak association between instant coffee and filtered coffee consumption and serum cholesterol concentrations found in various clinical trials. *In vitro* experimental studies indicate that cafestol and kahweol might increase serum cholesterol concentrations by suppressing bile acid synthesis, increasing several acyl transferase enzymes, and downregulating LDL receptors.

Long-term intake of boiled coffee and French-press coffee raises total and LDL cholesterol concentrations. For patients with high serum cholesterol who are heavy coffee consumers, a shift from boiled coffee to filtered coffee or no coffee may be clinically important. However, for the general population with normal cholesterol concentrations who are moderate coffee consumers, giving up coffee intake would not lower the risk of cardiovascular diseases significantly (Wei et al., 1995).

REFERENCES

Ahola, I., Jauhiainen, M., & Aro, A. (1991). The hypercholesterolaemic factor in boiled coffee is retained by a paper filter. *Journal of Internal Medicine, 230,* 293–297.

al Kanhal, M. A. (1997). Lipid analysis of *Coffea arabica* Linn. beans and their possible hypercholesterolemic effects. *International Journal of Food Science & Nutrition, 148,* 135–139.

Arnesen, E., Forde, O.H., & Thelle, D.S. (1984). Coffee and serum cholesterol. *British Medical Journal (Clinical Research Edition), 288,* 1960.

Aro, A., Kostiainen, E., Huttunen, J. K., Seppala, E, & Vapaatalo, H. (1985). Effects of coffee and tea on lipoproteins and prostanoids. *Atherosclerosis, 57,* 123–128.

Aro, A., Pietinen, P., Uusitalo, U., & Tuomilehto, J. (1989). Coffee and tea consumption, dietary fat intake and serum cholesterol concentration of Finnish men and women. *Journal of Internal Medicine, 226,* 127–32.

Aro, A., Teirila, J., & Gref, C. G. (1990). Dose-dependent effect on serum cholesterol and apoprotein B concentrations by consumption of boiled, nonfiltered coffee. *Atherosclerosis, 83,* 257–261.

Aro, A., Tuomilehto, J., Kostiainen, E., Uusitalo, U., & Pietinen, P. (1987). Boiled coffee increases serum low density lipoprotein concentration. *Metabolism, 36,* 1027–1030.

Bak, A. A., & Grobbee, D. E. (1989). The effect on serum cholesterol levels of coffee brewed by filtering or boiling. *New England Journal of Medicine, 321,* 1432–1437.

Bak, A. A., & Grobbee, D. E. (1991). Caffeine, blood pressure, and serum lipids. *American Journal of Clinical Nutrition, 53,* 971–975.

Boekschoten, M. V., Engberink, M. F., Katan, M. B., & Schouten, E. G. (2003). Reproducibility of the serum lipid response to coffee oil in healthy volunteers. *Nutrition Journal, 4,* 8.

Brown, C. R., & Benowitz, N. L. (1989). Caffeine and cigarette smoking: Behavioral, cardiovascular, and metabolic interactions. *Pharmacology,Biochemistry, & Behavior, 34,* 565–570.

Burr, M. L., Gallacher, J. E., Butland, B. K., Bolton, C. H., & Downs, L. G. (1989). Coffee, blood pressure and plasma lipids: a randomized controlled trial. *European Journal of Clinical Nutrition, 43,* 7–83.

Burr, M. L., Limb, E. S., Sweetnam, P. M., Fehily, A. M., Amarah, L., & Hutchings, A. (1995). Instant coffee and cholesterol: A randomized controlled trial. *European Journal of Clinical Nutrition, 49,* 779–784.

Carson, C. A., Caggiula, A. W., Meilahn, E. N., Matthews, K. A., & Kuller, L. H. (1994). Coffee consumption: Relationship to blood lipids in middle-aged women. *International Journal of Epidemiology, 23,* 523–527.

Carson, C. A., Cauley, J. A., & Caggiula, A. W. (1993). Relation of caffeine intake to blood lipids in elderly women. *American Journal of Epidemiology, 138,* 94–100.

Christensen, B., Mosdol, A., Retterstol, L., Landaas, S., & Thelle, D. S. (2001). Abstention from filtered coffee reduces the concentrations of plasma homocysteine and serum cholesterol—A randomized controlled trial. *American Journal of Clinical Nutrition, 74,* 302–307.

Curb, J. D., Reed, D. M., Kautz, J. A., & Yano, K. (1986). Coffee, caffeine, and serum cholesterol in Japanese men in Hawaii. *American Journal of Epidemiology, 123*, 648–655.

D'Amicis, A., Scaccini, C., Tomassi, G., Anaclerio, M., Stornelli, R., & Bernini, A. (1996). Italian style brewed coffee: effect on serum cholesterol in young men. *International Journal of Epidemiology, 25*, 513–520.

Davis, B. R., Curb, J. D., Borhani, N. O., Prineas, R. J., & Molteni, A. (1988). Coffee consumption and serum cholesterol in the hypertension detection and follow-up program. *American Journal of Epidemiology, 128*, 124–136.

Dawber, T. R., Kannel, W. B., & Gordon, T. (1974). Coffee and cardiovascular disease. Observations from the Framingham study. *New England Journal of Medicine, 291*, 871–874.

de Roos, B., & Katan, M. B. (1999). Possible mechanisms underlying the cholesterol-raising effect of the coffee diterpene cafestol. *Current Opinion in Lipidology, 10*, 41–45.

de Roos, B., Van Tol, A., Urgert, R, Scheek, L. M., Van Gent, T., Buytenhek, R., Princen, H. M., & Katan, M. B. (2000). Consumption of French-press coffee raises cholesteryl ester transfer protein activity levels before LDL cholesterol in normolipidaemic subjects. *Journal of Internal Medicine, 248*, 211–216.

Donahue, R. P., Orchard, T. J., Stein, E. A., & Kuller, L. H. (1987). Lack of an association between coffee consumption and lipoprotein lipids and apolipoproteins in young adults: The Beaver County Study. *Preventive Medicine, 16*, 796–802.

Du, Y., Melchert, H. U., Knopf, H., Braemer–Hauth, M., Gerding, B., & Pabel, E. (1999). Association of serum caffeine concentrations with blood lipids in caffeine-drug users and nonusers—Results of German National Health Surveys from 1984 to 1999. *European Journal of Epidemiology, 20*, 311–316.

Folsom, A. R. (1984). Does dietary fat intake confound coffee lipids association? *CVD Epidemiology News Letter AHA, 35*, 53.

Forde, O. H., Knutsen, S. F., Arnesen, E., & Thelle, D. S. (1985). The Tromso Heart Study: Coffee consumption and serum lipid concentrations in men with hypercholestero-laemia: A randomized intervention study. *British Medical Journal (Clinical Research Edition), 290*, 893–895.

Fried, R. E., Levine, D. M., Kwiterovich, P. O., Diamond, E. L., Wilder, L. B., Moy, T. F., & Pearson, T. A. (1992). The effect of filtered-coffee consumption on plasma lipid levels. Results of a randomized clinical trial. *JAMA, 267*, 811–815.

Green, M. S., & Harari, G. (1992). Association of serum lipoproteins and health-related habits with coffee and tea consumption in free-living subjects examined in the Israeli CORDIS Study. *Preventive Medicine, 21*, 532–545.

Gross, G., Jaccaud, E., & Huggett, A. C. (1997). Analysis of the content of the diterpenes cafestol and kahweol in coffee brews. *Food & Chemical Toxicologgy, 35*, 54.

Haffner, S. M., Knapp, J. A., Stern, M. P., Hazuda, H. P., Rosenthal, M., & Franco, L. J. (1985). Coffee consumption, diet, and lipids. *American Journal of Epidemiology, 122*, 1–12.

Halvorsen, B., Ranheim, T., Nenseter, M. S., Huggett, A. C., & Drevon, C. A. (1998). Effect of a coffee lipid (cafestol) on cholesterol metabolism in human skin fibroblasts. *Journal of Lipid Research, 39*, 901–912.

Hofman, A. & Klein, F. (1983). Coffee and cholesterol. *New England Journal of Medicine, 309*, 1249.

Jacobsen, B. K., & Thelle, D. S. (1987a). The Tromso Heart Study: Food habits, serum total cholesterol, HDL cholesterol, and triglycerides. *American Journal of Epidemiology, 125*, 622–630.

Jacobsen, B. K., & Thelle, D. S. (1987b). The Tromso Heart Study: Is coffee drinking an indicator of a lifestyle with high risk for ischemic heart disease? *Acta Medica Scandinavica, 222*, 215–221.

Jansen, D., Nedeljkovic, S., Feskens, E. J., Ostojic, M. C., Gruijic, M. Z., et al. (1995). Coffee consumption, alcohol use, and cigarette smoking as determinants of serum total and HDL cholesterol in two Serbian cohorts of the Seven Countries Study. *Arteriosclerosis, Thrombosis, and Vascular Biology*, 15, 1793–1797.

Jee, S. H., He, J., Appel, L. J., Whelton, P. K., Suh, I., & Klag, M. J. (2001). Coffee consumption and serum lipids: A meta-analysis of randomized controlled clinical trials. *American Journal of Epidemiology*, *153*, 353–362.

Kark, J. D., Friedlander, Y., Kaufmann, N. A., & Stein, Y. (1985). Coffee, tea, and plasma cholesterol: The Jerusalem Lipid Research Clinic Prevalence Study. *British Medical Journal (Clinical Research Edition)*, *291*, 699–704.

Klatsky, A. L., Petitti, D. B., Armstrong, M. A., & Friedman, G. D. (1985). Coffee, tea and cholesterol. *American Journal of Cardiology*, *55*, 577–578.

Kovar, M. G., & Feinleib, M. (1983). Coffee and cholesterol. *New England Journal of Medicine*, *309*, 1249.

Lancaster, T., Muir, J., & Silagy, C. (1994). The effects of coffee on serum lipids and blood pressure in a U.K. population. *Journal of the Royal Society of Medicine*, *87*, 506–507.

Lindahl, B., Johansson, I., Huhtasaari, F., Hallmans, G., & Asplund, K. (1991). Coffee drinking and blood cholesterol—Effects of brewing method, food intake and life style. *Journal of Internal Medicine*, *230*, 299–305.

Miyake, Y., Kono, S., Nishiwaki, M., Hamada, H. Nishikawa, H., Koga, H., & Ogawa, S. (1999). Relationship of coffee consumption with serum lipids and lipoproteins in Japanese men. *Annals of Epidemiology*, *9*, 121–126.

Phillips, N. R., Havel, R. J., & Kane, J. P. (1981). Levels and interrelationships of serum and lipoprotein cholesterol and triglycerides. Association with adiposity and the consumption of ethanol, tobacco, and beverages containing caffeine. *Arteriosclerosis*, *1*, 13–24.

Pietinen, P., Aro, A., Tuomilehto, J., Uusitalo, U., & Korhonen, H. (1990). Consumption of boiled coffee is correlated with serum cholesterol in Finland. *International Journal of Epidemiology*, *19*, 586–590.

Post, S.M., de Wit, E. C., & Princen, H. M. (1997). Cafestol, the cholesterol-raising factor in boiled coffee, suppresses bile acid synthesis by down regulation of cholesterol 7 alpha-hydroxylase and sterol 27-hydroxylase in rat hepatocytes. *Arteriosclerosis Thrombosis & Vascular Biology*, *17*, 3064–3070.

Puccio, E. M., McPhillips, J. B., Barrett–Connor, E., & Ganiats, T. G. (1990). Clustering of therogenic behaviors in coffee drinkers. *American Journal of Public Health*, *80*, 1310–1313.

Ratnayake, W. M., Hollywood, R., O'Grady, E., & Stavric, B. (1993). Lipid content and composition of coffee brews prepared by different methods. *Food & Chemical Toxicology*, *31*, 263–269.

Rosmarin, P. C., Applegate, W. B., & Somes, G. W. (1990). Coffee consumption and serum lipids: A randomized, crossover clinical trial. *American Journal of Medicine*, *88*, 349–356.

Ruiz del Castillo, M. L., Herraiz, M., & Blanch, G. P. (1999). Rapid analysis of cholesterol-elevating compounds in coffee brews by off-line high-performance liquid chromatography/high-resolution gas chromatography. *Journal of Agricultural & Food Chemistry*, 47, 1525–1529.

Salvaggio, A., Periti, M., Miano, L., Quaglia, G., & Marzorati, D. (1991). Coffee and cholesterol, an Italian study. *American Journal of Epidemiology*, *134*, 149–156.

Sanguigni, V., Gallu, M., Ruffini, M. P., & Strano, A. (1995). Effects of coffee on serum cholesterol and lipoproteins: The Italian brewing method. Italian Group for the Study of Atherosclerosis and Dismetabolic Diseases, Rome II Center. *European Journal of Epidemiology*, *11*, 75–78.

Schwarz, B., Bischof, H. P., & Kunze, M. (1990). Coffee and cardiovascular risk: Epidemiological findings in Austria. *International Journal of Epidemiology, 19*, 894–898.

Shekelle, R. G. & Paul, O. (1983). Coffee and cholesterol. *New England Journal of Medicine, 309*, 1249.

Solvoll, K., Selmer, R., Loken, E. B., Foss, O. P., & Trygg, K. (1989). Coffee, dietary habits, and serum cholesterol among men and women 35 to 49 years of age. *American Journal of Epidemiology, 129*, 1277–1288.

Stensvold, I., Tverdal, A., & Foss, O. P. (1989). The effect of coffee on blood lipids and blood pressure. Results from a Norwegian cross-sectional study, men and women, 40 to 42 years. *Journal of Clinical Epidemiology, 42*, 877–884.

Strandhagen, E., & Thelle, D. S. (2003). Filtered coffee raises serum cholesterol: Results from a controlled study. *European Journal of Clinical Nutrition, 57*, 1164–1168.

Superko, H. R., Bortz, W., Williams, P. T., Albers, J. J., & Wood, P. D. (1991). Caffeinated and decaffeinated coffee effects on plasma lipoprotein cholesterol, apolipoproteins, and lipase activity: A controlled, randomized trial. *American Journal of Clinical Nutrition, 54*, 599–605.

Thelle, D. S. (1991). Coffee and cholesterol: what is brewing? *Journal of Internal Medicine, 230*, 289–291.

Thelle, D. S. (1995). Coffee, tea and coronary heart disease. *Current Opinions in Lipidology, 6*, 25–27.

Thelle, D. S., Arnesen, E., & Forde, O. H. (1983). The Tromso Heart Study. Does coffee raise serum cholesterol? *New England Journal of Medicine, 308*, 1454–1457.

Thelle, D. S., Heyden, S., & Fodor, J. G. (1987). Coffee and cholesterol in epidemiological and experimental studies. *Atherosclerosis, 67*, 97–103.

Thompson, W. G. (1994). Coffee: brew or bane? *American Journal of Medical Sciences, 308*, 49–57.

Tuomilehto, J., Tanskanen, A., Pietinen, P., Aro, A., Salonen, J. T., Happonen, P., Nissinen, A., & Puska, P. (1987). Coffee consumption is correlated with serum cholesterol in middle-aged Finnish men and women. *Journal of Epidemiology & Community Health, 41*, 237–242.

Urgert, R., Essed, N., van der Weg, G., Kosmeijer–Schuil, T. G., & Katan, M. B. (1997). Separate effects of the coffee diterpenes cafestol and kahweol on serum lipids and liver aminotransferases. *American Journal of Clinical Nutrition, 65*, 519–524.

Urgert, R., & Katan, M. B. (1996). The cholesterol-raising factor from coffee beans. *Journal of the Royal Society of Medicine, 89*, 618–623.

Urgert, R., & Katan, M. B. (1997). The cholesterol-raising factor from coffee beans. *Annual Review of Nutrition, 17*, 305–324.

Urgert, R., Kosmeijer–Schuil, T. G., & Katan, M. B. (1996). Intake levels, sites of action and excretion routes of the cholesterol-elevating diterpenes from coffee beans in humans. *Biochemical Society Transactions, 24*, 800–806.

Urgert, R., Meyboom, S., Kuilman, M., Rexwinkel, H., Vissers, M. N., Klerk, M. & Katan M. B. (1996). Comparison of effect of cafetiere and filtered coffee on serum concentrations of liver aminotransferases and lipids: Six-month randomized controlled trial. *British Medical Journal, 313*, 1362–1366.

Urgert, R., Weusten–van der Wouw, M. P., Hovenier, R., Lund–Larsen, P. G., & Katan, M. B. (1996). Chronic consumers of boiled coffee have elevated serum levels of lipoprotein(a). *Journal of Internal Medicine, 240*, 367–371.

Urgert, R., Weusten–van der Wouw, M. P., Hovenier, R., Meyboom, S., Beynen, A. C., & Katan, M. B. (1997). Diterpenes from coffee beans decrease serum levels of lipoprotein(a) in humans: results from four randomized controlled trials. *European Journal of Clinical Nutrition, 51*, 431–436.

van Dusseldorp, M., & Katan, M. B. (1990). The effect of coffee on serum cholesterol level. *Nederlands Tijdschrift Geneeskunde, 134*, 2325–2327.

van Dusseldorp, M., Katan, M. B., & Demacker, P. N. (1990). Effect of decaffeinated versus regular coffee on serum lipoproteins. A 12-week double-blind trial. *American Journal of Epidemiology, 132*, 33–40.

van Dusseldorp, M., Katan, M. B., van Vliet, T., Demacker, P. N., & Stalenhoef, A. F. (1991). Cholesterol-raising factor from boiled coffee does not pass a paper filter. *Arteriosclerosis Thrombosis, 11*, 586–593.

van Tol, A., Urgert, R., de Jong–Caesar, R., van Gemt, T., Scheek, L. M., de Roos, B., & Jatan, M. B. (1997). The cholesterol-raising diterpenes from coffee beans increase serum lipid transfer protein activity levels in humans. *Atherosclerosis, 132*, 251–254.

Wahrburg, U., Martin, H., Schulte, H., Walek, T., & Assmann, G. (1994). Effects of two kinds of decaffeinated coffee on serum lipid profiles in healthy young adults. *European Journal of Clinical Nutrition, 48*, 172–179.

Wei, M., Macera, C. A., Hornung, C. A., & Blair, S. N. (1995). The impact of changes in coffee consumption on serum cholesterol. *Journal of Clinical Epidemiology, 48*, 1189–1196.

Weusten–Van der Wouw, M. P., Katan, M. B., Viani, R., Huggett, A. C., Liardon, R., Liardon, R., Kund–Karsen, P. G., Thelle, D. S., Ahola, I., Aro, A., et al.(1994). Identity of the cholesterol-raising factor from boiled coffee and its effects on liver function enzymes. *Journal of Lipid Research, 35*, 721–733.

Zock, P. L., Katan, M. B., Merkus, M. P., van Dusseldorp, & Harryvan, J. L. (1990). Effect of a lipid-rich fraction from boiled coffee on serum cholesterol. *Lancet, 335*, 1235–1237.

Section III

Menstrual and Reproductive Effects

8 Menstrual Endocrinology and Pathology: Caffeine, Physiology, and PMS

Hoa T. Vo, Barry D. Smith, and Solmaz Elmi

CONTENTS

Biological, psychological, and social factors that may individually and interactively affect the menstrual cycle and related disorders have been subjected to considerable research over the past several decades. Concern with issues relating to women's health began in the mid-19th century in post–Industrial Revolution Europe and North America, when a new wave of feminism was breaking. Early work focused on normative experiences of women across the menstrual cycle. Thereafter, investigators began to focus on mood and behavioral changes during the cycle (Walker, 1997), and this focus eventually led to the identification and study of premenstrual syndrome (PMS).

Menarche occurs on average at age 12.34 in the United States (Anderson & Must, 2005) and continues until menopause, which occurs, on average, at age 51 (NIA, 2006). There is, of course, considerable individual variability in the menstrual cycle and a woman's experience of that cycle, with biological parameters and psychosocial experiences varying from woman to woman (James, 1997). The length of the menstrual cycle varies as a function of a number of biological and environmental factors (National Women's Health Information Center [NWHIC], 2004).

In some women, the cycle is associated with significant mood changes, often accompanied by physical symptoms, that can be debilitating and may result in functional impairment. Such symptomatology results from sensitivity to changes in the levels of reproductive hormones across the cycle, sometimes exacerbated by environmental stressors (Lustyk, Widman, Paschane, & Olson, 2004). When mood dysregulation and associated symptoms are substantial, a woman can meet diagnostic criteria for PMS. The present chapter reviews what is known about the menstrual cycle, PMS, and, particularly, the role of caffeine in the overall cycle and the disorder.

McLean and Graham (2002) examined the effects of menstrual functions on caffeine metabolism by comparing men and women. The authors suspect that there are sex differences in the rate at which caffeine is metabolized. However, results showed little difference in the pharmacokinetics of caffeine between the two sexes, and caffeine metabolism did not vary substantially from one phase of the menstrual cycle in women to another. The results of this relatively recent investigation notwithstanding, other studies have often demonstrated that caffeine metabolism is affected by menstrual physiology and that the drug may, in turn, alter symptomatology across the cycle (Balogh, Irmisch, Klinger, Splinter, & Hoffmann, 1987; Dalton, 1979; Rubinow, Hoban, & Grover, 1988; Schmidt et al., 2000).

CAFFEINE AND PMS: AN OVERVIEW

Although few researchers have examined gender differences in caffeine metabolism, there has been increasing interest in recent years in examining the effect of caffeine consumption on endocrinological (Khan–Sabir & Carr, 2004; Schmidt et al., 2000; Tsafriri, 1994), physiological (Balogh et al., 1987; Kaminori, Joubert, Otterstetter, Santaromana, & Eddington, 1999; Severino & Moline, 1988), psychological (Berlin, Jamuna, Schmidt, Adams, & Rubinow, 2001; Coppen & Kessel, 1963; Subhash & Shashi, 2002), and social (Miller, 2002; Parlee, 1973, 1974; Walker, 1995) parameters related to the menstrual cycle and premenstrual dysfunction. Researchers have examined the effect of caffeine on the output of various reproductive hormones, such as follicle-stimulating hormone (FSH), luteinizing hormone (LH), estrogen, and progesterone. Impact on menstrual cycle length and duration of menses has also been studied. Other work has investigated the interactions of caffeine consumption with personality traits and expectation biases, particularly as these relate to premenstrual dysfunction.

CAFFEINE: BIOLOGICAL AND ENVIRONMENTAL VARIABLES

Caffeine is a methylxanthine that acts primarily as an antagonist of adenosine A1 and A2 receptors to produce its basic biological effects. The downstream impact of adenosine receptor inhibition is reflected in a number of biological substrates, including some of those involved in regulating the menstrual cycle. These physiological effects of the drug interact with a number of biological and psychological factors potentially to alter its pharmacokinetics and pharmacodynamics and thereby its overall impact on body systems and behavior. The rate of caffeine absorption, for example, is slowed by the presence of food in the stomach (Institute of Medicine, 2001), and psychological stress can act to exacerbate certain effects of caffeine, such as increases in blood pressure (Lustyk et al., 2004).

Of particular interest in this chapter are the physiology and psychology of the menstrual cycle as these interact with the presence of caffeine in the body. Hormonal physiology changes systematically across the several phases of the cycle, and some studies suggest that these changes affect the processing of caffeine. In particular, elimination of the drug is approximately 25% slower during the luteal phase of the menstrual cycle when progesterone levels are highest (see later discussion), as compared with the follicular phase, when progesterone and estrogen levels are lower (Balogh et al., 1987; Institute of Medicine, 2001; James, 1997). Although this finding is consistent across studies, it remains unclear why progesterone level affects caffeine elimination rates.

Other specific variables that can also moderate the rate of clearance are: gender (slightly faster in women than in men; Kaminori et al., 1999), cigarette smoking (which can double clearance rate), and oral contraceptives (which decrease clearance rate; Kaminori et al., 1999; Patwardhan, Desmond, Johnson, & Schenker, 1980). These conditions can enter into complex interactions with baseline menstrual phase physiology to further affect caffeine elimination.

THE MENSTRUAL CYCLE

The menstrual cycle is divided into three phases, with the onset of menstrual bleeding designated as the beginning of the first phase. The three phases are: (a) the menstrual phase, Days 1 to 5; (b) the follicular phase (also called the preovulatory or proliferative phase), Days 5 to 13; and (c) the luteal (also called secretory) phase, Days 14 to 28 or 30 (Severino & Moline, 1988). Between the follicular and luteal phases, (around Day 13 or 14) ovulation takes place (Walker, 1997). A typical menses lasts from 3 to 5 days. The menstrual flow consists of blood and tissue from the uterus. A cycle begins on the first day of a period and typically lasts for 28 to 30 days. However, depending on individual differences, a cycle may last anywhere from 23 to 35 days (Khan–Sabir & Carr, 2004; NWHIC, 2004). The menstrual cycle is typically least regular around the extremes of reproductive life—menarche and menopause—due to anovulation and inadequate follicular development (Apter, Raisanen, Ylostalo, & Vihko, 1987; Fraser, Michie, Wide, & Baird, 1973; NWHIC, 2004).

The endocrinology of the menstrual cycle involves a series of phase-differentiated hormonal changes. During Days 1 to 6, follicle-stimulating hormone (FSH) and luteinizing hormone (LH) levels are increased relative to baseline. Estrogen and progesterone levels are low at this stage. Beginning approximately 8 days into the cycle, FSH levels decrease due to negative feedback at the level of the pituitary gland and estradiol levels increase due to previous stimulation by FSH at the level of the ovary (Tsafriri, 1994). One day before ovulation, a surge in LH occurs and FSH levels also increase and then begin to decrease toward baseline levels almost immediately. By the time ovulation occurs, LH and FSH are on the decline.

Progesterone and, to a lesser extent, estrogen are produced by the corpus luteum, which evolves under the influence of the pre-ovulatory surge in LH. LH and FSH are under negative feedback control by these ovarian hormones at the level of the pituitary gland. In the absence of fertilization, the corpus luteum degenerates and progesterone and estrogen levels subsequently fall. At Day 28 of the average menstrual cycle, estrogen and progesterone are at their lowest levels. Negative feedback on FSH is removed, and FSH secretion can again increase to trigger the onset of the next cycle.

During the follicular phase of the menstrual cycle, folliculogenesis ensues. It begins when a primordial follicle is recruited into a pool of developing follicles and typically terminates with ovulation (Khan–Sabir & Carr, 2004). Once menses begins, FSH levels decline due to the negative feedback of estrogen and the negative effects of inhibin produced by the developing follicle (Sawetawan et al., 1996; Tsafriri, 1994). FSH activates the aromatase enzyme in granulosa cells, which converts androgens to estrogen (Khan–Sabir & Carr, 2004). A decline in FSH levels leads to the production of a more androgenic microenvironment within adjacent follicles, contributing to the growth of a dominant follicle. The granulosa cells of the growing follicle also secrete a variety of peptides that may play an autocrine/paracrine role in the inhibition of development of the adjacent follicles.

After ovulation, the corpus luteum (a transient endocrine organ) secretes progesterone. This is then followed by a secondary rise in estrogen levels during the midluteal phase with a decrease at the end of the menstrual cycle. The secondary rise in estradiol parallels the rise of serum progesterone and 17-hydroxyprogesterone. Ovarian vein studies confirm that the corpus luteum is the site of steroid production during the luteal phase (Niswender & Nett, 1994). Of particular interest in this chapter is the question of how caffeine affects the menstrual cycle and how its pharmacokinetics is affected by changing menstrual physiology.

PREMENSTRUAL SYNDROME

The considerable interest in studying the menstrual cycle in the 1800s soon spread to investigations of a phenomenon called premenstrual syndrome (PMS). During its infancy, the study of PMS was primarily focused on methodological issues involving diagnosis and measurement (Endicott, 2000). Most work focused on such efforts as determining the symptoms that best differentiate PMS from other psychiatric disorders (e.g., depression, anxiety) and constructing questionnaires that would reflect the definition of the disorder (e.g., Backstrom & Carstensen, 1974; Backstrom & Mattson, 1975). Empirical studies of PMS then turned to the testing of early etiological theories, such as a progesterone deficiency hypothesis (Dalton, 1979; Wyatt, Dimmock, & O'Brien, 2000), which have received only minimal support (Schmidt, Grover, & Rubinow, 1994; Schmidt et al., 2000).

The current research definition of PMS in the United States was established at a 1983 workshop at the National Institutes of Mental Health (NIMH, 1983; Rubinow & Roy–Byrne, 1984). The basic diagnostic criterion is a difference of 30% between premenstrual and postmenstrual mood scores on The Daily Rating Form (DRF; Endicott, Schacht, & Halbreich, 1981) or The Self-Rating Scale for Premenstrual Tension Syndrome (PMTS-SR; Steiner, Haskett, & Carroll, 1980). The most common physical symptoms are abdominal bloating, headaches, muscle and joint pain, and breast tenderness

(Gotthell, Steinberg, & Granger, 1999). The behavioral and emotional symptoms most commonly observed in women with PMS are fatigue, poor concentration, mood lability, irritability, and depression (Dickerson, Mazyck, & Hunter, 2003).

An alternative definition is found in the *International Classification of Diseases* (*ICD*). According to the *ICD*-10, PMS is diagnosed if one or more of the following symptoms is experienced during the luteal phase and ends with the onset of menses: minor psychological discomfort, bloating or weight gain, breast tenderness, muscular tension, aches and pains (including headaches), poor concentration, or changes in appetite (WHO, 1992). Other frequently seen symptoms include depression, irritability, anger, and short temper (Endicott, 2000). Some symptoms that indicate severe forms of PMS can include moderate to severe depression, hot flashes, and sleep disturbances (Sullivan, 2003).

With some variability across studies, approximately 30 to 40% of women meet diagnostic criteria for premenstrual syndrome (ACOG, 2000; NWHIC, 2004). A recent cross-sectional, population-based study involving 1,395 women aged 15 to 49 yielded prevalence rates of 60.3% on a self-report measure, but only 25.2% when daily ratings and behavioral functional measures (interference with school, work, etc.) were used. The predominant premenstrual symptoms reported were irritability, abdominal discomfort, nervousness, headache, fatigue, and breast pain (Silva, Cigante, Carret, & Fassa, 2006). The authors especially noted that higher risk was present in women of higher socioeconomic and educational levels, those under 30 years of age, and Caucasians.

PREMENSTRUAL DYSPHORIC DISORDER

Although more than a quarter of women who menstruate have PMS, only about 3 to 8% of these experience premenstrual dysphoric disorder (PMDD; APA 2000; NWHIC, 2004). Although PMS is not included in the current *Diagnostic and Statistical Manual* (*DSM-IV*) as a formally recognized psychiatric disorder, PMDD is included in the appendix (APA, 1994). The designation is intended to alert diagnosticians to a combination of specific severe symptoms of PMDD that could mimic other psychiatric disorders, with the exception that the symptoms occur only in the premenstrual phase of the menstrual cycle. To meet diagnostic criteria for PMDD, patients must experience at least five symptoms associated with the disorder, and one of those symptoms must be dysphoric mood.

Much like PMS, PMDD is to be diagnosed using at least 2 months of prospective daily diaries, and the reported symptoms must occur during the late luteal phase of most menstrual cycles. The symptoms must also remit at or shortly after the onset of menses and completely resolve within a week of onset (Endicott, 2000). There must also be a clear interval of at least 7 to 10 days during each menstrual cycle when a woman feels well mentally and physically (Walker, 1997).

ETIOLOGY OF PMS AND PMDD

Several theories have addressed the etiology of PMDD and PMS. Collectively, they attempt to take into account physiological, psychological, and psychosocial components of the syndromes. These factors are hypothesized to interact with each other to cause the syndrome and to exacerbate its symptomatology.

Physiological Factors

The most basic factor in PMS and PMDD may be a genetic predisposition. Evidence suggests that genetic factors may be important in regulation of the hormonal substrates involved in premenstrual symptoms (FitzGerald et al., 1997; Li & Thompson, 2001). Monozygotic (MZ) twins have significantly higher concordance than do dizygotic (DZ) twins for heaviness of menstrual flow and menstrual pain (Silberg, Martin, & Heath, 1987). In addition, model-fitting provides support for the hypothesis that MZ twins display higher concordance for PMS than do DZ twins (Silberg et al., 1987; Condon, 1993). However, the exact expression of the genetic component and its role in the disorder are not yet well understood (Silberstein & Merriam, 2000).

The more proximal physiology of the menstrual disorders is concerned with the impact of cyclical variations in the levels of ovarian steroids. Although these reproductive hormones have been extensively investigated, their role in PMS remains unclear. One possibility is that the steroids are structurally or functionally anomalous in women with PMS, perhaps as a result of the genetic predisposition. However, it appears more likely that PMS patients are simply more sensitive to the effects of estrogen, progesterone, or both and that the steroids are normal (Schmidt et al., 2000).

We know that the ovarian steroids have complex signaling pathways that affect a substantial variety of organ systems and physiological substrates (NIAAA Working Group, 2005). Of particular interest is the neuroregulatory potential of these biochemicals, which exert influence in a number of brain structures, including the basal forebrain, hippocampus, caudate-putamen, midbrain raphe, and brainstem locus coeruleus. They interact in complex ways with neurotransmitters, including serotonin, and with neuropeptides, and these interactions may theoretically contribute to the mood changes that are symptomatic of PMS (Walker, 1995). It is important to note, however, that the complexities of ovarian steroid signaling have made definitive knowledge of their role in PMS elusive.

In addition, some researchers have noted the need to investigate the role of the pituitary hormones, FSH and LH, and have garnered evidence that the reproductive steroids modulate the activity of the hypothalamic–pituitary–adrenal (HPA) axis. Because the HPA axis is dysregulated in depression—a primary symptom of PMS—it may well be that the disorder involves, in part, the modulatory actions of the steroids. Indeed, recent work has shown that women with PMS, when symptomatic, exhibit an abnormal response to progesterone, though they do not show the pattern of HPA axis anomalies seen in major depression (Roca et al., 2003).

Consistent with the progesterone findings, a major current hypothesis is that the irritability, anxiety, tension, and mood swings characteristic of PMS are caused, in part, by a relative deficiency of progesterone (Munday, 1997), which affects amino acid levels and lipid metabolism (Merck Source, 2004). Research in this area has focused on the role of deficiencies in the anesthetic progesterone metabolites, especially allopregnanolone, in PMS. To study the effects of progesterone deficiency, Rapkin and colleagues (1997) examined the level of allopregnanolone in 36 PMS patients and controls and found that its serum concentration was lower in those with PMS than in controls during the luteal phase.

Furthermore, the authors hypothesize that diminished concentrations of allo-pregnanolone may lead to an inability to enhance gamma-aminobutyric acid (GABA)-mediated inhibition during states of altered central nervous system excitability, such as those accompanying ovulation and stress. The lowered metabolite levels could contribute to the mood symptoms seen in PMS. However, a meta-analysis of 14 randomized trials examining progesterone and progestogen therapy for PMS showed no overall difference in outcomes between progesterone and placebo (Wyatt et al., 2001). Clearly, further research is needed to evaluate the role of progesterone in PMS.

The role of estrogen has also been examined in a number of studies. Schmidt and colleagues (2000) studied 34 women, ages 44 to 55, with onset of depression coinciding with perimenopause, as confirmed by hormone measures and standardized diagnostic interviews. The women were randomly assigned to receive estrogen or placebo for 3 to 6 weeks. Using standardized symptom rating scales and structured interviews, the researchers confirmed that estrogen significantly boosted mood in 80% of the depressed women, as compared with only 20% on placebo. The degree of relief and the time required to achieve a therapeutic effect—about 3 weeks—were comparable to what is typically seen with antidepressant drugs. Among depression symptoms that improved with the hormone were early morning awakening, loss of enjoyment, sadness, and irritability. Among symptoms that failed to improve were sexual interest and disturbed sleep.

Furthermore, the authors found that blood concentrations of estrogen (estradiol) prior to the study and after hormone treatment did not predict therapeutic response. This suggests that the beneficial effects of estrogen are not mediated by correcting abnormally low levels of the hormone. Rather, Schmidt and colleagues (2000) suggest that some women may be especially sensitive to changing hormone levels. As with disorders like PMS and postpartum depression, such hormonal changes appear to be necessary, but not sufficient, to trigger perimenopausal depression. Although it remains uncertain whether excessive or deficient estrogen and progesterone cause PMS, it is clear that women with PMS tend to have exaggerated responses to normal changes in both hormones. Rapid shifts in these two hormones therefore facilitate the abnormal emotional and physical responses seen in women with PMS.

Personality and Psychopathology

Physiological factors do not constitute the only influences on the menstrual cycle and related disorders. Psychological and psychosocial factors have also been implicated by theory and research. The principal personality factor studied in connection with premenstrual disorder is neuroticism, which has been shown in a number of investigations to be correlated positively with a diagnosis of PMS (Berlin et al., 2001; Coppen & Kessel, 1963; Slade & Jenner, 1980). This association is, however, neither direct nor simple.

First, neuroticism is also associated with the occurrence of a number of other syndromes, including anxiety and somatoform disorders (Hettema, Prescott, & Kendler, 2004). In addition, neuroticism displays substantial heritability (Keller, Coventry,

Heath, & Martin, 2005; Beem et al., 2005), thereby complicating its correlation with PMS. Further research will thus be needed to understand more fully the role of neuroticism in PMS and to determine what other personality factors may also be involved, if any.

The premenstrual syndromes display substantial comorbidity with *DSM-IV* Axis I pathologies, including anxiety disorders (Kim, Gyulai, Freeman, Morrison, & Baldassano, 2004) and, particularly, depression. Subhash and Shashi (2002) suggest that 30 to 76% of women diagnosed with PMDD have a lifetime history of depression, as compared with 15% of women without PMDD. This finding is confirmed by a number of other studies (Halbreich, Endicott, & Lasser, 1985; Hart, Coleman, & Russell, 1987; Kim et al., 2004; Kornstein et al., 2005; Schuckit, Daly, Herrman, & Hineman, 1975; Wetzel, Reich, McClure, & Wild, 1975; Halbreich & Endicott, 1985; Hart et al., 1987; Roca, Schmidt, & Rubinow, 1999; Rubinow & Roy–Byrne, 1984).

This raises the question of whether PMS is an entirely separate diagnostic entity in which hormonal changes trigger cyclical depression or whether major depression is the primary disorder. Another possibility is that the co-occurrence of PMS and affective disorders simply reflects inadequate diagnostic differentiation (Haskett, Steiner, & Carroll, 1984).

Psychosocial Factors

Even though social learning theories of PMS are seen as the stepchild of this research field, the focus of this perspective on stereotypical beliefs and reporting biases may be important. For instance, some theorists attribute reported PMS symptoms to psychosocially biased perceptions based on culturally learned, stereotyped beliefs about menstruation (Paige, 1971; Parlee, 1973, 1974), rather than actual experiences. Additionally, Ruble (1977) showed that women who believed they were in the premenstrual phase reported more symptoms than women who believed otherwise, regardless of which actual cycle phase they were in. Although this social learning perspective cannot completely explain PMS, it does point to the need to examine the role of society and culture in the patient's experience of the disorder.

Accordingly, some investigators have evaluated the role of cultural factors in PMS. Many cultures convey very negative views of menstruation and, in particular, of premenstrual syndrome (Chrisler & Levy, 1990; Coutts & Berg, 1993; Walker, 1995). Accordingly, some work suggests that, indeed, sociocultural expectations can lead a woman to attribute irritable moods to PMS, even when the reported symptoms might not have any relationship to the menstrual cycle (Sullivan, 2003). In addition, Parlee (1974) has suggested that the MDQ measures stereotypical beliefs about psychological concomitants of menstrual changes. He also concluded that menarche brings with it a socialization process that leads the woman to expect negative premenstrual emotional experiences.

Other research, however, has shown that mood reports are unrelated to culturally biased preconceptions (Gallant, Hamilton, Popiel, Morokoff, & Chakraborty, 1991). Addressing this seeming dilemma, Miller (2002) provides an evolutionary perspective, suggesting that environmental contexts determine what behaviors are adaptive and dictate how premenstrual experiences should be perceived. For example, premenstrual changes in appetite involve increased carbohydrate cravings, which would be highly adaptive in a resource-poor environment because extra "fuel" is needed to build the uterine lining and thereby increase the probability of reproduction and species survival. An affluent society might, however, interpret this change in appetite as a symptom (Miller, 2002).

CAFFEINE AND THE MENSTRUAL CYCLE

Caffeine may affect menstrual physiology; in turn, the hormonal changes that characterize the course of the menstrual cycle may alter the pharmacokinetics of the drug. One effect of caffeine on the cycle is to decrease the duration of menses. In one investigation, urine samples and a daily symptom diary were employed to examine the effects of caffeine. It was found that women who consumed more than 300 mg of caffeine had less than one third of the risk of prolonged menses, as compared with those consuming less than that amount of the drug (Fenster et al., 1999). Additionally, the study showed that relatively heavy caffeine consumers had double the risk of experiencing short cycles (<24 days). Thus, heavy caffeine use was associated with longer menses and shorter cycles. At the same time, caffeine intake was not significantly related to an increased risk for anovulation, short luteal phase, or long follicular phase. Additional empirical work in this area is needed to further examine the effects of caffeine consumption on cycle length longitudinally.

Pharmacokinetic studies show that caffeine elimination is about 25% slower during the luteal phase when progesterone and estradiol concentrations are highest (Balogh et al., 1987; Institute of Medicine, 2001). Lane, Steege, Rupp, and Kuhn (1992) found the slower caffeine clearance during the luteal phase to be associated with proximity to onset of menstruation and also to increased levels of progesterone. In another study, 300 mg of caffeine was administered to 10 menstruating women during the follicular, ovulatory, and luteal phases of the menstrual cycle. The authors found no significant differences in the pharmacokinetic parameters of caffeine across the menstrual cycle phases (Kaminori et al., 1999). These findings again suggest that the slower luteal elimination rate is the result of the heightened level of progesterone.

Our interest in detecting differences in the rate of caffeine elimination across the menstrual cycle is that it may facilitate our understanding of the overall role and importance of caffeine elimination in PMS. Because caffeine elimination is slowest during the luteal phase, when PMS symptoms manifest and the production of ovarian steroids is at its highest, pharmacokinetic studies may lead to greater understanding of the physiological underpinnings of the disorder. Overall, there appears to be consistent support for the slower rate of caffeine clearance during the luteal phase, most likely due to increased levels of progesterone. The use of oral contraceptive steroids (OCS) may complicate this picture because these drugs have been shown to delay caffeine clearance substantially (Meyer & Zanger, 1997). Thus, assessment of OCS utilization is an important control in pharmacokinetic studies of caffeine in women.

The consumption of caffeine can also alter levels of the ovarian steroids. Some investigations have shown that drinking more than two cups of coffee daily boosts estrogen levels in women and can therefore potentially exacerbate such conditions as endometriosis and breast pain (Dickerson et al., 2003). Studies supporting this finding show that increased caffeine consumption is associated with heightened levels of estradiol during the early follicular phase (Lucero, Harlow, Barbieri, Sluss, & Cramer, 2001; Zeiner & Kegg, 1981). It thus seems clear that caffeine increases estradiol levels; however, further research is needed to determine the extent to which this change may be responsible for PMS symptoms.

THE ROLE OF CAFFEINE IN PREMENSTRUAL SYNDROME

Does caffeine contribute to or exacerbate PMS symptomatology? Studies addressing this question have thus far yielded quite mixed results. Anne Rossignol's group (Rossignol & Bonnlander, 1990; Rossignol, Bonnlander, Song, & Phillis, 1991; Rossignol, Zhang, Chen, & Xiang, 1989) completed a series of studies consistently showing a positive correlation between caffeine consumption and PMS symptomatology, but some other researchers have found no such relationship (Caan et al., 1993; Marks, Hair, Klock, Ginsburg, & Pomerleau, 1994; Vo, Rubinow, & Smith, in preparation).

Rossignol and colleagues (1989, 1990, 1991) suggest that caffeine is a major trigger for PMS symptoms. Among women in their studies with more severe symptoms, there was a relationship between consumption of caffeine-containing beverages and premenstrual syndrome. In fact, they suggest that the association between premenstrual symptoms and daily consumption of caffeine-containing beverages is dose dependent, with heavier consumption associated with more severe symptoms. In a study of 295 college sophomores, Rossignol (1985) found that caffeine-containing beverages are related to the presence and severity of premenstrual syndrome. In addition, a survey study of 841 participants revealed that consumption of caffeine-containing beverages was strongly related to the prevalence of PMS (Rossignol & Bonnlander, 1990).

The effect of caffeine consumption on PMS also seems to be prevalent cross culturally in the Rossignol studies. This was demonstrated in a study of Chinese women (Rossignol et al., 1989). The study examined level of consumption of tea using questionnaires for nursing students and women who worked in a tea factory. The questionnaires were distributed during classes (nursing students) and during routine physical examinations (tea factory workers). Women in both groups met criteria for premenstrual syndrome. Analysis using 188 nursing students and tea factory workers showed that tea consumption is strongly related to the prevalence of premenstrual syndrome and that the effects are dose dependent.

In another study, Rossignol and Bonnlander (1991) found evidence that 47 of 96 women with moderate or severe PMS demonstrated monthly patterns in caffeine consumption. The authors reported that women consumed more caffeine during the luteal phase and interpreted this to suggest that perhaps women with premenstrual syndrome self-medicate with caffeine in response to premenstrual symptoms, which in turn exacerbates their symptoms. However, it is notable that only approximately half of the women in their PMS sample showed the expected self-medication pattern of caffeine consumption.

The studies mentioned did not assess consumption of other foods containing caffeine, such as chocolate. In a final study, however, Rossignol and Bonnlander

(1991) did examine the association of junk food consumption with the prevalence and severity of PMS symptoms and found that, although no significant associations with junk food consumption in general were found, there was a significant association between chocolate consumption and the prevalence and severity of PMS.

One of the major methodological problems in these and some other studies is the failure to report in detail the procedures and criteria used in diagnosing PMS. Most of the studies published by Rossignol and colleagues, for example, do not provide diagnostic details. It appears that in some studies diagnosis followed a 2-month study of symptoms, while in others it is unclear whether or not this approach was employed. In addition, the authors do not report which symptoms they used to diagnose PMS and whether or not they determined that there was a 30% increase in defining symptoms in the premenstrual phase, as recommended by the NIMH Workshop group (see preceding discussion). It is also likely that they examined premenstrual symptoms dimensionally rather than categorically. These studies also used a retrospective, one-time questionnaire, which relies on potentially poor or biased memories.

Some other studies in this literature have used improved methodologies and reported details of their diagnostic procedures and criteria. Caan and colleagues (1993) and Vo and colleagues (in preparation) conducted their studies using 2 months of prospective data to diagnose PMS (based on a 30% increase in symptomatology) and recorded daily caffeine consumption using daily diaries, although the populations sampled in these two studies were somewhat different. Caan used a sample from the general population, and Vo investigated a college sample with limited age range (18 to 26). Despite their sampling differences, both studies failed to support Rossignol's results. They found no difference between participants in the PMS and control groups on level of caffeine consumption.

Caan and colleagues (1993) examined the association of caffeine and alcohol intake; in a sample of 102 women with PMS and a similar comparison group, they found no significant differences during the pre-and postmenstrual periods. They suggest that other environmental variables, rather than caffeine consumption, might be responsible for the experiences of PMS. Interestingly, Caan and colleagues found that women with PMS consumed fewer caffeinated beverages, but more decaffeinated coffee and herbal tea than controls. The authors suggested that perhaps knowledge of the media might have effects on the consumption behavior of those who know or think they have PMS, but they did not collect data to demonstrate specifically that this was responsible for the differences detected.

To further investigate the association between caffeine and experiences of premenstrual syndrome, Vo and colleagues (in preparation) collected daily ratings for PMS symptoms and daily caffeine consumption across two full menstrual cycles from 83 college-age participants and used the NIMH criteria to diagnose PMS. Results indicated that average consumption was higher during the follicular phase for control and PMS groups compared to level of consumption during the luteal phase, and normal volunteers reported higher levels of consumption than did the PMS group. Moreover, results indicated that normal volunteers consumed more caffeine on average during the luteal phase than did the PMS group.

These findings indicate that overall caffeine consumption is not associated with PMS symptomatology. More specifically, the data suggest that caffeine consumption is not a product of or responsive to PMS symptom experiences. Although there are some differences in specific findings, several studies are now consistent in showing that caffeine consumption is not associated with PMS (Caan et al., 1993; Marks et al., 1994; Vo et al., in preparation).

CONCLUSIONS

Overall, it appears that caffeine consumption is related to the physiology of the menstrual cycle and to related disorders, but the details of this relationship remain elusive. Evidence for increased levels of the reproductive hormones during the follicular phase in women who consume more than 100 mg of caffeine per day is quite consistent (Zeiner & Kegg, 1981; Lucero et al., 2001). Additionally, caffeine elimination is delayed during the luteal phase of the cycle but not during the follicular phase (Institute of Medicine, 2001; Fenster et al., 1999; Lane et al., 1992). It remains unclear why this occurs, though it may be due to the increased production of progesterone. Other environmental factors, such as the use of oral contraceptives, may also delay caffeine clearance, complicating the results of any studies in which OCS use is not assessed. A further issue is whether or not caffeine alters the length of the menstrual cycle. Further research is clearly needed; however, evidence to date suggests that the drug leads to longer menses and shorter cycle.

The other major issue with which this chapter is concerned is whether or not caffeine consumption is related to the prevalence and severity of premenstrual symptoms. Studies with better diagnostic procedures and improved controls suggest that it probably is not, though discrepancies in the literature certainly do exist. It appears that these inconsistencies may be due largely to differences in methodology. First, several symptom scales are available that assess somewhat different sets of symptoms. In addition, some authors do not report which of the approximately 20 symptoms they used as diagnostic criteria. Much as in research concerned with the influence of caffeine on fertility and pregnancy, it is possible that lower amounts of caffeine consumption (<300 mg/day) might not yield detectable effects on premenstrual syndrome, whereas consumption of more than 500 mg/day might have significant effects (compare chapter 9 in this book; Lucero et al., 2001).

Overall, it seems clear that considerable additional research, with careful attention paid to diagnostic methods and criteria, is needed before we can know with any certainty the nature of the association between caffeine and premenstrual syndrome. At this time, we can only conclude that caffeine consumption and pharmacokinetics are very likely related to aspects of the menstrual cycle, but no strong evidence indicates that consumption of the drug affects or is affected by PMS or PMDD.

REFERENCES

American College of Obstetricians and Gynecologists (2000) Clinical management guidelines for obstetrician–gynecologists. Practice bulletin number 15: Premenstrual syndrome. *Obstetrics & Gynecology, 95,* 1–9.

American Psychiatric Association. (2000). *Diagnostic and statistical manual of mental disorders,* 4th ed. text rev. Washington, D.C.: American Psychiatric Association.

Anderson, S. E., & Must, A. (2005). Interpreting the continued decline in the average age at menarche: results from two nationally representative surveys of U.S. girls studied 10 years apart. *Journal of Pediatrics, 147*, 753–760.

Apter, D., Raisanen, I., Ylostalo, P., & Vihko, R. (1987). Follicular growth in relation to serum hormonal patterns in adolescence compared with adult menstrual cycles. *Fertility & Sterility, 47*, 82–88.

Backstrom, T., & Carstensen, H. (1974). Estrogen and progesterone in plasma in relation to premenstrual tension. *Journal of Steroid Biochemistry, 5*, 257–260.

Backstrom, T., & Mattson, B. (1975). Correlation of symptoms in premenstrual tension to estrogen and progesterone concentrations in blood plasma. *Neuropsychobiology, 1*, 80–86.

Balogh, A., Irmisch, E., Klinger, G., Splinter, F. K., & Hoffmann, A. (1987). Elimination of caffeine and metamizol in the menstrual cycle of the fertile female. *Zentralblatt fur Gynakologie, 109*, 1135–1142.

Beem, A. L., Geus, E. J., Hottenga, J. J., Sullivan, P. F., Wilemsen, G., Slagboom, P. E., & Boomsma, D. I. (2005). Combined linkage and association analyses of the 124-bp allele of marker D2S2944 with anxiety, depression, neuroticism and major depression. *Behavior Genetics, 24*, 1–10.

Berlin, R. E, Jamuna, D. R., Schmidt, P. J., Adams, L. F., & Rubinow, D. R. (2001). Effects of the menstrual cycle on measures of personality in women with premenstrual syndrome: A preliminary study. *Journal of Clinical Psychiatry, 62*, 337–342.

Caan, B., Duncan, D., Hiatt, R., Lewis, J., Chapman, J., & Armstrong, M. A. (1993). Association between alcoholic and caffeinated beverages and premenstrual syndrome. *Journal of Reproductive Medicine, 38*, 630–636.

Chrisler, J. C., & Levy, K. B. (1990). The media construct a menstrual monster: A content analysis of PMS articles in the popular press. *Women and Health, 16*, 89–104.

Condon, J. T. (1993). The premenstrual syndrome: A twin study. *British Journal of Psychiatry, 162*, 481–486.

Coppen, A., & Kessel, N. (1963). Menstruation and personality, *British Journal of Psychiatry, 109*, 711–721.

Coutts, L. B., & Berg, D. H. (1993). The portrayal of the menstruating women in menstrual product advertisements. *Health Care for Women International, 14*, 179–191.

Dalton, K. (1979). *The premenstrual syndrome and progesterone therapy*. London: Heinemann Medical Books

Dickerson, L. M., Mazyck, P. J., & Hunter, M. H. (2003). Premenstrual syndrome. *American Family Physician, 67*, 1743–1752.

Endicott, J. (2000). History, evolution, and diagnosis of premenstrual dysphoric disorder. *Journal of Clinical Psychiatry, 61*(suppl 12), 5–8.

Endicott, J., Schacht, S., & Halbreich, U., & Nee, J. (1981). Premenstrual changes and affective disorders. *Psychosomatic Medicine, 43*, 519–529.

Fenster, L., Quale, C., Walker, K., Windham, G. C., Elkin, E. P., Benowitz, N., & Swan, S. H. (1999). Caffeine consumption and menstrual function. *American Journal of Epidemiology, 149*, 550–557.

FitzGerald, M., Malone, K. M., Li, S., Harrison, W. M., McBride, P. A., Endicott, J., Cooper, T., & Mann, J. J. (1997). Blunted serotonin response to femfluramine challenge in premenstrual dysphoric disorder. *American Journal of Psychiatry, 154*, 556–558.

Fraser, I. S., Michie, E. A., Wide, L., & Baird, D. T. (1973). Pituitary gonadotropin and ovarian function in adolescent dysfunctional uterine bleeding. *Journal of Clinical Endocrinology & Metabolism, 37*, 407–414.

Gallant, S., Hamilton, J., Popiel, D., Morokoff, P., & Chakraborty, P. K. (1991). Daily moods and symptoms: Effects of awareness of study focus, gender, menstrual cycle phase and day of week, *Health Psychology, 10*, 180–189.

Gotthell, M., Steinberg, R., & Granger, L. (1999). An exploration of clinicians' diagnostic approaches to premenstrual symptomatology. *Canadian Journal of Behavior Science, 31*, 254–262.

Halbreich, W., & Endicott, J. (1985). Relationship of dysphoric premenstrual changes to depressive disorders. *Acta Psychiatr. Scand.*, 71, 331–338.

Halbreich, U., Endicott, J., & Lesser, J. (1985). The clinical diagnosis and classification of premenstrual changes. *Canadian Journal of Psychiatry, 30*, 489–497.

Hart, W., Coleman, G., & Russell, J. (1987). Assessment of premenstrual symptomatology: A re-evaluation of the predictive validity of self report. *Journal of Psychosomatic Research, 31*, 183–190.

Haskett, R. F., Steiner, M., & Carroll, B. J. (1984). A psychoendocrine study of premenstrual tension syndrome. A model for endogenous depression? *Journal of Affective Disorders, 6*, 191–199.

Hettema, J. M., Prescott, C. A., & Kendler, K. S. (2004). Generic and environmental sources of covariation between generalized anxiety disorder and neuroticism. *American Journal of Psychiatry, 161*, 1581–1587.

Institute of Medicine. (2001). *Caffeine for the sustainment of mental task performance: Formulations for military operations*. Washington, D.C.: National Academy Press.

James, J. E. (1997). *Understanding caffeine: A biobehavioral analysis*. Thousand Oaks, CA: Sage Publications.

Kaminori, G. H., Joubert, A., Otterstetter, R., Santaromana, M., & Eddington, N. D. (1999). The effect of the menstrual cycle on the pharmacokinetics of caffeine in normal, health eumenorrheic females. *European Journal of Clinical Pharmacology, 55*, 213–222.

Keller, M. C., Coventry, W. L., Heath, A. C., & Martin, N. G. (2005). Widespread evidence for nonadditive genetic variation in Cloniger's and Eysenck's personality dimensions using a twin plus sibling design. *Behavior Genetics, 35*, 707–721.

Khan–Sabir, N., & Carr, B. R. (2005, March 1). The normal menstrual cycle and the control of ovulation. www.endotext.org, Female, Reproductive Endocrinology Section, R. Rebar (Ed.) Retrieved, February 17, 2006, from www.endotext.org/female/female3/femaleframe3.htm.

Kim, D. R., Gyulai, L., Freeman, E. W., Morrison, M. F., Baldassano, C., & Dube, B. (2004). Premenstrual dysporic disorder and psychiatric comorbidity. *Archives of Women in Mental Health, 7*, 37–47.

Kornstein, S. G., Harvey, A. T., Rush, A. J., Wisniewski, S. R., Trivedi, M. H., Svikis, D. S., McKensie, N. D., Bryan, C., & Harley, R. (2005). Self-reported premenstrual exacerbation of depressive symptoms in patients seeking treatment for major depression. *Psychological Medicine, 35*, 683–692.

Lane, J. D., Steege, J. F., Rupp, S. L., & Kuhn, C. M. (1992). Menstrual cycle effects on caffeine elimination in the human female. *European Journal of Clinical Pharmacology, 43*, 543–546.

Li, J., & Thompson, D. S. (2001). Treating premenstrual dysphoric disorder using serotonin agents. *Journal of Women's Health & Gender-Based Medicine, 10*, 745–750.

Lucero, J., Harlow, B. L., Barbieri, R. L., Sluss, P., & Cramer, D. W. (2001). Early follicular phase hormone levels in relation to patterns of alcohol, tobacco, and coffee use. *Fertility & Sterility, 76*, 723–729.

Lustyk, K. B., Widman, L., Paschane, A. E., & Olson, K. C. (2004). Physical activity and quality of life: Assessing the influence of activity frequency, intensity, volume, and motives. *Behavior Medicine, 30*, 124–131.

Marks, J. L., Hair, C. S., Klock, S. C., Ginsburg, B. E., & Pomerleau, C. S. (1994). Effects of menstrual phase on intake of nicotine, caffeine, and alcohol and nonprescribed drugs in women with late luteal phase dysphoric disorder. *Journal of Substance Abuse, 6*(2), 235–243.

McLean, C., & Graham, T. E. (2002). Effects of exercise and thermal stress on caffeine pharmacokinetics in men and eumenorrheic women. *Journal of Applied Physiology, 93*(4), 1471–1478.

Merck Source. 2004. Harvard Health Website www.mercksource.com/pp/us/cns/cns_home.jsp.

Meyer, U. A., & Zanger, U.M. (1997). Molecular mechanisms of genetic polymorphisms of drug metabolism. *Annual Review of Pharmacology and Toxicology, 37*, 269–296.

Miller, L. (2002). Premenstrual dysphoric disorder. *Psychiatric Times*, June 1, pg. 54. Available online at www.web4.infotrac.galegroup.com.

Munday, M. R. (1997). A comprehensive evaluation of premenstrual syndrome. *American Journal of Natural Medicine, 4*, 6–20.

National Institute on Aging (n.d.) Age page. Retrieved February 17, 2006, from www.niapublications.org/agepages/menopause.asp.

National Women's Health Information Center. (2004). Frequently asked questions about menstruation and the menstrual cycle. Available at www.4woman.gov.

NIMH premenstrual syndrome workshop guidelines. (1983). National Institute of Mental Health, (not published), Rockville, MD.

Niswender, G. D., & Nett, T. M. (1994). The corpus luteum and its control in infraprimate species. In E. Knobil & J. D. Neill, (Eds.), *The physiology of reproduction*, 2nd ed., vol. 1 (p. 781). New York: Raven Press.

Paige, K. (1971). Effects of oral contraceptives on affective fluctuations associated with the menstrual cycle. *Psychosomatic Medicine, 33*, 515–537.

Parlee, M. B. (1973). The premenstrual syndrome. *Psychological Bulletin, 80*, 454–465.

Parlee, M. B. (1974). Stereotypical beliefs about menstruation: A methodological note on the Moos MDQ and some new data. *Psychosomatic Medicine, 36*, 229–240.

Patwardhan, R. V., Desmond, P. V., Johnson, R. F., & Schenker, S. (1980). Impaired elimination of caffeine by oral contraceptive steroid. *Journal of Laboratory & Clinical Medicine, 95*, 603–608.

Rapkin, A. J., Morgan, M., Goldman, L., Brann, D. W., Simone, D., & Mahesh, V. B. (1997). Progesterone metabolite allopregnanolone in women with premenstrual syndrome. *Obstetrics & Gynecology, 90*, 709–714.

Roca, C. A., Schmidt, P. J., Altemus, M., Deuster, P., Sanaceau, M. A., Putnam, K, & Rubinow, D. R. (2003). Differential menstrual cycle regulation of hypothalamic–pituitary–adrenal axis in women with premenstrual syndrome and controls. *Journal of Clinical Endocrinology & Metabolism, 88*, 3057–3063.

Roca, C. A., Schmidt, P. J., & Rubinow, D. R. (1999). A follow-up study of premenstrual syndrome. *Journal of Clinical Psychiatry, 60*, 763–766.

Rossignol, A. M. (1985). Caffeine-containing beverages and premenstrual syndrome in young women. *American Journal of Public Health, 75*, 1335–1337.

Rossignol, A. M., & Bonnlander, H. (1990). Caffeine-containing beverages, total fluid consumption, and premenstrual syndrome. *American Journal of Public Health, 80*, 1106–1109.

Rossignol, A. M., Bonnlander, H., Song, L., & Phillis, J. W. (1991). Do women with premenstrual symptoms self-medicate with caffeine? *Epidemiology, 2*, 403–408.

Rossignol, A. M., Zhang, J., Chen, Y., & Xiang, Z. (1989). Tea and premenstrual syndrome in the People's Republic of China. *American Journal of Public Health, 79*, 67–69.

Rubinow, D. R., Hoban, M. C., & Grover, G. N. (1988). Changes in plasma hormones across the menstrual cycle in patients with menstrually related mood disorder and in control subjects. *American Journal of Obstetrics & Gynecology, 158*, 11–15.

Rubinow, D. R., & Roy–Byrne, P. (1984). Premenstrual syndromes: Overview from a methodologic prespective. *American Journal of Psychiatry, 141*, 163–172.

Ruble, D. N. (1977). Menstrual syndrome: A reinterpretation. *Science, 197*, 291–292.

Sawetawan, C., Carr, B. R., McGee, E., Bird, I. M., Hong, T. L., & Rainery, W. E. (1996). Inhibin and activin differentially regulate androgen production and 17-a-hydroxylase expression in human ovarian thecal-like tumor cells. *Journal of Endocrinology, 148*, 213–221.

Schmidt, P. J., Grover, G. N., & Rubinow, D. R. (1993). Alprazolam in the treatment of premenstrual syndrome, a double-blind, placebo-controlled trail. *Archives of General Psychiatry, 50*, 467–473.

Schmidt, P. J., Nieman, L., Danaceau, M. A., Tobin, M. B., Roca, C. A., Murphy, J. H., & Rubinow, D. R. (2000). Estrogen replacement in perimenopause-related depression: A preliminary report. *American Journal of Obstetrics and Gynecology, 183*, 414–420.

Schuckit, M., Daly, V., Herrman, G., & Hineman, S. (1975). Premenstrual symptoms and depression in a university population. *Diseases of the Nervous System, 36*, 516–517.

Severino, S., & Moline, M. L. (1988). *Premenstrual syndrome: A clinician's guide.* New York: The Guilford Press.

Silberg, J. L., Martin, N. G., & Heath, A. C. (1987). Genetic and environmental factors in primary dysmonorrhea and its relationship to anxiety, depression, and neuroticism. *Behavior Genetics, 17*, 363–83.

Silberstein, S. D. & Merriam, G. R. (2000). Physiology of the menstrual cycle. *Cephalalgia, International Journal of Headache, 20*, 148–154.

Silva, C. M., Cigante, D. P., Carret, M. L., & Fassa, A. G. (2006). Population study of premenstrual syndrome. *Revista de Saude Publica, 40*, 47–56.

Slade, P., & Jenner, F. A. (1980). Attitudes to female roles, aspects of menstruation and complaining of menstrual symptoms. *British Journal of Social and Clinical Psychology, 19*, 109–113.

Steiner, M., Haskett, R. F., & Carroll, B. J. (1980). Premenstrual tension syndrome: The development of research diagnostic criteria and new rating scales. *Acta Psychiatrica Scandinavica, 62*, 177–190.

Subhash, C. B., & Shashi, K. B. (2002). Diagnosis and treatment of premenstrual dysphoric disorder. *American Family Physician, 66*, 1239–1248.

Sullivan, M. G. (2003). Severe menopausal symptoms linked to severe PMS. *Clinical Psychiatry News, 31*, 52–53.

Tsafriri A. L. (1994). Nonsteroidal regulators of ovarian function. In E. Knobil & J. D. Neill (Eds.), *The physiology of reproduction*, 2nd ed., vol. 1 (pp. 817–860). New York: Raven Press.

Vo, H. T., Rubinow, D. R., & Smith, B. D. (in preparation). The effect of caffeine on premenstrual syndrome.

Walker, A., (1995). Theory and methodology in premenstrual syndrome research. *Social Science and Medicine, 41*, 793–800.

Walker, A. (1997). *The menstrual cycle.* London: Routledge.

Wetzel, R., Reich, T., McClure, J., & Wald, J. (1975). Premenstrual affective syndrome and affective disorder. *British Journal of Psychiatry, 127*, 219–221.

WHO. (1992). *The ICD-10 classification of mental and behavioral disorders: Clinical descriptions and diagnostic guidelines.* Geneva, Switzerland: WHO.

Wyatt, K. M, Dimmock, P. W., & O'Brien, P. M. (2000). Premenstrual syndrome. In S. Barton (Ed.), *Clinical evidence*, 4th issue (pp. 1121–1133). London: BMJ Publishing Group.

Wyatt, K. M. Dimmock, P. W., Jones, P. M., Obhrai, M., & O'Brien, P. M. (2001). Efficacy of progesterone and progestogens in management of premenstrual syndrome: Systemic review. *British Medical Journal, 323,* 776–780.

Zeiner, A. R., & Kegg, P. S. (1981). Effects of sex steroids on ethanol pharmacokinetics and autonomic reactivity. *Progress in Biochemical & Pharmacology, 18,* 130–142.

9 Effects of Caffeine Intake on Female Fertility: A Critical Review

Kate Northstone and Jean Golding

CONTENTS

There appears to be a rising trend in recent years in the number of couples struggling to conceive. A wide variety of factors has been suggested and hence investigated as contributing to the apparent decline in fertility levels; caffeine has been one of them. Fifteen studies evaluating the possible detrimental effects of caffeine consumption on female fertility have been published to date. This review provides a critical appraisal of these papers.

INTRODUCTION

Despite concerns that fertility levels are decreasing (Carlsen, Giwercman, Keiding, & Skakkebaek, 1992) (particularly declining male reproductive health), Joffe (2000) has reported recently that, in fact, in Britain, rising trends are evident. Despite this, the study of infertility is important because the implications of the one in six couples who seeks specialist help (Hull et al., 1985) is wide reaching. Many exposures have been implicated as having detrimental effects on male and female fertility, but many of these have yet to be firmly established. In this chapter, we review the evidence in regard to caffeine in the 15 relevant studies:

Alderete, Eskenazi, and Sholtz, 1995
Bolumar, Olsen, Rebagliato, Bisanti, and European Study in Infertility and
 Subfecundity, 1997
Caan, Quesenberry, and Coates, 1998
Christiansen, Oechsli, and van den Berg, 1989
Curtis, Savitz, and Arbuckle, 1997
Florack, Zielhuis, and Rolland, 1994
Grodstein, Goldman, Ryan, and Cramer, 1993
Hakim, Gray, and Zucar, 1998
Hatch and Bracken, 1993
Jensen et al., 1998
Joesoef, Beral, and Bramer, 1990
Olsen, 1991
Stanton and Gray, 1995
Wilcox, Weinberg, and Baird, 1988
Williams, Manson, Goldman, Mittendorf, and Ryan, 1990

As we will show, study methodologies and reported results varied widely; further research is needed.

In the past, animal literature has been extensively reviewed (Grice, 1984; Purves & Sullican, 1993). It is unrealistic, however, to attempt to extrapolate findings obtained in laboratory animals to humans. Varying effects have been shown in such a setting, due to differences in metabolic pathways across animal species (Bonati, Latini, Tognoni, Young, & Garattini, 1985). As such, it will not be regarded here. Male fertility is more easily quantified than female fertility: it can be more directly measured by examining sperm counts, density, and motility. In fact, the literature points to a positive effect of caffeine on male fertility caused by its apparent ability to stimulate sperm motility (Aitken, Best, & Richardson, 1983; Garbers, First, Sullivan, & Hardy, 1971).

Although female fertility is harder to diagnose, it is the subject of the bulk of the epidemiological literature, primarily using time to pregnancy data rather than clinical outcomes. The effects of caffeine consumption have previously been reviewed in terms of reproduction (Dlugosz & Bracken, 1992; Golding, 1995; Leviton, 1995); however, although encompassing fertility, pregnancy outcomes including spontaneous abortion, birth weight, gestational length, and congenital malformations have also been examined, with fertility possibly lost in this broad subject

Examining time to pregnancy is a useful marker for couple fertility in retrospective epidemiological studies, but as te Velde, Eijkemans, and Habbema (2000) state, "It does not enable conclusions as to which link of the reproductive chain [including spermatogenesis, oogenesis, coitus, transportation, fertilization, and implantation] is affected." However, a substantial literature exists on the use of time to pregnancy in epidemiological studies, its appropriateness, and possible sources of bias (Baird, Wilcox, & Weinberg, 1986; Basso, Juul, & Olsen, 2000; Joffe, 1989; Joffe, Villard, Li, Plowman, & Vessey, 1993; Olsen, Juul, & Basso, 1998; Weinberg, Baird, & Wilcox, 1994). These are summarized later.

Time to pregnancy, usually measured in terms of menstrual cycles, allows assessment of "fecundability." This is the probability of conceiving a pregnancy within each given cycle and represents the combined ability of males and females to conceive and sustain a pregnancy. Time to pregnancy is also commonly used to identify infertile, or at least subfertile, couples. Couples are conventionally deemed to be infertile in a clinical setting if they have failed to conceive within 12 months of trying. Many retrospective studies use this dichotomy (<12 months vs. ≥12 months) as the main outcome variable of interest when investigating environmental effects on fertility, but it has a number of pitfalls. As Baird et al. (1986) discuss, "It does not reflect the range of fecundability that exists in a population [and] is also insensitive to short term effects."

Quite possibly a more appropriate measure is to record the number of cycles needed to achieve pregnancy from the time the couple decides to attempt conception. This prospective method is somewhat idealistic. Great effort is required in setting up such a study; selection bias is almost inevitable and insufficient numbers of participants are often enrolled, resulting in reduced statistical power. Participants may also modify their behavior to reduce any possibly harmful exposures if they are aware of their low fertility or the hypothesis being tested. The alternative is to recruit participants after the event (i.e., during pregnancy) and use self-reported recall to gather information on time to pregnancy. This method is subject to bias and might raise questions of validity. However, it has been reported to be fairly accurate (Joffe et al., 1993).

Nevertheless, studies executed in this manner will fail to include those who ultimately do not conceive. Accidental, unplanned, and mistimed pregnancies are unlikely to be included (this is also true for prospective studies) and these are most likely to occur in the more fertile couples, thus biasing the sample further. Therefore, time to pregnancy does not necessarily reflect the probability of conception in the population as a whole.

The consumption of caffeine (trimethylxanthine) is a universally accepted habit; it is the most commonly consumed drug in the world. The primary sources of caffeine are tea and coffee, but it is also available through other dietary sources, including cola beverages and chocolate and nondietary sources via nonprescription drugs such as cold or flu remedies (Barone & Roberts, 1996; Graham, 1978).

The amount of caffeine available in coffee and tea varies widely. It depends not only on the content of the natural plants from which the products are derived (Grice, 1984; Jensen et al., 1998) but also on the way in which the drinks are brewed. Levels of caffeine in coffee are also affected by the processes of roasting and grinding the beans (Barone & Roberts, 1996; Bunker & McWilliams, 1979; Leonard, Watson, & Mohs, 1987). In today's society, where coffee shops are springing up on every corner, a multitude of different coffee drinks is available, such as espressos and cappuccinos. Add to this the wide variation in serving sizes and the considerable within-person variation (with different amounts consumed at weekends compared to weekdays and seasonality effects), the measurement of an individual's caffeine intake is particularly difficult to establish.

In epidemiological studies, caffeine intake is almost always estimated from the actual number of drinks consumed ascertained via questionnaires or dietary diaries. Different studies have used varying estimates for the caffeine content of tea and coffee. The majority disregard further sources and so may well underestimate the actual amounts consumed.

Caffeine is known to have a variety of behavioral and physiological effects. However, moderate intake is not believed to cause any considerable harm (Leonard et al., 1987). Nevertheless, due to its unsurpassable level of consumption in the Western world, caution may be warranted with respect to certain biological systems until the evidence of proof shows otherwise.

The human reproductive system has received significant attention with respect to the outcome of pregnancy and caffeine intake during pregnancy. The majority of published studies have reported a negative effect of caffeine consumption on pregnancy outcome. Increased levels of caffeine intake have been associated with spontaneous abortion (Dlugosz et al., 1996; Fenster, Eskanazi, Windham, & Sean, 1991; Infante–Rivard, Fernandez, & Gaulthier, 1993), lower birth weight (Caan & Goldhaber, 1989; Fenster, Eskenazi, Windham, & Swan, 1991; Fortier, Marcoux, & Beaulac–Baillargeon, 1993), and possibly, preterm delivery (Caan & Goldhaber; Olsen, Overvard, & Frische, 1991). Meanwhile, the literature on caffeine intake and fertility has reached no firm conclusions.

For there to be a causal mechanism between an exposure and an outcome, the occurrence of the exposure precedes the outcome and that exposure must be a necessary component for the outcome to occur. In reality, a component is all that the exposure is—often one of several. In epidemiological studies, a causal effect of an exposure—in this case caffeine—is rarely able to be concluded. Instead, we must assign the risk of the outcome, given the exposure.

Stratification enables the investigator to test the effects of one exposure within subgroups of another simultaneously measured exposure. However, if small numbers are found within any stratum, the question of statistical power is raised and if the numbers of each stratum vary significantly, the precision of any estimates of effect size must also be questioned.

A wide variety of variables that may be risk factors for increased time to pregnancy, including demographic, social, lifestyle and prior medical history factors, should be considered as potential confounders or at least mediating factors. Coital frequency is undoubtedly a major determinant of the chance of conception; however, it is unreliably reported and varies with time.

Other environmental or biological factors that appear to have an effect on fertility might occur through altering sexual libido. Many other factors have been cited as being associated with decreased fertility, including active (Hull et al., 2000) and passive (Argood, Duckitt, & Templeton, 1998) smoking, alcohol consumption (Jensen et al., 1998), maternal (Menken, Trussell, & Larsen, 1986) and paternal (Ford et al., 2000) age, and previous birth control (Vessey, Wright, McPherson, & Wiggins, 1978), together with a host of environmental and occupational exposures.

One of the most important is smoking, which substantially increases the rate at which caffeine is eliminated from the body (Parsons & Neims, 1978). Smokers are also significantly more likely to consume higher levels of caffeine (Klesges, Ray, & Klesges, 1994). It may also be important to consider the male partner's consumption of caffeine. Marshburn, Sloan, and Hammond (1989) have reported a deleterious effect of combined smoking and coffee drinking on sperm viability and motility.

There are always limitations to an epidemiological study. They are purely observational and as a result one cannot attribute cause but only report any evident association between an exposure and the outcome of interest. Nevertheless, a well-designed and executed study could have public health implications if the results reflect a causal relationship. Indeed, some studies did make recommendations based on their results. With this in mind, we will review the current literature in terms of the design and analytic methods used in each study. Epidemiological publications on the relationship between caffeinated beverages and female fertility were identified by searching MEDLINE and BIDS from 1980 to present, using a variety of keywords (caffeine, coffee, tea, caffeinated beverages, fertility, sub/infertility, time to pregnancy/conception, fecundity). We also supplemented our search through citations in relevant articles. Only publications in peer-reviewed journals were considered.

We have split this review into several sections: study design; outcome measure; exposure measures; possible confounders, power and sample size; and reported results and conclusions. Table 9.1 provides a summary of the studies under review.

REVIEW OF LITERATURE

STUDY DESIGN, ELIGIBILITY, AND EXCLUSION

Prospective Studies

Five of the published studies investigating the effects of caffeine on female fertility were prospective (Caan et al., 1998; Florack et al., 1994; Hakim et al., 1998; Jensen et al., 1998; Wilcox et al., 1988) and enrolled 221 American female volunteers who were planning to become pregnant (although only 104 gave information about exposures after enrollment). They entered the study at the time they stopped birth control and were originally investigated for very early pregnancy loss. Florack et al. enrolled 260 women who were planning to become pregnant from a mail-out to 7,000 Dutch nonmedical hospital workers. The date of commencing a pregnancy attempt over a 12-month period was obtained by personal interview. The authors stated that 155 (60%) had already begun trying for a pregnancy prior to enrollment and 56 (36%) of these had been trying for over a year.

Caan et al. (1998) followed 210 volunteers in America who had been trying to conceive for no more than 3 months. A further American study by Hakim et al. (1998) investigated reproductive health in 124 women employed in two semiconductor plants. Participants were eligible for study if they were of reproductive age, had not been sterilized, and were not using oral contraceptives or intrauterine devices, although it was not actually stated whether they intended to become pregnant. The last prospective study, conducted in Denmark by Jensen et al. (1998), recruited 430

TABLE 9.1
Summary of Studies Investigating Effects of Caffeine on Female Fertility

Study	Participants	Measure of exposure	Outcome measure	Main result
Prospective				
Wilcox et al., 1988	104 women trying to conceive	Interview at enrollment, 3 mths, and 6 mths; current consumption of coffee (brewed and instant), tea, and soda	Fecundability; time to conception ($\leq$ vs. >12 mths)	Reduction in fertility
Florack et al., 1994	260 women trying to conceive	Average daily consumption of coffee, tea, and cola	Fecundability; urine samples monthly	No significant associations
Caan et al., 1998	210 women trying to conceive	Number of cups of coffee, tea, cola at end of each month	Fecundability	No significant associations
Hakim et al., 1998	124 women trying to conceive	Number of cups of coffee, tea, cola at end of each month	Fecundability; urine samples daily	No significant associations
Jensen et al., 1998	430 couples trying to conceive	Number of cups of coffee, tea, cola, chocolate beverages, and chocolate bars at end of each month	Fecundability; semen sample at enrollment	No significant associations
Retrospective				
Joesoef et al., 1990	2,817 women had live birth; 1,818 infertile women	Current average daily consumption of coffee, decaff coffee, tea, and weekly consumption of cola	Mean time to pregnancy (mths); fecundability	No significant associations
Williams et al., 1990	3,100 women had live birth	Number of cups of coffee per day in first trimester of pregnancy	Fecundability; time to pregnancy ($\leq$ vs. >12 mths)	Reduction in fertility
Grodstein et al., 1993	3,833 women had live birth; 1,050 infertile women	Average daily consumption of coffee, tea, and cola	Primary diagnosis of infertility	Association with tubal disease and endometriosis

Study	Sample	Caffeine measure	Outcome	Result
Stanton & Gray, 1995	2,501 pregnancies to 1,430 women	Average daily consumption of coffee, tea, and cola prepregnancy in first month of pregnancy	Fecundability; time to pregnancy (≤ vs. >12 mths)	Reduction in fertility only in nonsmokers
Bolumar et al., 1997	3,187 women	Number of cups of coffee, tea, cola at time of stopping birth control	Time to pregnancy (≤ vs. >9.5 mths)	Reduction in fertility
Curtis et al., 1997	2,607 pregnancies to 1,277 couples	Number of cups of coffee, tea, cola when trying to become pregnant	Fecundability	No significant associations
Christiansen et al., 1989	6,303 pregnant women	Usual consumption of caffeinated drinks prepregnancy	Difficulty in becoming pregnant	Reduction in fertility
Olsen, 1991	10,866 pregnant women	Asked in last trimester how many cups of coffee or tea consumed prepregnancy	Time to pregnancy (≤ vs. >12 mths)	Reduction in fertility only in smokers
Hatch & Bracken, 1993	1,909 pregnant women	Average daily consumption of coffee, tea, and cola	Fecundability; time to pregnancy (≤ vs. >12 mths)	Reduction in fertility
Alderete et al., 1995	1,341 pregnant women	Average daily consumption of coffee, tea, and cola prepregnancy	Time to pregnancy (≤ vs. >3, 6, 12 mths)	No significant associations

female trade union members, aged 20 to 35, living with a partner, and with no reproductive experience, who intended to discontinue contraception to become pregnant.

One aspect of a prospective study of time to pregnancy that needs to be considered is measuring the time the woman was at risk of becoming pregnant *prior* to enrollment. This would need to be taken into account in some manner for the outcome measure to be accurate. Three of the preceding studies appear to have done this by approaching participants before they discontinued contraceptive methods (Caan et al., 1998; Jensen et al., 1998; Wilcox et al., 1988). However, Hakim et al. (1998) did not clearly state the point in the process of deciding and actively trying to become pregnant at which participants were enrolled. In the study by Florack et al. (1994), it is not clear whether the authors took into account the number of months during which the participants had already been actively trying to become pregnant prior to enrollment. Indeed, by commencing the study in this way, considerable bias is introduced because the partners who were very fertile would be differentially omitted (having already conceived).

Retrospective Studies

Of the retrospective studies, four enrolled participants during pregnancy (Alderete et al., 1995; Christiansen et al., 1989; Hatch & Bracken, 1993; Olsen, 1991). The remainder considered women who had already given birth (Bolumar et al., 1997; Curtis et al., 1997; Grodstein et al., 1993; Joesoef et al., 1990; Stanton & Gray, 1995; Williams et al., 1990). Two of these also included a sample of infertile women (Grodstein et al; Williams et al., 1990). The timing of data collection varied among those studies performed during pregnancy. Christiansen et al. interviewed 6,303 women in early pregnancy, although the precise time was not specified. In the Danish study by Olsen, which aimed to study the impact of social conditions on the outcome of pregnancy, a questionnaire was administered at 36 weeks' gestation. But it was not confirmed what time span had elapsed between administration and actual completion. In the event, data were obtained from 10,866 eligible women after exclusions were made for those who had received infertility treatment.

Hatch and Bracken (1993) performed personal interviews, 80% of which were completed by the 15th week of pregnancy. No comment was made on the remaining 20%. The original aim of the study was to examine future pregnancy outcome in those who had prior induced abortions. Analysis was restricted to 1,909 women who were married for the first time and did not conceive while using birth control. Women in the study by Alderete et al. (1995) were participating in child and health development studies in San Francisco, so there were a number of eligibility criteria for the substudy: primigravidas with regular menses who had not used hormones other than oral contraceptives and had used contraception since marriage. The authors gave no indication as to when data were collected in pregnancy.

Recollection of time to pregnancy is likely to be better as soon after the event as possible (i.e., while the woman is pregnant) if accurate reports are to be gathered. However, this method is still subject to digit preference, which is an important phenomenon when asking participants of any study to recall an interval of time.

Of those studies whose participants were enrolled after pregnancy, none specified the timing of data collection with respect to any of the pregnancies under scrutiny. Curtis et al. (1997) asked participants in the Ontario Farm Family Health Study about *all* pregnancies that had occurred over the past 30 years, resulting in 2,607 planned pregnancies to 1,277 couples. Participants were asked to recall information pertinent to each pregnancy. Unplanned pregnancies were excluded. Planned pregnancies in which fertility drugs had been used were also excluded as were those in which the date of trying to conceive was greater than 1 year before the date of marriage. Using the Reproductive Health Study, Stanton and Gray (1995) obtained information on 2,501 pregnancies to 1,430 women not practicing contraception over the previous 10 years (those who had used infertility drugs were excluded).

Bolumar et al. (1997) using The European Multicenter Study on risk factors for infertility collected data by personal interview from 6,630 women aged 25 to 44 on their first and most recent pregnancies. Data were obtained from 3,010 women postpartum who were participants in the study by Williams et al. (1990). Joesoef et al. (1990) enrolled two study groups: 2,817 women delivering a live-born child as a result of a planned pregnancy and 1,818 women who had presented with primary infertility. Finally, Grodstein et al. (1993) enrolled 2,097 couples. These were women attending one of seven infertility clinics; the control group consisted of 4,023 women recruited from those who were admitted for the delivery of a live birth in the hospitals adjoining the infertility clinics. This case-control study was originally intended to examine contraceptive practices and the relationship with the woman's ability to conceive.

Asking women to recall time intervals that occurred up to 30 years previously is obviously open to error and, as mentioned earlier, digit preference—particularly when reporting on multiple events. In time to pregnancy studies, exclusions based on various criteria are particularly important to prevent or reduce sample and recall bias. This is especially relevant in retrospective studies. For prospective studies, clear statements of eligibility are equally vital to maintaining the validity of the study.

OUTCOME MEASURES

The majority of the published studies reviewed here used fecundability (the probability of conceiving within a given menstrual cycle) as the outcome. However, some used the time taken to pregnancy (generally taken as the time elapsing between ceasing protected intercourse and conception), measured in months, in conjunction with this. Only one study used a clinical diagnosis of infertility (Grodstein et al., 1993).

All five prospective studies examined fecundability as their main outcome (Caan et al., 1998; Florack et al., 1994; Hakim et al., 1998; Jensen et al., 1998; Wilcox et al., 1988). The latter followed their group for 6 months and those who were not pregnant within that time were telephoned 1 and 2 years after enrollment. They reported the fecundability ratio (per-cycle probability of pregnancy for exposed and unexposed, expressed as a ratio), using information on menstrual bleeding recorded daily, for each given cycle. They also examined the proportion of women who had not conceived within 12 months of trying.

Florack et al. (1994) enrolled 104 participants who had not yet actively started trying to conceive and 155 who had. For the latter group, the "date of commencing a pregnancy attempt" was obtained. Participants recorded their menstrual periods for 12 months and if their period was 5 or more days later than expected, they collected early morning urine samples to be tested in a laboratory. Fecundability ratios were then used. Similarly, Hakim et al. (1998) used fecundability ratios gleaned from daily records of vaginal bleeding and urine samples that were collected daily. Data collection ceased on detection of a clinically recognized pregnancy.

Jensen et al. (1998) had a maximum follow-up period of 6 months and women recorded menstrual bleeding daily. Unlike all other studies, the women's partners gave a semen sample at enrollment and once in every cycle. It was not specified how pregnancy was determined. Caan et al. (1998) followed their sample for 12 months and reported fecundability ratios, although they failed to report how menstrual cycle information was collected and how pregnancy was determined.

Of the six retrospective studies that enrolled women after pregnancy (Bolumar et al., 1997; Curtis et al., 1997; Grodstein et al., 1993; Joesoef et al., 1990; Stanton & Gray, 1995; Williams et al., 1990), four used time to pregnancy in months as their outcome. Only Joesoef et al. considered the mean time to pregnancy; the remainder used a dichotomous variable (Bolumar et al.; Curtis et al.; Grodstein et al.; Stanton & Gray; Williams et al.). Bolumar et al. used a cutoff of 9.5 months and the others employed a cutoff at 12 months. Four also examined fecundability (Bolumar et al.; Joesoef et al.; Stanton & Gray; Williams et al.).

Grodstein et al. (1993) differed from all other studies by using an actual diagnosis of primary infertility due to ovulatory failure, tubal disease, cervical factors, endometriosis, or idiopathic fertility. They also had a set of controls who had delivered live births. It is hard to elicit from the paper whether women diagnosed with one form of infertility were compared just to the controls or to the controls and the remaining cases (who were also infertile).

With the exception of Christiansen et al. (1989), all the studies involving pregnant women (Alderete et al., 1995; Hatch & Bracken, 1993; Olsen, 1991) measured time to pregnancy. All used a cutoff point of 12 months, but, in addition, Alderete et al. used 3- and 6-month time points. Christiansen et al. asked their participants whether they had difficulty becoming pregnant.

The major difficulty immediately obvious when attempting to compare distinct time to pregnancy studies is the study sample: those who are trying to become pregnant; those who are already pregnant; and those who have delivered. By considering only conception as reported by the participant as the outcome, those pregnancies that resulted in early miscarriage may be missed and indeed will probably result in what appears to be a longer waiting time. Similarly, by following a group of women attempting to conceive and then clinically diagnosing pregnancy, miscarriage may follow later.

An important aspect of any epidemiological study is the representativeness of the sample. By encompassing all those who conceived, investigators would be including nulliparous and multiparous women, whose previous fertility has already been proven. Investigators need to determine whether they evaluate the ability of a woman to produce a live birth or merely the ability to conceive.

The prospective studies under scrutiny here stopped following their participants once a pregnancy had been clinically diagnosed, although these pregnancies would not necessarily have resulted in live births. The retrospective studies primarily used samples of women who had given birth or who were in the latter half of pregnancy. Both methods have their disadvantages and realistically are not directly comparable. One would imagine that any couple from the general population wanting to conceive wants to produce a baby, not test their reproductive function. Therefore, any conclusions drawn from these studies that lend themselves to public health advice would need to be generalizable to the whole population—that is, those wanting a child.

MEASUREMENT OF EXPOSURE

The first study by Wilcox et al. (1988) investigating the possible effects of caffeine on female infertility appears to have set the precedent for the way in which caffeine intake is measured in later studies. The authors asked their participants how much coffee (brewed and instant), tea (nonherbal and iced), and caffeinated soft drinks they consumed. It was not clear whether this was asked on a daily, weekly, or monthly basis, although participants reported a monthly intake. They assumed that the caffeine content of brewed coffee, instant coffee, tea, and soft drinks was 100, 65, 50, and 40 mg, respectively. This was taken from a report by Lecos (1984).

A further six studies used the same estimates of caffeine content (Curtis et al., 1997; Grodstein et al., 1993; Hakim et al., 1998; Jensen et al., 1998; Stanton & Gray, 1995; Williams et al., 1990), all quoting Wilcox et al. (1988) as their reference. However, none of these distinguished between brewed and instant coffee. Jensen et al. used the same estimates for tea and coffee but attributed 100 mg of caffeine to 0.25 L of cola, as given by Bunker and McWilliams (1979). Unlike in previous studies, this group also considered chocolate beverages and chocolate bars as sources of caffeine with the content of each 25 and 12.5 mg (for a 50-g bar), respectively. In the mutlicenter study of Bolumar et al. (1997), the same estimates as those of Wilcox were also used for tea and cola drinks, but they estimated each person's caffeine intake from coffee as dependent on the country from which he or she came: 130 mg in Denmark and 115 mg elsewhere.

Caan et al. (1997) and Hatch and Bracken (1993) also estimated levels of caffeine intake, but assigned different values to the caffeine content of drinks. Caan et al. gave regular coffee 104 mg; decaffeinated coffee 3 mg; tea 36 mg; decaffeinated tea 0 mg; regular sodas 40 mg and diet caffeinated sodas 52 mg, quoting their source as Bunker and McWilliams (1979). However, they took into account serving sizes, assigning half the amounts to small servings and 1.5 times the amount to large servings. Hatch and Bracken also quoted Bunker and McWilliams, but attributed 107 mg to a 5-oz cup of coffee, 34 mg to a 5-oz cup of tea, and 47 mg to a 12-oz serving of cola.

The remaining four studies used a simple count of the number of cups of coffee consumed per day (Alderete et al., 1995; Christiansen et al., 1989; Olsen, 1991; Williams et al., 1990). Alderete et al. also asked about daily tea consumption. A variety of classifications were used to test the effects of caffeine and/or coffee consumption. These are summarized in Table 9.2.

TABLE 9.2
Classifications of Caffeine Exposure

Study	Caffeine intake	Other intake	Country of study
Prospective			
Wilcox et al., 1988	Median intake per month (3,150 mg) used as cutoff between lower and higher caffeine consumers. Also categorized as mg/month: <501; 201–3000; 3001–5000; 5001–7000; >7000	Coffee and noncoffee sources considered separately	U.S.
Florack et al., 1994	None	Cups of caffeinated drinks per day: <3; 3–7; >7	Holland
Caan et al., 1998	Daily intake (mg): ≤10.4; 10.5–106.8; >106.8	Servings per day of coffee, decaff coffee, tea, and soda: 0; 0.1–0.5; >0.5	U.S.
Hakim et al., 1998	Daily intake (mg): 0–25; 26–100; 101–300; ≥301	None	U.S.
Jensen et al., 1998	Daily intake (mg): 0–299; 300–699; ≥700	Coffee and noncoffee sources considered separately	Denmark
Retrospective			
Joesoef et al., 1990	As Wilcox, where median intake = 4200mg/month	Number of cups per day of coffee, decaff coffee, tea and cola: <1; 1–3; 4–6; >7	U.S. and Canada
Williams et al., 1990	None	Number of cups of coffee per day: 0; 1; 2; 3; ≥4	U.S.
Grodstein et al., 1993	Monthly intake (g): 0–3; 3.1–5; 5.1–7; >7	None	U.S. and Canada
Stanton & Gray, 1995	Daily intake (mg): 0; 1–150; 151–300; ≥301	None	U.S.
Bolumar et al., 1997	Daily intake (mg): 0–100; 101–300; 301–500; ≥501	Cups of coffee per day: 0; 1–2; 3–4; ≥5	Denmark, Germany, Italy, Poland, Spain

Study	Daily intake	Cup/source categories	Country
Curtis et al., 1997	Daily intake (mg): 0; 1–100; 101–300; 301–500; ≥501	Cups of coffee per day: 0; 1–2; 3–4; 5–6; ≥6 Cups of tea per day: 0; 0–1; 2–3; >3 Cups of cola per day: 0; 1; 2; >3	Canada
Christiansen et al., 1989	None	Number of cups of coffee per day: < 1; 1-3; 4-6; > 7	U.S.
Olsen, 1991	None	Number of cups of coffee/tea per day: 0–3; 4–7; ≥8 (2 cups tea ≡ 1 cup coffee)	Denmark
Hatch & Bracken, 1993	Daily intake (mg): 0; 1–150; 151–300; ≥301	Caffeine from each source: Coffee: none (0); light (1–150); moderate (151–300); high (≥300) Tea: none (0); light (1–50); moderate (51–100); high (≥100) Cola: none(0); light (1–50); moderate (51–150); high (≥151)	U.S.
Alderete et al., 1995	None	Cups of coffee per day: <1; 1–3; >3	U.S.

Studies that use the same estimates of caffeine intake are probably not directly comparable. Particularly, the study by Jensen et al. (1998), which used the same estimates as those of Wilcox et al. (1988), was an American study compared to theirs, which was based in Denmark. It is clear that different levels of exposure are apparent in different countries (Bolumar et al., 1997). However, the estimates used by Wilcox et al. and their followers were taken from a report published in 1984. It is possible that these are now out of date and the more recent reports may indeed have under- or overestimated actual caffeine intake. Nevertheless, any future studies that use more up-to-date estimates of caffeine content will make direct comparisons with previous research difficult.

As with the outcome measures used in these studies, the measures of exposure are open to recall bias and, to some extent, digit preference. Participants have been urged to recall a typical day's consumption as far back as 30 years ago and acceptable levels of recollection are a necessity. This is also subject to within-person variation and, as previously discussed, precise intake of caffeine is particularly hard to estimate considering differences in serving sizes, brands of drinks consumed, and brewing methods. None of these factors was sufficiently taken into account in any analyses reviewed here. It is highly likely that the bulk of analyses investigating caffeine intake are imprecise. However, with consistency in estimation across studies and appropriate categorizations and classifications used in analyses, satisfactory results can be obtained.

The two studies that reported caffeine intake during pregnancy, as opposed to the time interval of interest (when attempting to become pregnant), are immediately open to criticism (Hatch & Bracken, 1993; Williams et al., 1990). It has been reported that many women reduce their caffeine (coffee) intake during pregnancy (Fenster, Esemazi, Windham, & Swan, 1991) or at least those experiencing nausea do so (Wen, Sju, Jacobs, & Brown, 2001). These investigators are likely to have underestimated caffeine intake among participants who were affected by this phenomenon.

CONFOUNDERS

As briefly mentioned in the introduction, a large number of factors have been shown to be associated with fertility. Table 9.3 summarizes the factors that have been taken into account in the studies under review and shows that some of those studies have failed to consider these. This is important because they may contribute to any evident association between caffeine and fertility. The majority of studies adjusted for the number of previous pregnancies experienced by the women, female alcohol consumption, and some measure of socioeconomic status. All studies took into account female smoking, primarily by adjustment in multivariate analysis, although some stratified their sample (Alderete et al., 1995; Florack et al., 1994; Hakim et al., 1998; Jensen et al., 1998; Williams et al., 1990).

Categorization of all variables that are also examined needs to be considered. As with caffeine, to identify a biologic effect, a dose response needs to be ascertained. It is often not enough to dichotomize smokers from nonsmokers. The effects seen in heavy smokers are likely to be stronger than those in lighter smokers.

TABLE 9.3
Possible Confounding Factors Examined by Each Study

Study	Smoking	Coital freq.	Age	Age at menarche	Alcohol consumption	Marijuana use	Weight/height/BMI	Male caffeine consumption	Parity/gravidity	Ethnicity	Education/SES/employment status	Previous miscarriage	Previous birth control	Religion	Exercise	Number of sexual partners	Occupational exposures	Medical drug use	Previous history of infertility	History of disease of repro. organs
Wilcox et al., 1988	X	X	X	X	X	X	X	X												
Florack et al., 1994	X		X	X					X	X							X	X		
Caan et al., 1998	X																			
Hakim et al., 1998	X	X	X	X					X	X	X								X	
Jensen et al., 1998	X		X	X	X								X							X
Joesoef et al., 1990	X	X	X	X	X	X	X		X			X	X							
Williams et al., 1990	X		X	X	X		X		X											
Grodstein et al., 1993	X		X	X	X				X					X	X	X	X			
Stanton & Gray, 1995	X		X	X					X	X	X	X	X						X	
Bolumar et al., 1997	X	X	X	X					X			X	X							X
Curtis et al., 1997	X		X	X			X	X		X	X		X				X			
Christiansen et al., 1989	X								X	X										
Olsen, 1991	X		X	X					X	X										
Hatch & Bracken, 1993	X								X				X							
Alderete et al., 1995	X		X	X	X					X	X		X							

Of those studies that stratified their sample by smoking behavior, four looked at smoking versus not smoking (Alderete et al., 1995; Hakim et al., 1998; Jensen et al., 1998; Williams et al., 1990). Florack et al. (1994) looked at increasing doses of smoking (1 to 9, 10 to 19, ≥20 cigarettes per day) by coffee consumption (none, one to three, more than three cups per day). Interestingly, in response to a letter from Leviton (1996) about their study, Stanton and Gray (1995) did not consider smoking to be a confounder. However, they were concerned about the possible interaction between caffeine and smoking because smoking accelerates caffeine metabolism, thus reducing the possible biologic effects of caffeine. Leviton (1996) was critical of their subset analysis because Stanton and Gray only found an effect of caffeine on time to conception in nonsmokers, but no overall effect was evident. This is in contrast to findings in the other studies.

Given what we have stated about coital frequency, it is surprising that only three studies measured this (Jensen et al., 1998; Joesoef et al., 1990; Wilcox et al., 1988). Similarly only two studies considered the male partner's consumption of caffeine (Curtis et al., 1997; Wilcox et al.). In fact, hardly any male partner information was collected and, although the woman sustains any pregnancy, a host of male-mediated factors have an impact on the conception of that pregnancy.

POWER AND SAMPLE SIZE

The statistical power of a study represents the ability of that study to detect a significant difference between exposed and nonexposed participants and the outcome of interest. It depends on the size of the sample, proportion of the population exposed, and significance level chosen. For example, a study with a power of 80% would be 80% sure of detecting a defined difference as being statistically significant at a set significance level. Baird et al. (1986) have previously demonstrated the sample sizes required to detect differences in time to pregnancy studies with differing power and for different proportions of exposed versus unexposed at a significance level of 0.05 (two-tailed).

The authors of only three of the studies under review passed comment on the power of their studies (Caan et al., 1998; Florack et al., 1994; Hakim et al., 1998). The remainder merely commented that their study population was large (Alderete et al., 1995; Bolumar et al., 1997; Christiansen et al., 1989; Williams et al., 1990) or small (Wilcox et al., 1988), or did not appear to consider it (Curtis et al., 1997; Grodstein et al., 1993; Hatch & Bracken, 1993; Jensen et al., 1998; Joesoef et al., 1990; Olsen, 1991; Stanton & Gray, 1995).

Hakim et al. (1998) acknowledged their small sample size of 124 but stated that "analyzing all observed menstrual cycles increased the power of the study." However, to some extent, this may violate assumptions of independence and may not increase the power. Florack et al. (1994) also acknowledged that the power of their study may have been limited in detecting small differences, but claimed that this did not explain the fact that their findings were "more consistent with no effect or a small positive influence than with a positive influence." Similarly, Caan et al. (1998) stated that their lack of sufficient statistical power did explain the lack of association they reported.

A large sample size can increase the power of a study, provided an appropriate number of participants have the exposure and the outcome of interest. To test any dose–response effects of caffeine, a sufficient number would need to be present in the two extreme groups of exposure. Ideally, the reference category for investigating such effects would be an intake of zero. However, to achieve reliable point estimates, this group would need to be of sufficient size. Only five studies used zero consumption as baseline (Bolumar et al., 1997; Curtis et al., 1997; Hatch & Bracken, 1993; Stanton & Gray, 1995; Williams et al., 1990). The remainder included zero consumption in their lowest consumption categories, primarily due to the small numbers who did not consume any caffeine or coffee.

Figure 9.1a shows the proportions of each sample under review falling within the lowest categories for coffee or caffeine consumption. The proportions ranged

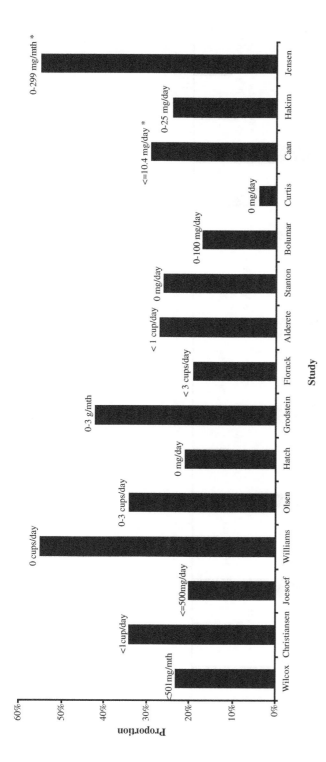

FIGURE 9.1 Proportion of sample within highest caffeine/coffee exposure group.

* Based on number of cycles, not number of participants

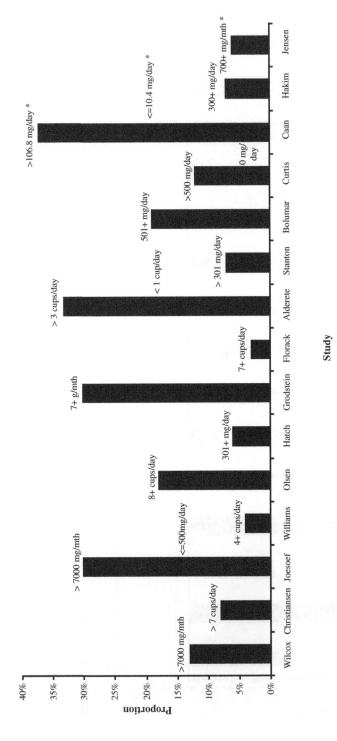

FIGURE 9.1 (Continued).

* Based on number of cycles, not number of participants

from 4 to 55%. Figure 9.1b shows the proportions of each sample under review falling within the highest categories for coffee or caffeine consumption; these proportions ranged from 3 to 34%. Small numbers within a category (such as the 3% of the population in the Florack et al., 1994, study) would result in wide confidence intervals, hence reducing the confidence we would have in the estimate of effect.

REPORTED RESULTS AND CONCLUSIONS FROM THE STUDIES

Seven studies found no statistically significant evidence to suggest that caffeine intake or coffee consumption had a detrimental effect on time to conception (Alderete et al., 1995; Caan et al., 1998; Curtis et al., 1997; Florack et al., 1994; Hakim et al., 1998; Jensen et al., 1998; Joesoef et al., 1990). The majority of them were prospective (Caan et al.; Florack et al.; Hakim et al.; Jensen et al.). Table 9.4 summarizes the main statistical results obtained by each study.

Although performing a retrospective study, Joesoef et al. (1990) were content with their measures of outcome and exposure. The distribution of time to pregnancy was similar to that reported in other studies and their study also reported similar significant associations with other factors and time to pregnancy to those in the literature. Alderete et al. (1995) did not observe a deleterious effect of coffee consumption, though they acknowledge that they may have underestimated the effects of caffeine because they only measured coffee consumption and no other sources of caffeine.

The retrospective survey by Curtis et al. (1997) reported no association between caffeine consumption and decreased fertility, although they state that their study had one major limitation: The average time between questionnaire administration and date of conception was 9 years. They admit that this "may have led to substantial misclassification of caffeine exposure." Also, because their study sample was restricted to an occupational group of farm workers, they may not have been representative of the general population and the couples under study may have had more than one pregnancy, potentially violating statistical independence.

Caan et al. (1998) showed a decrease in fertility with caffeine intake and coffee consumption, but this failed to reach significance. However, they did show a significant increase with the consumption of tea, although very few women consumed high levels and they concede that this could be a spurious finding. The authors recommended that "future research should focus on separating out individual caffeinated and noncaffeinated beverages."

Hakim et al. (1998) also showed a nonsignificant decreased risk of conception with coffee consumption and suggest that there may be an association with lower levels of caffeine consumption than had previously been reported. Their recording of caffeine could have been improved because they updated caffeine consumption on a monthly basis, but they had the opportunity to ask participants to record daily intake in their diaries. Despite these limitations, the authors recommended that women wanting to become pregnant reduce their caffeine intake.

The most recent prospective study (Jensen et al., 1998) found no adverse effects of caffeine on fecundability. Although nonsignificant, reduced point estimates were

TABLE 9.4
Main Statistical Results

Study	Main statistical results
Prospective	
Wilcox et al., 1988	Adjusted fecundability ratio for highest caffeine concentration: 0.51 (95% CI: 0.33, 0.75)
Florack et al., 1994	Adjusted fecundability ratio for >700 mg/day compared to lowest intake: 0.6 (95% CI: 0.3–0.97); 400–700 mg/day compared to lowest intake: 1.6 (95% CI: 1.0, 2.4)
Caan et al., 1998	Overall adjusted fecundability ratios compared to ≤10.4 mg/day for 10.5–106.8 mg/day: 1.08 (95% CI: 0.65, 1.81); for >106.8 mg/day: 1.09 (95% CI: 0.63, 1.89)
Hakim et al., 1998	Adjusted fecundability ratios compared to 0–25 mg/day for 26–100 mg/day: 1.13 (95% CI: 0.51, 2.49); for 101–300 mg/day: 0.48 (95% CI: 0.26, 1.35); for ≥301 mg/day: 0.83 (95% CI: 0.34, 2.01)
Jensen et al., 1998	Adjusted fecundability raio compared to nonsmokers consuming <300 mg/day for nonsmokers consuming 300–700 mg/day: 0.88 (95% CI: 0.60, 1.31); for nonsmokers consuming ≥700 mg/day: 0.63 (95% CI: 0.25, 1.60)
Retrospective	
Joesoef et al., 1990	Adjusted fecundability ratio for 700 mg/mth compared to ≤500 mg/mth: 1.03 (95% CI: 0.92, 1.16)
Williams et al., 1990	Adjusted fecundability ratio for 4+ cups coffee/day compared to none: 0.81 (95% CI: 0.67, 0.97)
Grodstein et al., 1993	Relative risk of tubal infertility for >7 g caffeine/mth compared to <3 g/mth: 1.5 (95%CI: 1.1, 2.0); relative risk of endometriosis for 5.1–7 g caffeine/mth compared to <3 g/mth: 1.9 (95%CI: 1.2, 2.9); >7 g caffeine/mth compared to <3 g/mth: 1.6 (95% CI: 1.1, 2.4)
Stanton & Gray, 1995	Odds ratio for taking >12 mths to conceive in nonsmokers consuming ≥301 mg compared to nonsmoking nonconsumers: 2.65 (95% CI: 1.38. 5.07)
Bolumar et al., 1997	Adjusted odds ratio for taking ≥9.5 mths to conceive consuming ≥500 mg/day: 1.45 (95% CI: 1.03, 2.04)
Curtis et al., 1997	Fecundability ratio for ≥100 mg/day compare to ≤100 mg/day: 0.98 (95% CI: 0.91, 1.07); any coffee drinking compared to no coffee drinking: 0.92 (95% CI: 0.84, 1.00)
Christiansen et al., 1989	Adjusted relative risk for difficulty in becoming pregnant, >7 cups of coffee/day: 1.96
Olsen, 1991	Odds ratio for taking ≥1 year to conceive in smokers consuming 8+ cups of coffee per day: 1.35 (95% CI: 1.02, 1.48)
Hatch & Bracken, 1993	Adjusted odds ratio for taking ≥1 year to conceive compared to no caffeine consumption; 1–150 mg: 1.39 (95% CI: 0.90, 2.13); 151–300 mg: 1.88 (95% CI: 1.13, 3.11); >300 mg: 2.24 (95% CI: 1.06, 4.73)
Alderete et al., 1995	Adjusted odds ratios ranged from 1.0–1.2 for nonsmoking consumers compared to nonsmoking nonconsumers

Note: Fecundability ratio: per-cycle probability of pregnancy for exposed and unexposed expressed as a ratio.

found in smoking and nonsmoking women who consumed the equivalent of three or more cups of coffee per day. However, only 460 couples were involved in total and only a small proportion had high caffeine intake. In spite of their lack of associations, the authors also suggested that women wanting to become pregnant—in particular, nonsmokers—may benefit from reduced caffeine intake.

Florack et al. (1994) showed that moderate caffeine intake did not have an adverse effect on fecundability in females; in fact, they found a nonsignificant positive association. However, theirs was one of the few studies to investigate caffeine intake of the partner. Males drinking more than seven cups of coffee per day had reduced fecundability. They conclude that the significant effects reported by others are probably partly due to additional factors that, in turn, are associated with consumption of caffeine.

Only one prospective study showed a significant reduction in fertility with increased caffeine intake. Wilcox et al. (1988) reported that women consuming the equivalent of over one cup of coffee per day were half as likely to conceive, per cycle, compared to those drinking less. A dose response with caffeine intake was also evident. The authors advocate caution when interpreting these results and they recommend that future studies be prospective in design in order to collect the best possible data.

The results reported by Christiansen et al. (1989) were given in a letter to *Lancet* in response to the Wilcox et al. 1988 study. A preliminary analysis of their data showed a dose-related effect of coffee consumption and "reported difficulties becoming pregnant." They acknowledge that their data are less refined than their predecessors' but stated that their data were based on a much larger population.

The results by Williams et al. (1990) were also in a letter to *Lancet*. They were prompted to examine their data after the conflicting results published by Wilcox et al. (1988) and Joesoef et al. (1990). In their sample, the authors found that women consuming at least four cups of coffee per day were 81% as likely to conceive, per cycle, as those who were nonconsumers. However, they used consumption during the first trimester of pregnancy as a proxy for consumption during the time when pregnancy was attempted. They argued that this misclassification would actually "underestimate the true risk of exposure" if women reduced their intake during pregnancy, but there is no evidence that this is a reliable proxy for intake prior to conception.

Olsen (1991) found no association between coffee intake and an increased risk of subfecundity when restricting the sample to nonsmokers. However, in nonsmokers, high consumers (eight or more cups per day) of coffee had significantly increased risk of taking more than 1 year to conceive. The author states that this significant association "may ... have public health implications if it reflects a causal relation."

In the study by Hatch and Bracken (1993), no significant association was seen between total caffeine intake and reduced fertility. However, after adjusting for the last method of birth control, parity, and smoking, there was an apparent association. Low (1 to 150 mg/day) to moderate (151 to 300 mg/day) levels of caffeine intake were associated with a 10% reduction in the per-cycle probability of conception; the highest level of intake (≥301 mg/day) was associated with a 27% reduction.

Elevated but nonsignificant odds ratios were evident for heavy intake of coffee and cola, but not for tea, leading the authors to believe that the overall association reported could not be accounted for by any individual type of drink. The authors conclude their paper by commenting that their "study adds to the evidence that caffeine intake [or other component] may be related to a reduction in fertility among females."

The only study that looked at clinical diagnoses of primary fertility (Grodstein et al., 1993) found a significant increased risk of tubal infertility and endometriosis with the higher levels of caffeine intake and a nonsignificant elevated risk of fertility due to cervical factors. Grodstein and colleagues specify that "further investigation of the biologic influence of caffeine on the reproductive system is needed."

Stanton and Gray (1995) stratified their sample by smoking behavior and only found a significant effect of caffeine intake in nonsmokers consuming more than 300 mg per day. However, their study included all pregnancies to their participants over a 10-year period and they acknowledge that "the relation between caffeine and fecundity merits further research given the prevalence of caffeine consumption in women of childbearing age." They also recommend that women considering pregnancy avoid high levels of caffeine intake.

The most recent study finding significant effects is that by Bolumar et al. (1997), who reported increased odds ratios of taking at least 9.5 months to conceive in those who consumed more than 500 mg of caffeine per day. This effect was stronger in smokers. Nevertheless, they concluded that a more specific study is needed to rule out the effect of caffeine intake in relation to other job- and life-related stress variables.

POSSIBLE MECHANISMS OF ANY DETRIMENTAL CAFFEINE EFFECT

The nature of the biological mechanisms involved with any detrimental effect of caffeine on female infertility is currently uncertain. Indeed, only five studies discussed the possible biological plausibility of how caffeine could interfere with fertility (Bolumar et al., 1997; Grodstein et al., 1993; Hatch & Bracken, 1993; Jensen et al., 1998; Stanton & Gray, 1995). Other studies have shown an association between increased caffeine use and spontaneous abortion (Joffe, 1989; Wilcox, Weinberg, & Baird, 1990). If spontaneous abortion occurs early in pregnancy, the woman may not even be aware that she had been pregnant, resulting in what would appear to be a longer waiting time to pregnancy.

Two studies (Jensen et al., 1998; Stanton & Gray, 1995) quoted Lane et al., who demonstrated varying levels of caffeine metabolism throughout the menstrual cycle (Lane, Steege, Rupp, & Kuhn, 1992). Both Jensen et al. (1998) and Stanton & Gray (1995) reported "reduced clearance during the luteal phase, resulting in greater accumulation during the period of implantation and early embryonic development." Fenster et al. (1999) stated that consumers of high levels of caffeine were at a greater risk of short cycle lengths, which may reflect underlying endocrine patterns.

Caffeine could detrimentally affect female infertility by directly influencing ovulation through alterations in hormone levels, as Hatch and Bracken (1993) and Bolumar et al. (1997) discuss. They referred to a study that noted that coffee consumption was associated with reduced levels of estrogens (Petridou et al., 1992).

Caffeine is reported to act as a smooth muscle relaxant and as such could prolong the time taken for the conceptus to travel from the fallopian tube to the uterus (Leonard et al., 1987), thus affecting the process of implantation. Tannic acid, a component of tea, has also been put forward as a possible factor. According to Cramer (1990), tea is a richer source of tannin than coffee is. The author of the letter to *Lancet* in response to the Joesoef et al. (1990) study postulates that this could account for the observation in that study that there was a significant adverse effect of tea.

Wilcox et al. (1988) showed that a greater effect was seen with recent caffeine consumption on the per-cycle probability of conception than with previous consumption. This suggests that any adverse effects of caffeine are transient and reversible.

SUMMARY

A total of 15 published epidemiological studies were found in the literature evaluating the possible detrimental effects of caffeine (or coffee) consumption on female fertility:

Alderete et al., 1995
Bolumar et al., 1997
Caan et al. 1998
Christiansen et al. 1989
Curtis et al., 1997
Florack et al., 1994
Grodstein et al., 1993
Hakim et al., 1998
Hatch and Bracken, 1993
Jensen et al., 1998
Joesoef et al., 1990
Olsen, 1991
Stanton and Gray, 1995
Wilcox et al., 1988
Williams et al., 1990

Seven of these found an overall association between increased caffeine intake and a significant reduction in fertility, measured as time to pregnancy (Bolumar et al., 1997; Caan et al. 1998; Christiansen et al. 1989; Florack et al., 1994; Wilcox et al., 1988; Williams et al., 1990); one further study found such an association only in smokers (Olsen, 1991); and another only in nonsmokers (Stanton & Gray, 1995). Grodstein et al. (1993) reported an association between specific primary diagnoses of infertility and caffeine intake. The remaining six studies reviewed here found no significant associations with caffeine intake and time to pregnancy in females (Alderete et al., 1995; Caan et al.; Florack et al.; Hakim et al., 1998; Jensen et al., 1998; Joesoef et al., 1990).

Generally, the results reviewed here are weak and inconsistent. Discrepancies can be attributed to differences in the measure of caffeine/coffee intake and time to conception data, both of which are imprecise in some studies. The large variations in study methodology also make comparisons difficult. Five of the studies were prospective (Caan et al., 1998; Hakim et al., 1998; Jensen et al., 1998; Olsen, 1991; Wilcox et al., 1988) and it is of particular interest that only one of them reported a significant association between caffeine intake and decreased fertility (Wilcox et al.), compared to seven out of the ten retrospective studies (Bolumar et al., 1997; Christiansen et al. 1989; Grodstein et al., 1993; Hatch & Bracken, 1993; Olsen; Stanton & Gray, 1995; Williams et al., 1990).

Kennedy, van Molcke, and Harmatx (1991) recommend that reports of caffeine intake should be "confirmed by biochemical means." This is expensive and time consuming and, because caffeine has a relatively short half-life, is unlikely to be reliable. Nevertheless, future studies should attempt to consider the differences between persons in cumulative exposure and individual metabolism. The studies of time to pregnancy can be useful provided that estimates of prepregnancy caffeine consumption are good; however, it is essential that several sources of bias are accounted for before making any conclusive statements based on the results obtained.

ACKNOWLEDGMENTS

We would like to thank Maureen Brennan for obtaining some of the papers and Clare Bell for her valuable comments on the manuscript.

REFERENCES

Aitken, R. J., Best, F., & Richardson, D. W. (1983). Influence of caffeine on the movement characteristics, capacity and ability to penetrate cervical mucus of human spermatozoa. *Journal of Reproductive Fertility, 67*, 19–27.

Alderete, E., Eskenaz, I. B., & Sholtz, R. (1995). Effect of cigarette smoking and coffee drinking on time to conception. *Epidemiology, 6*, 403–408.

Argood, C., Duckitt, K., & Templeton, A. A. (1998). Smoking and female infertility: A systematic review and meta-analysis. *Human Reproduction, 13*, 1532–1539.

Baird, D. D., Wilcox, A. J., & Weinberg, C. R. (1986). Use of time to pregnancy to study environmental exposures. *American Journal of Epidemiology, 124*, 470–480.

Barone, J. J., & Roberts, H. R. (1996). Caffeine consumption. *Food & Chemical Toxicology, 34*, 119–129.

Basso, O., Juul, S., & Olsen, J. (2000). Time to pregnancy as a correlated of fecundity: Differential persistence in trying to become pregnant as a source of bias. *International Journal of Epidemiology, 29*, 856–861.

Bolumar, F., Olsen, J., Rebagliato, M., Bisanti, L. & the European Study in Infertility and Subfecundity. (1997). Caffeine intake and delayed conception: A European multi-center study on infertility and subfecundity. *American Journal of Epidemiology, 145*, 324–334.

Bonati, M., Latini, R., Tognoni, G., Young, J.F., & Garattini, S. (1985). Interspecies comparison of *in vivo* caffeine pharmacokinetics in man, monkey, rabbit, rat and mouse. *Drug Metabolism Review, 15*, 1355–1383.

Bunker, M. L., & McWilliams, M. (1979). Caffeine content of common beverages. *Journal of the American Dietetic Association, 74*, 28–32.

Caan, B., Quesenberry, C. P., & Coates, A. O. (1998). Differences in fertility associated with caffeinated beverage consumption. *American Journal of Public Health, 88,* 270–274.

Caan, B. J., & Goldhaber, M. K. (1989). Caffeinated beverages and low birth weight: A case-control study. *American Journal of Public Health, 79,* 1299–1300.

Carlsen, E., Giwercman, A., Keiding, N., & Skakkebaek, N. E. (1992). Evidence for decreasing quality of semen during the past 50 years. *British Medical Journal, 305,* 609–613.

Christiansen, R. E., Oechsli, F. W., & van den Berg, B. J. (1989). Caffeinated beverages and decreased fertility. *Lancet, 1,* 378.

Cramer, D. W. (1990). Caffeine and infertility (letter). *Lancet, 1,* 742.

Curtis, K. M., Savitz, D. A., & Arbuckle, T. E. (1997). Effects of cigarette smoking, caffeine consumption and alcohol intake on fecundability. *American Journal of Epidemiology, 146,* 32–41.

Dlugosz, L., Belanger, K., Hellenbrand, K., Holford, T. R., Leaderer, B., & Bracken, M. B. (1996). Maternal caffeine consumption and spontaneous abortion: A prospective cohort study. *Epidemiology, 7,* 150–155.

Dlugosz, L., & Bracken, B. (1992). Reproductive effects of caffeine: A review and theoretical analysis. *Epidemiology Reviews, 14,* 83–100.

Fenster, L, Eskanazi, B., Windham, G. C., & Swan, S. H. (1991a). Caffeine consumption during pregnancy and spontaneous abortion. *Epidemiology, 2,* 168–174.

Fenster, L., Eskenazi, B., Windham, G. C., & Swan, S. H. (1991b). Caffeine consumption during pregnancy and fetal growth. *American Journal of Public Health, 81,* 458–461.

Fenster, L., Quale, C., Waller, K., Windham, G. C., Elkin, E. P., Benowitz, N., & Swan, S. H. (1999). Caffeine consumption and menstrual function. *American Journal of Epidemiology, 149,* 550–557.

Florack, E. I. M., Zielhuis, G. A., & Rolland, R. (1994). Cigarette smoking, alcohol consumption and caffeine intake and fecundability. *Preventive Medicine, 23,* 175–180.

Ford, W. C. L., North, K., Taylor, H., Farrow, A., Hull, M. G. R., Golding, J., & the ALSPAC Study Team. (2000). Increasing paternal age is associated with delayed conception in a large population of fertile couples: Evidence for declining fecundity in older men. *Human Reproduction, 15,* 1703–1708.

Fortier, I., Marcoux, S., & Beaulac–Baillargeon, L. (1993). Relation of caffeine intake during pregnancy to intrauterine growth retardation and preterm birth. *American Journal of Epidemiology, 137,* 931–940.

Garbers, D. L., First, N. L., Sullivan, J. J., & Lardy, H. A. (1971). Stimulation and maintenance of ejaculated bovine spermatazoan respiration motility by caffeine. *Biology of Reproduction, 5,* 336–339.

Golding, J. (1995). Reproduction and caffeine consumption—A literature review. *Early Human Development, 43,* 1–14.

Graham, D. (1978). Caffeine: Its identity, dietary sources, intake and biological effects. *Nutrition Review, 36,* 97–102.

Grice, W. D. (1994) Influence of ingested caffeine on animal reproduction. In P. B. Dows (Ed.), *Caffeine: Perspectives from recent research.* Berlin: Springer–Verlag.

Grodstein, F., Goldman, M. B., Ryan, L., & Cramer, D. W. (1993). Relation of female infertility to consumption of caffeinated beverages. *American Journal of Epidemiology, 137,* 1353–1360.

Hakim, R. B., Gray, R. H., & Zacur, H. (1998). Alcohol and caffeine consumption and decreased fertility. *Fertility & Sterility, 70,* 632–637.

Hatch, E. E., & Bracken, M. B. (1993). Association of delayed conception with caffeine consumption. *American Journal of Epidemiology, 138,* 1082–1092.

Hull, M. G. R., Glazener, C. M. A., Kely, N. J., Conway, D. I., Foster, P. A., & Hinton, R. A. (1985). Population study of causes, treatment and outcome of infertility. *British Medical Journal*, *291*, 1693–1697.

Hull, M. G. R., North, K., Taylor, H., Farrow, A., Ford, W. C. L, Golding, J., & the ALSPAC Study Team. (2000). Delayed conception and active and passive smoking. *Fertility & Sterility*, *74*, 725–733.

Infante–Rivard, C., Fernandez, A., & Gaulthier, R. (1993). Fetal loss associated with caffeine intake before and during pregnancy. *JAMA*, *270*, 2940–2943.

Jensen, T. K., Henriksen, T. B., Hjollund, N. H. I., Schieke, T., Kolstad, H., Giwercman, A., Ernst, E., Bonde, J. P., Skakkebaek, N. E., & Olsen, J. (1998). Caffeine intake and fecundability: A follow-up study among 430 Danish couples planning their first pregnancy. *Reproductive Toxicology*, *12*, 289–295.

Jensen, T. K., Hjollund, N. H. I., Henriksen, T. B., Scheike, T., Kolstad, H., & Giwercman, A. (1998). Does moderate alcohol consumption affect fertility? Follow-up study among couples planning first pregnancy. *British Medical Journal*, *317*, 1389–1394.

Joesoef, M. R., Beral, V. O., & Cramer, D. W. (1990). Are caffeinated beverages risk factors for delayed conception? *Lancet*, *335*, 136–137.

Joffe, M. (1989). Feasibility of studying subfertility using retrospective self-reports. *Journal of Epidemiology & Community Health*, *43*, 268–274.

Joffe, M. (2000). Time trends in biological fertility in Britain. *Lancet*, *355*, 1961–1965.

Joffe, M., Villard, L., Li, Z., Plowman, R., & Vessey, M. (1993). Long-term recall of time to pregnancy. *Fertility & Sterility*, *60*, 99–104.

Kennedy, J. S., van Molcke, L. L., & Harmatz, J. J. (1991). Validity of self-reports of caffeine use. *Journal of Clinical Pharmacology*, *31*, 677–680.

Klesges, R. C., Ray, J. W., & Klesges, L. M. (1994). Caffeinated coffee and tea intake and its relationship to cigarette smoking. An analysis of the Second National Health and Nutrition Examination Survey (NHANES II). *Journal of Substance Abuse*, *6*, 407–418.

Lane, J. D., Steege, J. F., Rupp, S. L., & Kuhn, C. (1992). Menstrual cycle effects on caffeine elimination in the human female. *European Journal of Clinical Pharmacology*, *43*, 543–546.

Lecos, C. (1984). The latest caffeine scorecard. *Consumer Review*, *67*, 35–36.

Leonard,T. K., Watson, R. R., & Mohs, M. E. (1987). The effects of caffeine on various body systems: A review. *Journal of the American Dietetic Association*, *87*, 1048–1053.

Leviton, A. (1995). Does caffeine consumption increase the risk of reproductive adversities? *JAMA*, *50*, 20–22.

Leviton, A. (1996). Re: Effects of caffeine consumption on delayed conception. *American Journal of Epidemiology*, *144*, 800–801.

Marshburn, P. B., Sloan, C. S., & Hammond, M. G. (1989). Semen quality and association with coffee consumption, cigarette smoking, and ethanol consumption. *Fertility & Sterility*, *52*, 162–165.

Menken, J., Trussell, J., & Larsen, U. (1986). Age and infertility. *Science*, *233*, 1389–1394.

Olsen, J. (1991). Cigarette smoking, tea and coffee drinking and subfecundity. *American Journal of Epidemiology*, *133*, 734–739.

Olsen, J., Juul, S., & Basso, O. (1998). Measuring time to pregnancy. Methodological issues to consider. *Human Reproduction*, *13*, 1751–1756.

Olsen, J., Overvad, K., & Frische, G. (1991). Coffee consumption, birth weight and repro-ductive failures. *Epidemiology*, *2*, 370–374.

Parsons, W. D., & Neims, A. H. (1978). Effect of smoking on caffeine clearance. *Clinical Pharmacology & Therapeutics*, *24*, 40–45.

Petridou, E., Katsouyanni, K., Spannos, E., Skalkidis, Y., Panagiotopoulou, K., & Trichopoulos, D. (1992). Pregnancy estrogens in relation to coffee and alcohol intake. *Annals of Epidemiology, 2*, 241–247.

Purves, D., & Sullivan, F. M. (1993) Reproductive effects of caffeine: Experimental studies in animals. In S. Garantti (Ed.), *Caffeine, coffee and health.* New York: Raven Press.

Stanton, C. K., & Gray, R. H. (1995). Effects of caffeine consumption on delayed conception. *American Journal of Epidemiology, 142*, 1322–1329.

te Velde, E. R., Eijkemans, R., & Habbema, H. D. F. (2000). Variation in couple fecundity and time to pregnancy, an essential concept in human reproduction. *Lancet, 355*, 1928–1929.

Vessey, M. P., Wright, N. H., McPherson, K., & Wiggins, P. (1978). Fertility after stopping different methods of contraception. *British Medical Journal, 4*, 265–267.

Weinberg, C. R., Baird, D. D., & Wilcox, A. J. (1994). Sources of bias in studies of time to pregnancy. *Statistics in Medicine, 13*, 671–681.

Wen, W., Shum, X. O., Jacobs, D. R., & Brown, J. E. (2001). The associations of maternal caffeine consumption and nausea with spontaneous abortion, *Epidemiology, 12*, 38–42.

Wilcox, A., Weinberg, C., & Baird, D. (1988). Caffeinated beverages and decreased fertility. *Lancet, 2*, 1453–1455.

Wilcox, A. J., Weinberg, C. R., & Baird, D. D. (1990). Risk factors for early pregnancy loss. *Epidemiology, 1*, 382–385.

Williams, M. A., Manson, R. R., Goldman, M. B., Mittendorf, R., & Ryan, K. S. (1990). Coffee and delayed conception. *Lancet, 2*, 1603.

Section IV

Mood and Performance and Psychopathology

10 Effects of Caffeine on Mood

Hendrik J. Smit and Peter J. Rogers

CONTENTS

INTRODUCTION

After water, tea and coffee are the two most widely consumed beverages worldwide (Gilbert, 1984); thus, the physical and/or financial costs involved in tea and coffee making must somehow be outweighed by benefits in order to choose these drinks over water and also to support a rapid worldwide spread of their use during the last millennium. Further strength for this argument lies in the fact that the discovery of tea and coffee is recorded in a range of legends almost invariably referring to the invigorating, energizing or counterfatiguing effects of the two plants, or, as we know today, of caffeine (coffee: Wellman, 1961; tea: various sources, e.g., Campbell, 1995; Segal, 1996; see also chapter 2). Indeed, in the scientific literature, an almost "natural" focus has been on effects on mood and performance, with typical and reliable effects on alertness and attention reported (e.g., Smit & Rogers, 2000).

However, the vast range of publications on this topic has still not produced a clear and detailed picture of these effects and the factors explaining individual differences. This chapter attempts to clarify this by bringing together the most relevant and more recently published research on the effects caffeine has on mood, concentrating on the effects of ecologically relevant doses of caffeine. It is an in-depth account of various detailed effects of caffeine on mood. It also challenges the way in which most caffeine research has been conducted to date by looking at the issue from a different angle and discusses the pros and cons of the various approaches that some "aware" scientists have implemented in their research.

BACKGROUND

Although Hirsh (1984) warns against a general definition of caffeine as a central nervous system (CNS) stimulant, this definition is still used today (e.g., Hindmarch, Quinlan, Moore, & Parkin, 1998). Maybe a driving force behind this definition is a certain level of general appeal because the effects of caffeine go well beyond an excitation of the CNS. The current view is that, considering the wide range of bodily functions on which caffeine and adenosine show antagonistic effects (blood pressure, renin release, catecholamine release, urine output, CNS activity, lipolysis, respiration, and intestinal peristalsis; James, 1991), caffeine's main mode of action is that of competitively blocking adenosine receptor sites (see Fredholm, Bättig, Holmén, Nehlig, & Zvartau, 1999, for a review). Caffeine-induced changes in these bodily functions are likely to be experienced as subjective symptoms, thereby (directly or indirectly) changing the caffeine consumer's mood state.

However, several factors are known to modify the effects of caffeine. First of all, large differences in caffeine discrimination and subjective effects have been found between subjects (e.g., Mumford et al., 1994), and also very large inter- and intraindividual variations in caffeine clearance (e.g., Balogh, Harder, Vollandt, & Staib, 1992). These differences could reflect individual changes and differences in caffeine metabolism (Lader, Cardwell, Shine, & Scott, 1996), which in turn is known to be influenced by, for example, the use of oral contraceptives, pregnancy, diet, age, disease (Yesair, Branfman, & Callahan, 1984), and tobacco use (Benowitz, Hall, & Modin, 1989).

Secondly, the "food context" in which caffeine is consumed can influence its absorption rate. There are indications that the fat and polyphenols in chocolate inhibit the uptake of caffeine (Czok, 1974), thus making these contextual factors an important issue for consideration. In addition, it has been reported that sugars antagonize some excitatory effect of methylxanthines (Chauchard, Mazoué, & Lecoq, 1945) by inhibiting gastric emptying (Chvasta & Cooke, 1971), as do several food-borne acids (Hunt & Knox, 1969). Typically, Mumford et al. (1996) and Liguori, Hughes, and Grass (1997) have shown remarkable differences in magnitude of drug effect and peak plasma time (PPT) for caffeine in cola, coffee, chocolate, and gelatine capsules.

Thirdly, because subjective effects can easily be affected by expectations and attitudes (e.g., Flaten & Blumenthal, 1999; Lotshaw, Bradley, & Brooks, 1996), researching the effects of caffeine on mood is more complicated when using real-life caffeine-containing food and drinks. This does not, however, devalue research on drinks such as tea and coffee; rather, it adds to the ecological validity of the findings. Finally, perhaps the most important determinant of an individual's response to caffeine is his or her habitual level of caffeine consumption. Indeed, the "withdrawal reversal" hypothesis predicts that positive mood effects occur only in regular caffeine consumers who are acutely caffeine withdrawn (e.g., James, 1998; James & Rogers, 2005; Rogers, Richardson, & Elliman, 1995) and must therefore represent a relief of withdrawal symptoms (see also later discussion).

Thus, various factors can affect caffeine uptake and caffeine metabolism, reported subjective effects, and mood after the consumption of caffeine or caffeine-containing foods and drinks.

MEASUREMENT OF MOOD

The measurement of mood is by no means straightforward. The choice among a 5-, 7-, or 9-point Likert scale or a 100-mm visual-analogue scale (VAS) is possibly of lesser practical importance when administering mood questionnaires than are the experimental design and instructions to participants. Even the use of "validated" mood or subjective symptoms questionnaires (e.g., the Profile of Mood States [POMS; Lorr & McNair, 1988]) does not guarantee results. Indeed, some researchers have failed to find effects of caffeine on mood using such scales (e.g., Landolt, Werth, Borbély, & Dijk, 1995; Lieberman, Wurtman, Emde, Roberts, & Coviella, 1987; Smith, Whitney, Thomas, Perry, & Brockman, 1997). Various factors appear to add noise to the data when administering mood questionnaires. These include:

- use of irrelevant or ambiguous mood descriptors
- lack of motivation due to the length or layout of the questionnaire
- insufficient or unclear instructions for filling out mood questionnaires
- learned responses through repetitions (not randomizing) of mood adjectives
- attitudes of participant towards filling out questionnaires in general
- experimental set-up and general instructions
- individual differences in the projection of intensity on the line or category scales
- differences in definitions of one particular mood adjective
- confusion regarding differences in definition between similar mood adjectives (e.g., "tired" and "fatigued")

Our experience of mood measurement in caffeine research is that each group of participants tested will make a variable reduction technique such as principal component analysis (PCA) produce slightly different mood dimensions, possibly due to small individual differences in definitions of some mood adjectives used or possibly because of the variation in these descriptors caused by design of the study. This is shown very clearly when one compares the PCA outcomes of the three relatively similar studies reported in Smit, Cotton, Hughes, and Rogers (2004). Typically, energetic arousal, tense arousal and hedonic tone are dimensions of mood as proposed by Thayer (1989). Energetic arousal, a mood dimension formerly named "high positive affect" (see Thayer, 1978), comprises mood adjectives such as "active," "elated," "enthusiastic," "excited," "peppy," and "strong" versus "drowsy," "dull," "sleepy," and "sluggish."

All of our studies (e.g., Smit, Cotton, et al., 2004; Smit, Gaffan, & Rogers, 2004; Smit & Rogers, 2000) found a similar construct explaining most of the variance in the mood data, comprising the adjectives "clearheaded," "revitalized," "alert," and "energetic" versus "tired" and "fatigued." Likewise, tense arousal ("negative affect") is typically constructed of adjectives such as "tense," "angry," "nervous," "jittery," "distressed," "anxious," and "frustrated" versus "calm," "relaxed," and "placid." Hedonic tone (also the "pleasantness" dimension) constitutes items that seem more related to "well-being": "happy," "content," "friendly," and so on versus items such as "sad," "depressed," and "gloomy." The mood constructs "energetic arousal," "tense arousal," and "hedonic tone" will be used hereafter to describe the effects of caffeine on mood reported in the literature.

EXPERIMENTAL EVIDENCE

Actual experimental evidence of the effects of caffeine has been documented in hundreds, possibly thousands, of publications covering probably more than 100 years of research. Typically, these papers differ in various aspects: sample size, methodology, but also age groups, gender, nationality, nature of the treatments (e.g., coffee vs. decaf coffee; caffeine vs. placebo in capsules), etc. Our aim here is to review a good sample of more recent and important published research contributing to the understanding of effects of caffeine on mood. This literature is discussed later with further details given in Table 10.1.

EFFECTS OF CAFFEINE ON MOOD

Much research has been carried out to investigate the effects of caffeine, using various experimental designs, doses, and vehicles.

In a series of caffeine self-administration experiments, Liguori, Hughes, and Oliveto (1997) found that 17 mg caffeine/8 oz cola increased hedonic tone and energetic arousal, and decreased tense arousal, irritability, stomach problems, and feelings of "confusion" compared to placebo. Cola containing 33 mg/8 oz (vs. placebo) increased energetic arousal and hedonic tone and feeling "talkative" and "motivated to work." In general, caffeine-containing cola drinks were rated as more stimulating compared to the placebo cola. Another experiment, comparing 33 and 100 mg caffeine/8 oz cola or coffee to placebo, showed that caffeine increased energetic arousal, hedonic tone, confidence, impatience, and feeling "motivated to work" and decreased "nausea/vomiting" and marginal decreased headache scores.

Crucially, compared to 33 mg caffeine, 100 mg caffeine (across vehicles) showed increased ratings for energetic arousal, stomach problems, "hunger/appetite," and feeling "talkative." However, the vehicles differed: compared to coffee, cola showed increased ratings for "shaky/weakness" without providing any Vehicle × Dose

TABLE 10.1
Overview of Recent Caffeine Research Discussed in This Chapter

Year	Double-blind?	ws/bs[a]	N	Caff. consumption (mg/day)[b]	Caff. administration	Withdrawal	Mood measure	Caff. vs. placebo?	Effects	Ref.
2001	Y	ws	16	Equivalent to 0–3 cups of coffee/day	300 mg slow release over 50 h of continued wakefulness	None?	Bond and Lader VAS	Y	Cf. placebo, drowsiness DECR with SRC for up to 30 h of sleep deprivation, and confusion DECR for up to 37 h	Beaumont et al.
1994	Y	ws	12	480.3 (300–732)	Day 1: db deprivation condition (3 × 0- or 3 × 100-mg capsules, one each at 10:00, 14:00, and 18:00h) Day 2: db caff. condition (1 × 0- or 1 × 300-mg capsule, at 9:00h, after baseline measures) Counterbalancing 2 conditions on 2 days, creating 4	By virtue of deprivation condition; no caff from midnight at start of Day 1 to noon on Day 2. Therefore, withdrawal is overnight or 33 h	POMS, 10 item mood VAS	Y	Abstinence effects: Ss showed higher headache scores in the deprived condition; cf. nondeprived condition. Headache ratings in the deprived condition were highest at baseline on Day 2. Also, Ss reported being sign more disoriented following caff. administration cf. placebo. Acute effects: Day 2 Dose × Time interactions for VAS "stimulated" and POMS "arousal" and "vigor." Main caff dose effects on VAS "alert," "sleepy," "sluggish," and POMS "arousal," "fatigue," and "vigor." Caff DECR "sleepy," "sluggish," and "fatigue" and	Brauer et al.

(continued)

TABLE 10.1 (Continued)
Overview of Recent Caffeine Research Discussed in This Chapter

Year	Double-blind?	ws/bs[a]	N	Caff. consumption (mg/day)[b]	Caff. administration	Withdrawal	Mood measure	Caff. vs. placebo?	Effects	Ref.
					conditions: PP, PC, CP & CC				INCR "alert," "arousal," and "vigor" cf. placebo. Day 1 Deprived × Day 2 Dose × Time interactions for VAS "anxious" and POMS "elation," "friendliness," and "positive mood."	
1997	Y	ws	12	100–1000	100 mg or placebo in capsule at 9:45, 13:45, and 17:45 (300 mg in total); caff on Days 1–4 and 7–11; placebo on Days 5–6 and 12–13	Overnight (in lab)	VAS (50 items)	Y	Cf. caff, placebo INCR "headache," "miserable," "sedated," "sleepy," "tired," "unmotivated," "yawning" and DECR "alert," "anxious," "energetic," "self-confident." No clear differences between different placebo days or placebo periods. Cf. placebo, caff postplacebo DECR "miserable," "sleepy," "tired," "unmotivated," "yawning," and INCR "jittery" and "self-confident."	Comer et al.
1999	I : Y	ws	15	241 ± 30	1 × 300 mg + 2 × 0 mg, or 3 × 100 mg in capsules spread	Overnight (no caff allowed in diet other	Caff. withdrawal Qu. POMS	Y	Only effects found for (both) active doses vs. placebo. Placebo INCR "headache," "headache/poor	Evans & Griffiths

(continued)

				out over the day; 1 × 300 dose built up over 4 days from 3 × 100 starting dose for everyone Final dose adminis- tration of 9 (1 × 300 mg) or 5 days (3 × 100 mg) + 2 days placebo; sequence run 3 times	than provided by researchers)			mood," "tiredness," "flu-like symptoms," "fatigue" and DECR "vigor," "activity/alertness," and "friendly."
II: Y	ws	17	277 ± 27	100, 300, or 600 mg/day, building up from 100 with 50 mg/day for higher doses Final dose maintained for 7 days, followed by placebo for 2 days; dose administration in 2 capsules spread out over the day	Overnight (no caff allowed in diet other than provided by researchers)	Caff. withdrawal Qu, POMS	Y	Drug × Dose interactions for: "headache," "headache/poor mood," "activity/alertness," "tiredness," "vigor," "fatigue," "confusion–bewilderment," "friendly," "total mood disturbance." Placebo substitution INCR "tiredness." Dose-related caff. withdr symptoms: "headache/poor mood" INCR when placebo was substituted for 600 mg/day; "activity/alertness" DECR after the 300 and 600 mg caff doses;

TABLE 10.1 (Continued)
Overview of Recent Caffeine Research Discussed in This Chapter

Year	Double-blind?	ws/bs[a]	N	Caff. consumption (mg/day)[b]	Caff. administration	Withdrawal	Mood measure	Caff. vs. placebo?	Effects	Ref.
III: Y		ws	19	294 ± 65	Baseline = 300 mg/day for 7 days, then lower dose for 2 days (0, 25, 50, 100, 200, or 300 mg/day) followed by baseline dose, etc. until all lower doses had been taken; dose administration in 2 capsules spread out over the day	Overnight (no caff allowed in diet other than provided by researchers)	Caff. withdrawal Qu, POMS	Y	"headache" INCR after each active dose but with increasing sign with increasing dose. No overall effects of drug, but dose substitution effects for "activity/alertness," "tiredness," "fatigue," "total mood disturbance"; Drug × Dose substitution effects for "headache" and "vigor." Two-day maintenance dose of 300 mg did not differ from 200 mg. "Headache" and "headache/poor mood" only INCR with the placebo substitution. "Activity/alertness" scores were DECR cf. to maintenance dose for 0 and 25 mg/day. "Tiredness" scores INCR when the maintenance dose was substituted for 0, 25, 50, and 100 mg caff.	

	IV	n	Dose	Procedure	Abstinence	Measure	Sig	Results	Reference	Year
ws	IV: Y	25	263 ± 32	Baseline = 2 × 0 mg/day for 7 days, then 2 × 150 mg/day for 1, 3, 7, or 14 consecutive days, followed by baseline duration etc. until Ss had been exposed to all durations	Overnight (no caff. allowed in diet other than provided by researchers)	Caff. withdrawal Qu, POMS	Y	"activity/alertness" after 3 days of caff.; similar + INCR "headache" after 7 days of caff.; similar, minus "activity/alertness" effects, after 14 days of caff. Across all 4 experiments, placebo after 300 mg/day maintenance dose INCR "headache," "headache/poor mood," "tiredness," "fatigue," "confusion–bewilderment," "total mood disturbance" and DECR "activity/alertness," "vigor," and "friendly."		
ws	Y	11	555 ± 84	Ad lib 125 and 0 (placebo) mg in capsule with every cup of decaf coffee to replace their normal coffee	Overnight; no dietary caff. other than prescribed for each condition on day of testing	11 item, 6-point mood Qu	Y	Negative affect (tense arousal) showed a Dose × Time interaction, indicating that caff INCR tense arousal during midmorning and afternoon. No effects of caff. on early mornings and evenings on tense arousal. No effects of caff on positive affect (energetic arousal) or "tired."	Green & Suls	1996
ws	Unknown	20	6.4 cups of coffee/day (3–16)	0, 1.5, 3, and 6 mg/kg in decaf coffee	12 h	STAI, coffee effects and mood Qu	Y	Highest caff. dose tended to INCR state anxiety cf. to the 2 lower doses; dose effects were found for "the coffee activated me," "the	Hasenfratz & Bättig	1994

(continued)

TABLE 10.1 (Continued)
Overview of Recent Caffeine Research Discussed in This Chapter

Year	Double-blind?	ws/bs[a]	N	Caff. consumption (mg/day)[b]	Caff. administration	Withdrawal	Mood measure	Caff. vs. placebo?	Effects	Ref.
									coffee was strong," and "the coffee was good" and for the mood adjectives "sleepy," "awake," "dull," and "active," as well as for their combined "factor" score "wakefulness." "Nervousness" was reduced after 1.5 mg/kg dose but not after any of the other treatments. No correlations were found with habitual coffee consumption.	
2005	Y	ws	49	373 ± 45	1.2 mg/kg predose + 1.2 mg/kg or placebo after 4, 6, or 8 h, in 250 ml lemon squash	4, 6, or 8 h	4 item, bipolar 9-point mood Qu	Y	Only 8 h caff. abstinence showed INCR energetic mood and hedonic tone cf. placebo.	Heatherley et al.
1999	Y	Unknown	12	112.5 (50–150)	0 or 5 mg/kg body weight, capsules (= 350 mg in 70-kg person)	Overnight (>12 h)	POMS, mood grid, total score of self-report Qu	Y	Caff. vs. placebo: mood grid: INCR arousal, no effects of pleasantness. POMS: INCR vigor and DECR fatigue on vigor/activity and fatigue/inertia. No effects of any of the other subscales. SRQ	Herz

Year		Design	N	Prior caffeine	Dose	Deprivation	Measures		Findings	Reference
1998	N	ws	19	Unknown	0 or 300 mg/coffee, tea, or water (3 × 0 or 100 mg per condition, spread out over the day)	Overnight	LARS, STAI	Y	showed Ss scored higher on caff-related symptoms if they had received caff. cf. placebo. No interactions with daily caff cons or gender were found. Ss receiving a different compound at learning and retrieval were in different moods. Ss who received the same compound twice were in similar moods, except that Ss who received caff at both sessions were higher in vigor/activity at the learning session than at the retrieval session. 5 mg/kg caff neither produced any facilitation (or harm) to learning or memory, nor induced dissociative (SDM) effects.	Hindmarsch et al.
1994	N	bs	120	5.3 ± 1.8 cups of coffee	Ad lib 56 and 2 (placebo) mg/cup, and alternating, 3 days each	No dietary caff other than prescribed for each condition	8-item subjective effects Qu inc. "awake," "awake,"	N	Caffeinated drinks gave lower "sedation" ratings on the LARS cf. decaffeinatedl drinks, as acute and chronic effects. Acutely, this effect included a Time × Caff dose interaction. STAI was unaffected. No effects of continued caff consumption. Subjective "wakefulness" scores were DECR with decaf cf. caff. coffee during the first 3 days after	Höfer & Bättig

(continued)

TABLE 10.1 (Continued)
Overview of Recent Caffeine Research Discussed in This Chapter

Year	Double-blind?	ws/bs[a]	N	Caff. consumption (mg/day)[b]	Caff. administration	Withdrawal	Mood measure	Caff. vs. placebo?	Effects	Ref.
					condition after 3 days habitual baseline Alternating condition had 2 days decaf, 1 day caff		"nervous," "sleepy," "stressed," "dull"		baseline and in the alternating group. Decaf coffee DECR and caff coffee (alternating group only) INCR "problems falling asleep." Sleep duration DECR after the caff days in the alternating group. No effects on "sleeping through," "awakening," and "overall sleep quality." Decaf INCR headache, in decaf group and on decaf days in alternating group. Upon caff use, headache scores reverted back to baseline. Also, decaf INCR "nausea" on first days of abstinence, but in alternating group this effect was stronger on 2nd days of abstinence. Decaf coffee (both groups) DECR "well-being," "day exciting," and "general indisposition" INCR. No other effects.	

Year	Design	N	Dose	Regimen	Deprivation	Measures	Sig	Results	Reference
2000	ws	10	333 (184–477)	1/2 subject's daily average 7–8 a.m., then 1/2 subject's daily average 2–3 p.m.	Overnight (>13 h)	POMS, caff withdr Qu	Y	Placebo vs. caff INCR heavy feelings in arms and legs, and DECR "alert/attentive/observant," "ability to concentrate," "energy/active," "vigor," and "friendliness."	Jones et al.
1996	bs	40	360.3	PPCCC, CPPCC (caff = 500 mg, capsule) P = placebo, C = caff, 1 cap/day on 5 cons. days, at 9 a.m.	Overnight (no caff before 1st trial in morning, and not during rest of experiment)	16 mood item VAS, bodily symptoms scale, sleep ratings scale, STAI	N	Withdr: 27 Ss reported tiredness and lethargy, followed by cerebral fullness, which developed into a diffuse throbbing headache in 18 Ss. Quality of sleep ratings INCR during withdr, then dropped again after caff readministration. Ss fell asleep faster during withdr, returning back to baseline values after caff readmin. Feeling sleepy on awakening INCR during withdr and reverted below baseline on resumption of caff. Mood: drowsiness INCR when placebo was administered but DECR beyond baseline when caff was reintroduced on Day 4. Clearheadedness DECR when placebo was administered but INCR when caff was reintroduced. Lethargy INCR during withdrawal (d2–d3; energetic INCR when caff was reintroduced.	Lader et al.

(continued)

TABLE 10.1 (Continued)
Overview of Recent Caffeine Research Discussed in This Chapter

Year	Double-blind?	ws/bs[a]	N	Caff consumption (mg/day)[b]	Caff administration	Withdrawal	Mood measure	Caff. vs. placebo?	Effects	Ref.
									Mood factor 1 (sedation) elevated slightly during withdrawal (d2–d3) but decreased markedly when caff was reintroduced. Bodily symptoms: tiredness INCR during 1st 24 h of withdr (d1–d2), but DECR at 48 h of withdr. Levels dropped further when caff was reinstated, i.e., Ss felt more alert (d3–d4). Ss felt less able to concentrate after 48 h of withdr and INCR after caff readmin (d3–d4). Withdrawal of caff was related to intake on only a few variables. Resumption showed many corr with physiol and psychol variables, particularly bodily symptoms. The higher the caff intake, the greater the unpleasant mood and bodily feelings (during withdrawal), and the more the reversal on resumption.	

1997	N	ws	16	547 (127–1,245)	Abstain (withdrawal) / ad lib	Overnight (12–28 h), only in withdrawal group	POMS, Caff Withdr Inventory	Y	Caff vs. withdr: INCR vigor-activity, well-being, desire to socialize/talkativeness, ability to concentrate, energy/active, content/satisfied, and DECR fatigue–inertia, light headed/dizzy, drowsy/sleepy, yawning, lethargy/fatigued/tired/sluggish, muzzy/foggy/not clearheaded, headache, flu-like feelings, heavy arms and legs.	Lane
1997a	I: Y	ws	8	157	0, 17, or 33 mg/8 oz cola, self-admin	On placebo days in sampling period	Behavior checklist, POMS, cola sheet stimulant effects rating	Y	Withdrawal symptoms (headache, drowsiness, fatigue) in 2 out of 8 Ss when 17 mg → placebo. Withdrawal symptoms (headache, drowsiness, fatigue) in 4 out of 8 Ss when 33 mg → placebo. 33 mg vs. placebo: INCR talkative, motivated to work, stimulated/active/energetic/excited, well-being, cola stimulant effect and cola liking. 17 mg vs. placebo: INCR well-being, friendliness, vigor scales and cola liking; DECR anxiety and confusion scales, and anxious/tense/nervous,	Liguori et al.

(continued)

TABLE 10.1 (Continued)
Overview of Recent Caffeine Research Discussed in This Chapter

Year	Double-blind?	ws/bs[a]	N	Caff consumption (mg/day)[b]	Caff administration	Withdrawal	Mood measure	Caff. vs. placebo?	Effects	Ref.
									irritable/frustrated/angry/cross, stomach upset/-ache. 33 mg vs. placebo: INCR ratings of vigor, alert/attentive/able to concentrate, anxious/tense/nervous, stimulated/active/energetic/ excited, cola stimulant effect and cola liking, and DECR ratings of confusion, depressed and fatigued/tired predicted INCR relative amounts of caffeinated cola drunk. Drowsiness did not and headache did only marginally predict INCR relative amounts of caffeinated cola drunk. 17 mg vs. placebo: INCR ratings of friendliness, vigor, motivation to work, nausea/vomiting, stimulated/active/energetic/excited, strong/vigor/energy, cola stimulant effect and cola liking, and DECR ratings.	

(continued)

II: Y	ws	16 579	0 or 33 mg/8 oz cola, self-admin	On placebo days in sampling period	Behavior checklist, cola sheet stimulant effects rating	Y	drowsy/sleepy, fatigued/tired, and headache predicted INCR relative amounts of caffeinated cola drunk Withdrawal symptoms (headache, drowsiness) in 2 out of 16 Ss when caff → placebo. Caff vs. placebo: INCR active/energetic/excited, confident, motivated to work, well-being, cola stimulant effect; DECR drowsy/sleepy, fatigued/tired, headache, lazy/sluggish/slow_moving, and stomach upset/-ache. Caff vs. placebo: INCR ratings of active/energetic/excited, anxious/tense/nervous, confident, mot to work, cola stimulant effect and cola liking, and DECR ratings of fatigued/tired, lazy/sluggish/slow moving predicted INCR relative amounts of caffeinated cola drunk. Drowsiness did not and headache did only marginally predict INCR relative amounts of caffeinated cola drunk.

TABLE 10.1 (Continued)
Overview of Recent Caffeine Research Discussed in This Chapter

Year	Double-blind?	ws/bs[a]	N	Caff consumption (mg/day)[b]	Caff administration	Withdrawal	Mood measure	Caff. vs. placebo?	Effects	Ref.
1997b	Y	ws	11	632	0 vs. 33 mg/8 oz and 100 mg/8 oz cola; 0 vs. 33 mg/8 oz and 100 mg/8 oz coffee	On placebo days in sampling period	Behavior checklist, cola and coffee sheet stimulant effects rating	Y	Sampling period, across conditions: caff vs. placebo: INCR active/energetic/excited, alert/attentive/able to concentrate, confident, frequent urination, impatience, motivated to work, stronger/more vigorous/more energy, well-being, DECR drowsy/sleepy, fatigued/tired, lazy/sluggish/slow moving, nausea/vomiting. Marg. DECR headache. Sampling period, across caff sampling days: 100 mg vs. 33 mg caff: INCR hunger/appetite, talkative, upset stomach/ache, stronger/more vigor/more energy. Sampling period, across vehicle: cola vs. coffee: INCR shaky/weakness (cola > coffee). No Vehicle × Dose interactions.	Liguori & Hughes

Only looking at commonly used doses only (cola 33 mg/dose, coffee 100 mg/dose): sampling period, across conditions: caff vs. placebo: INCR motivated to work, DECR drowsy/sleepy, lazy/ sluggish/slow moving.

Sampling period, cola 33 mg/dose vs. placebo: INCR confident, well-being, DECR upset stomach/-ache.

Sampling period, coffee 100 mg/dose vs. placebo: INCR active/energetic/excited, alert/ attentive/able to conc, more talkative, stronger/more vigorous/more energy.

In general, caff intake was predicted by increased energetic arousal and well-being.

Caff-containing drinks had higher "stimulant effects" ratings cf. placebos.

Caff-containing drinks had higher liking scores cf. placebos.

(continued)

TABLE 10.1 (Continued)
Overview of Recent Caffeine Research Discussed in This Chapter

Year	Double-blind?	ws/bs[a]	N	Caff consumption (mg/day)[b]	Caff administration	Withdrawal	Mood measure	Caff. vs. placebo?	Effects	Ref.
1997c	Y	ws	13	456	400 mg caff through 2 vehicles of diet cola, decaf coffee, or capsules containing 200 mg each	2 days or more	POMS, VAS (5 drug-related; 1 alert/energetic), behavior checklist	Y	Peak plasma time (PPT): capsules (67 min) > coffee or cola (40 min). Area under time action curve (AUT): cola > capsules > coffee. Subjective effects of caff vs. placebo at PPT: INCR anxious/tense/nervous, vigor, alert, jittery/tremulous, drug effect, high, good effect, bad effect, liking of drug; DECR drowsy/sleepy and fatigued/tired. Subjective caff effects showing a peak in the data were: tension–anxiety scale, drug effect, high, good effect, bad effect, liking of drugs. Time to peak was usually 85–110 min and did not sign. differ across caff vehicles. Coffee 77–115; cola 83–98; caps 93–130 min. AUT showed same effects as PPT.	Liguori et al.

| 1994 | Y | ws | 30 | (2–7 cups of coffee/day) | 0 or 200 mg in cup of decaf coffee + 0 or 50 mg in cup of decaf coffee later during the experimental session (50 min post-test to maintain relatively constant level of plasma caff | 12 h preceding study | POMS | Y | Fatigued Ss reported lowest levels of vigor cf. to well rested Ss. All Ss felt more energetically in the caff cond cf. placebo cond. Similarly, feelings of fatigue were DECR by caff, in particular for the fatigued Ss. In the caff cond, Ss reported to be less angry. No changes in depression or tension. | Lorist et al. |
| 1995 | N | ws | 188 | 50–500 | 0, 1, and 3 mg/kg as caff citrate in orange juice | 12 h | 10 item segmented bipolar mood VAS | Y | At 3 mg/kg Ss perceived their energy level as higher following caff ingestion. However, anxiety and mood were unaffected. Ss reported DECR energy throughout the day following caff, with highest energy reported at 11 a.m. and the lowest at 8 p.m., suggesting that caff was less likely to seem "energizing" to Ss in the evening cf. morning. But because precaff energy patterns were essentially similar, it is more likely to reflect a pattern towards decreased perceived energy. Pre-caff (deprived) mood effect was similar in TOD trend to nondominant hand strength. | Miller et al. |

(continued)

TABLE 10.1 (Continued)
Overview of Recent Caffeine Research Discussed in This Chapter

Year	Double-blind?	ws/bs[a]	N	Caff consumption (mg/day)[b]	Caff administration	Withdrawal	Mood measure	Caff. vs. placebo?	Effects	Ref.
1995	Y	ws	9	686 mg (>500 or >5 cups of 5-oz coffee was criterion)	0, 50, or 100% of daily intake, capsules (each condition was done twice)	33.5 h	10 item mood VAS (last 24 h and now as separate Qu)	Y	Withdr effects in the 0% caff condition on headache, sluggish, and tired-sleepy. The higher the prob of earning coffee, the more responses were made, but this was unrelated to caff dose. No. of responses for coffee was unaffected by caff dose condition, and amount of coffee Ss earned was unrelated to caff dose condition. Amount of earned coffee consumed was stable across caff dose condition.	Mitchell et al.
1994	I: N II: N	ws ws	7	330(112–489)	I: 200 and 300 mg vs. 0, capsules II: 178, 100, 56, 32, 18, 10, 5.6, 1.8, 1 mg	No caff during experiment	I: adverse subjective effects II: anecdotal information on basis for discriminat ion ability	N Y	I: No adverse effects II: Basis for discrimination involved similar changes in mood and behavior (e.g., INCR feelings of energy, motivation to work, and alert).	Mumford et al.

III: Y	n/a		III: 178 mg (smallest discriminable dose by least sensitive subj and largest dose tolerated by most sensitive subj) vs. 0 mg (placebo) 5 times each, once a day, a.m.		III: subjective ratings	Y	Onset of effects was approx 21 min (10–45). Minimum discriminable dose varied between Ss (1.8–178 mg). III: Individual effects of 178 mg caff on all measures, group effects on well-being, magnitude of drug effect, energy, affection for loved ones, motivation to work, self-confidence, social disposition, alert, concentration (INCR), sleepy and muzzy (DECR). Magnitude of drug effect was max after 1 h post-test. Clear relationship between subject sensitivity to discriminative effects (II) and subject sensitivity to changes in subj effects (III).
1993	bs	Y	50 ≤300 mg	0, 150, 300, or 600 mg/70 kg, after 49 h sleep deprivation; caff admin in artificially sweetened lemon juice drink	72 h preceding study	Stanford sleepiness scale, POMS, 8 item mood VASs, 4 item physical symptoms VASs	Y	SSS scores INCR from 1.6 (9 a.m. Day 1) to 4.8 (6 a.m. Day3). All doses of caff then reduced SSS values cf. placebo 1 and 2 h after drug admin. POMS: sleep deprivation INCR tension, anger, depression, fatigue, and confusion, and DECR vigor. Magnitude of change was largest for vigor and fatigue. Caff admin	Penetar et al

(continued)

TABLE 10.1 (Continued)
Overview of Recent Caffeine Research Discussed in This Chapter

Year	Double-blind?	ws/bs[a]	N	Caff consumption (mg/day)[b]	Caff administration	Withdrawal	Mood measure	Caff. vs. placebo?	Effects	Ref.
									INCR vigor, and DECR fatigue and confusion. Sign main effect for dose was observed for the vigor scores, and a sign Dose × Time interaction for vigor, fatigue, and confusion. These effects lasted for 2 h.	
									VAS: sleep deprivation INCR sleepiness and irritability, and DECR alertness, energy levels, confidence, and talkativeness. Caff doses reversed sleep deprivation effects in ratings of alertness for 2 h, energy levels for 12 h, confidence for 2 h, sleepiness for 12 h, and talkativeness for 2 h. Caff INCR anxiety for 2 h and jittery/nervousness for 12 h. No caff effects for heart pounding, headache, sweatiness, or upset stomach.	
									Drug detection: low dose was detected 88% of the time, medium	

Year									Results	Authors
1998	N	ws	31	603 (290–2000)	0 and 250 mg, capsule 4 h before arriving at the laboratory. 2 conditions with at least 1 day in between	Overnight	POMS, Caff Withdr Inventory	Y	83%, and high 92%. Also, 3 Ss said "yes" at both 60 and 120 min after placebo. Deprivation INCR fatigue/inertia, sleepy and yawning, and DECR vigor/activity cf. caff. No effects on headache.	Phillips-Bute & Lane
2000	I: N	ws	17	339 (110–534)	No drink, hot water, tea (37.5 and 75 mg), coffee (75 and 150 mg); doses prepared from black tea and instant coffee	Overnight	UWIST mood adjective Qu, LARS	Y (caff vs. H₂O)	No Time × Treatment interactions. Caff beverages INCR energetic arousal and hedonic tone, and DECR sedation cf. hot water. Coffee gave lower "sedation" ratings cf. tea. Energetic arousal INCR with 1 dose vs. 2 doses.	Quinlan et al.
	II: N	ws	15	351 (185–635)	Hot water, decaf tea containing 5, 30, 55, 105, or 205 mg caff	24 h	UWIST mood adjective Qu, LARS	Y	Caff and caff dose DECR sedation (all doses but 50 mg), and INCR energetic arousal in U-shaped dose–response curve. No effects on hedonic tone or tense arousal.	
1998	Y	bs	64	453 (200–1000)	PPP, CPP, CCP and CCC (C = caff 1.2 mg/kg = 84 mg/70 kg) in novel fruit juices	Overnight (>14 h)	Mood ratings (22 7-point scales)	N	Mood was divided into two factors: energetic moods and tense moods. Energetic mood: treatment effect but no Treatment × Time interaction. From the graph it	Robelin & Rogers

(continued)

TABLE 10.1 (Continued)
Overview of Recent Caffeine Research Discussed in This Chapter

Year	Double-blind?	ws/bs[a]	N	Caff consumption (mg/day)[b]	Caff administration	Withdrawal	Mood measure	Caff. vs. placebo?	Effects	Ref.
									seems that the CCC condition was only stat sign after the 3rd morning session cf. PPP. No effects on tense mood or other separate mood states. H & Ö Qu: evening-type Ss tended to consume more caff than morning-type Ss.	
1997	Y	ws	20	379 (218–500)	Placebo or average daily intake in 2 capsules 3rd session caff/placebo was determined by random selection of each of the Ss' previous multiple-choice form outcomes	10 h preceding study (overnight)	POMS, caff withdr Qu	Y	POMS: caff produced marginally lower scores on the fatigue scale and the individual. Items "peeved," "grouchy," "fatigued," and "exhausted" cf. placebo, and marginally higher scores on "shaky." Sign effects of caff were found on "worn out," "alert," and "helpful." CWQ: caff produced sign lower scores on "headache" and "flu-like feelings" cf. placebo, but sign higher scores on "upset stomach" and "well-being."	Schuh & Griffiths

1996	Y	bs	120	Unknown	600 mg slow-release, oral, capsule	17 h	Bond and Lader VAS	Y	Two reports of caff-related adverse effects (nausea, hand tremor) and 1 of placebo-related adverse effects (acute fatigue), all within 4 h of drug admin. Caff INCR only 1 alertness item cf. placebo, "sleepy-awake," 5 h post-test cf. placebo, with similar marginal effects at 2 and 10 h post-test.	Sicard et al.

Ratings for "drowsy/sleepy," "lethargy/fatigue," and "heavy feeling" were marginally lower after caff cf. placebo whereas "energy/active" and "jittery/shaky" were marginally higher. Level of COP was negatively correlated with level of "headache" and positively with "alert." Multiple regression showed that only "headache" accounted for most of the COP variance in the placebo condition, simultaneously indicating that "headache" is the only sign item in this equation (COP = crossover point on drug-or-money form).

(continued)

TABLE 10.1 (Continued)
Overview of Recent Caffeine Research Discussed in This Chapter

Year	Double-blind?	ws/bs[a]	N	Caff consumption (mg/day)[b]	Caff administration	Withdrawal	Mood measure	Caff. vs. placebo?	Effects	Ref.
									Caff DECR "calmness" and INCR "alertness" scores in the caff group at 2, 5, and 10 h post-test cf. baseline. No effect in placebo group or on "contentedness." Caff vs. placebo: no effects on "sleep quality," "wakings during the night," "quality of awakening in the morning," and "overall rating of the night." Habitual caff users and low caff metabolizers, but also smokers (not occasional or nonusers) showed a decrease in the quality of sleep onset. Calmness inversely correlates with circulating caff, as were sleep onset latency, quality of sleep onset, and overall rating of the post-test night cf. pretest night. Also, INCR in sleep onset latency correlated with the AUC of caff kinetics.	

Year		Design	N	Dose		Duration	Measures		Results	Authors
1992	Y	ws	62	235 mg ± 126 (<100–500/600)	0 or average daily intake, capsules	2 days?	BDI, STAI, symptoms checklist-90-R, POMS, caff withdr Qu	Y	Mood: placebo generated more reported headaches (52% of Ss) than baseline (2%) and caff (6%). BDI, STAI, and POMS: more Ss with abnormal scores in placebo cond cf. baseline and caff. More Ss took medication (all analgesics) during placebo period cf. caff period (13 vs. 2%). Caff dose CORR placebo–caff diff for drowsy/sleepy (p = 0.033), yawning (p = 0.006), and headache (p = 0.033) on CWQ; insomnia BDI (p = 0.049). Interview comments 1 year later re: caff period—none; re: placebo period—headache, flu-like, fatigue, glum, lack of concentration, depressed, vomiting.	Silverman et al.
1992	Unknown	n/a	15	>100 mg (433; 161–1,228)	178 mg and down	No caff outside lab	Self-report Qu	Y	Lowest discriminable dose (LDD): 18 mg—1 S; 32 mg—1 S; 56 mg—2 Ss; 100 mg—4 Ss; 178 mg—1 S. Onset of discrimination varied between 15 and 45 min. Group effects at LDD: relative to placebo, caff DECR ratings of "sleepy" and "foggy/hazy/not clear headed" and INCR ratings of "alert," "motivation to work,"	Silverman & Griffiths

(continued)

TABLE 10.1 (Continued)
Overview of Recent Caffeine Research Discussed in This Chapter

Year	Double-blind?	ws/bs[a]	N	Caff consumption (mg/day)[b]	Caff administration	Withdrawal	Mood measure	Caff. vs. placebo?	Effects	Ref.
									"energy/active," "trembling/shaky/jittery," "anxious/nervous," "desire to talk to people," "self-confidence," "well-being," "concentration," and "heart pounding." Individual differences: 1 subj indicated that caff DECR "trembling/shaky/jittery"; 1 subj indicated that caff DECR "motivation to work"; and another subj indicated that caff DECR "concentration." No effects on performance tasks.	
2000	Y	ws	23	26 (<100) and 340 (>200)	0, 12.5, 25, 50, 100 mg, capsule	Overnight (>13 h)	13 mood item VAS	Y	Mood construct energetic arousal: Treatment × Time: P = 0.016, mainly 100 mg effect. Feeling "bored" was prevented by all doses at the end of testing. Caff increased thirst in low caff consumers in a dose-dependent manner, but not in high caff consumers.	Smit & Rogers

Year									Results	Reference
1999	N	bs	144	Unknown	2 × 100 mg (breakfast and midmorning) conditions were 1 of 4 combinations of breakfast/no breakfast, caff/no caff. Caff admin in coffee	Overnight	18 item mood VAS	Y	Consumption of breakfast was associated with highly significantly greater positive mood prior to starting the test, for all scales. No differences in baseline scores. Those who had had breakfast felt calmer after they had completed the tests. Caff consumption led to greater post-test alertness.	A. P. Smith et al.
1994a	I: N	bs	24	Unknown	I: 0 or 4 mg/kg in 150 ml decaf coffee with fried, cereal or no breakfast	I: overnight (also CHO withdr)	18 bipolar mood ratings	Y	I: 2 h post-test, the cooked bf group felt more contented, interested, sociable, and outward-going cf. the other 2 bf groups. No effects of caff were found.	A. P. Smith et al.
	II: N	bs	48	Unknown	II: 0 or 4 mg/kg in 150 ml decaf coffee with fried or no breakfast	II: overnight (also CHO withdr)	18 bipolar mood ratings	Y	II: 1 h post-test, caff INCR alertness, and Caff × Breakfast interaction: Ss given bf and caff felt more friendly than bf and no caff. Little effect of caff in the non-bf group. 2 h post-test, breakfast INCR feeling quick-witted and proficient. Caff INCR feeling alert, attentive, proficient, happy, friendly, interested, sociable, and outward going.	

(continued)

TABLE 10.1 (Continued)
Overview of Recent Caffeine Research Discussed in This Chapter

Year	Double-blind?	ws/bs[a]	N	Caff consumption (mg/day)[b]	Caff administration	Withdrawal	Mood measure	Caff. vs. placebo?	Effects	Ref.
1994b	N	bs	48	Unknown	0 or 3 mg/kg in 150 ml decaf coffee	Overnight (also CHO withdr)	18 bipolar mood ratings	Y	Unlike paper (20), here we have some trait differences between groups: caff/decaff groups differed sing in trait anxiety, higher scores in caff group. Although caff manipulation was double blind, those receiving caff had stronger withdrawal-like symptoms: more drowsy, feeble, lethargic, dreamy, and depressed (but ANCOVA used on post-test measures). Mood: 90 min post-test no-meal group felt more bored cf. meal group; Meal × Caff interaction: 90 min post-test, no-meal Ss felt more elated when not given caff cf. meal Ss not given caff, they felt less elated. 3 h post-test, meal vs. no-meal INCR feeling strong, proficient, and outward going. 3 h post-test Meal × Caff interactions: no-meal + caff group felt more feeble than no-meal no caff, and	A. P. Smith, Maben, et al.

| 1994 | Y | ws | 11 | 357 (129–2548) | Individual average daily dose or placebo | During 2-day testing trials | BDI, POMS, caff withdr Qu | Y | the opposite effect was seen in the meal groups. Caff had little effect on how elated the no-meal group felt, but greatly INCR elation in meal group. 9 (82%) of Ss showed evidence of caff withdrawal during the placebo period. Seven (64%) showed sign INCR in ratings of fatigue or depression, or DECR in ratings of vigor (from BDI and POMS). 8 (73%) of the Ss reported functional impairment in normal daily activities during the placebo (caff withdr period). In contrast, 1 subj reported functional impairment during the caff period. | Strain et al. |

(continued)

TABLE 10.1 (Continued)
Overview of Recent Caffeine Research Discussed in This Chapter

Year	Double-blind?	ws/bs[a]	N	Caff consumption (mg/day)[b]	Caff administration	Withdrawal	Mood measure	Caff. vs. placebo?	Effects	Ref.

[a] ws or bs refers to caff manipulation only.
[b] Unless specified otherwise.

Notes: ws = within subjects (related samples)
bs = between subjects (independent samples)
Ss = subjects (participants)
INCR = increase(d)
DECR = decrease(d)
caff = caffein(ated)
withdr = withdrawn, withdrawal
vs. = versus
cf. = compared to
bf = breakfast
Qu = question(naire)
sign = significant, significance
BDI = Beck Depression Inventory
POMS = Profile of Mood States
VAS = visual analogue scales
LARS = Line analogue rating scale
STAI = State-Trait Anxiety Inventory
UWIST = University of Wales Institute of Science & Technology

interactions. When differences between ecologically valid vehicle–dose combinations (33 mg/8 oz cola and 100 mg/8 oz coffee) were analyzed, cola increased ratings for hedonic tone and feeling "confident" and decreased scores on stomach problems. Coffee, on the other hand, showed a much larger effect on energetic arousal (Liguori & Hughes, 1997).

Tea and coffee seem to be more similar in their subjective effects when using similar caffeine contents (Hindmarch et al., 1998) or when corrected for differences in caffeine dose (Quinlan et al., 2000). Generally, compared to placebo or hot water, tea and coffee increase scores for energetic arousal and hedonic tone. Double caffeine doses also increased energetic arousal, but not hedonic tone. It appears from these studies that lower doses of caffeine have a positive effect on hedonic tone, whereas slightly higher doses of caffeine (coffee or tea) have a more profound effect on energetic arousal. Although the effects found could, in fact, partly represent expectancy effects of the various drinks, the findings also indicate that coffee, tea, and cola are equally stimulating and reinforcing, thereby contrasting conventional wisdom and apparently confirming the legendary accounts of coffee and tea.

Clearly, although the previous studies have an advantage of being more "ecologically" valid, abandoning expectation effects with regard to the caffeine vehicle provides a more objective way of researching the effects of caffeine. Double-blind dose–response studies in which caffeine is administered in a novel drink or in capsules do more than that; they also compare the effects of different doses over a period of one to several hours. Investigating the effects of 0, 1.5, 3, and 6 mg/kg in high coffee consumers, using a decaf coffee vehicle, Hasenfratz & Bättig (1994) found that the highest caffeine dose tended to increase state anxiety compared to the two lower doses. Dose-related effects were found for energetic arousal, whereas "nervousness" was reduced after the 1.5 mg/kg dose but not after any of the other treatments. No correlations were found with habitual coffee consumption.

Smit and Rogers (2000) investigated the effects of a range of caffeine doses varying between 12.5 and 100 mg and found that the mood construct "energetic arousal" explained most of the variance in the mood data. The largest effect on this construct was shown by 100 mg caffeine; the other conditions provided a relatively flat, shallow dose–response curve. Also, feeling "bored" toward the end of the test session was prevented by all active doses compared to placebo. Although no effects of caffeine on tense moods or "overall mood" were reported (Dose × Time interaction was not significant), "overall mood" did increase compared to placebo 60 minutes after the test, but only for the 25- and 100-mg caffeine doses (Smit & Rogers, 2000; unpublished results).

Quinlan et al. (2000) showed that caffeine improved energetic arousal in a U-shaped dose–response curve (doses used: 0, 25, 50, 100, and 200 mg in decaf tea). No effects were found on hedonic tone or tense arousal. In another dose–response study, Miller, Lombardo, and Fowler (1995) found that caffeine at a level of 3 mg/kg increased energetic arousal, but anxiety and hedonic tone were unaffected. Participants also reported a decrease in energy throughout the day following caffeine, with highest energy levels reported at 11 a.m. and lowest at 8 p.m., suggesting that caffeine was less likely to seem "energizing" to participants in the evening compared to mornings.

Brauer, Buican, and de Wit (1994) reported increased scores over 3 hours post-test on energetic arousal of 300 mg caffeine in capsules compared to placebo. Similar effects at 5 mg/kg were found by Herz (1999). Again, no effects were found in hedonic tone or any other mood (sub)scales compared to placebo (0 mg/kg). Also, the self-report questionnaire showed that participants scored higher on caffeine-related symptoms (total score on questionnaire items; see Rush, Sullivan, & Griffiths, 1995) if they had received caffeine compared to placebo. Although these are fairly high caffeine doses, they have some ecological validity in that a substantial part of the population consumes high amounts of caffeine.

These results show a reliable effect of caffeine on energetic arousal, albeit with a fairly flat and/or inverted-U dose–response relationship. The fact that several of these studies did *not* find effects on hedonic tone for the lower doses could be related to the absence of expectation effects or the fact that these effects are easily overlooked in the types of analyses used (usually ANCOVA repeated measures, where a small effect of one dose simply does not produce a treatment effect or a Treatment × Time interaction). Possibly, other types of experimental designs might provide clearer answers.

Of all of the research performed on the effects of caffeine on mood and performance to date, possibly the most interesting is that which focuses on differences in sensitivity to the (subjective) effects of caffeine. Silverman and Griffiths (1992) established a reliable lowest discriminable dose (LDD) of 18 mg caffeine contained in a capsule in one subject; 32 mg in one; 56 mg in two; 100 mg in four; and 178 mg again in one subject. One subject even reported subjective effects at 10 mg.

The onset of discrimination varied between 15 and 45 minutes and was based on decreased ratings of "sleepy" and "foggy/hazy/not clear headed" and increased ratings of energetic arousal, tense arousal, hedonic tone, "motivation to work," "desire to talk to people," "self-confidence," "concentration," and "heart pounding" (significant group effects at LDD, relative to placebo). On an individual level, one subject indicated that caffeine decreased "trembling/shaky/jittery"; another indicated that caffeine decreased "motivation to work" and a third person indicated that caffeine decreased "concentration."

Also, Mumford et al. (1994) showed a 100-fold difference in "reliable" discrimination threshold (1.7 to 178 mg caffeine) between participants in a similar experiment in which discrimination was anecdotally but consistently based on perceived increases in energetic arousal and feelings such as "motivation to work." Onset of these effects occurred at around 21 (10 to 45) minutes after administration. Using 178 mg caffeine (the smallest discriminable dose by the least sensitive subject and the largest dose tolerated by the most sensitive subject) in the next phase of the study, all participants showed significant individual and group increases in energetic arousal, hedonic tone, "magnitude of drug effect," "motivation to work," and feelings of "affection for loved ones," "self-confidence," "social disposition," and "concentration" compared to placebo. The "magnitude of drug effect" was shown to peak 1 hour after the test.

The latter appears to confirm peak plasma time (PPT) of caffeine found elsewhere (James, 1991), although the vehicle in which caffeine is delivered appears to affect caffeine uptake from the digestive tract greatly, as indicated by differences in reported PPTs for caffeine after consumption of cola (median 120; range 60 to 120 minutes), chocolate (120; 60 to 180 minutes), and capsules (30; 30 to 90 minutes) (Mumford et al., 1996).

However, Liguori, Hughes, and Grass (1997) found caffeine PPT values substantially different from those of Mumford et al. (1996). Cola gave a mean PPT for caffeine of 39 ± 5 minutes (mean ± s.d.), capsules 67 ± 7 minutes, and coffee 42 ± 5 minutes. Interestingly, they also investigated participants' subjective effects at caffeine PPT rather than using generally fixed post-test time points for testing. The results showed that 400 versus 0 mg caffeine (placebo) increased scores on tense arousal, energetic arousal, and items or scales "jittery/tremulous," "drug effect," "high," "good effect," "bad effect," and "liking of drug." These effects did not depend on the vehicle used (cola, coffee, or capsule). No effects were found for items or scales "confident," "dizzy/light headed/faint," "headache," "lazy/sluggish/slow moving," "motivated to work," "anger–hostility," or "confusion–bewilderment" or those related to hedonic tone.

These results suggest that very low doses of caffeine (e.g., the 17 mg caffeine/8 oz condition in Liguori, Hughes, & Oliveto, 1997) make people feel more relaxed and at ease, whereas the effects of higher caffeine concentrations are more stimulating by nature, inducing a "physical arousal rather than an emotional arousal" (Herz, 1999). This notion would explain why medium to higher levels of caffeine can help combat effects of sleep deprivation (Beaumont et al., 2001; Lorist, Snel, & Kok, 1994; Penetar et al., 1993; see later discussion), and deprive people of good quality sleep (e.g., Sicard et al., 1996). Investigating the effects of two subsequent doses of 300 mg slow-release caffeine (SRC) on 64-hour sleep deprivation, Beaumont et al. found that participants felt less drowsy with SRC than with placebo for up to 30 hours of sleep deprivation and less confused for up to 37 hours.

Lorist et al. (1994) tested the restorative effects of 200 mg caffeine + a 50-mg maintenance dose administered during testing, compared to placebo (caffeinated decaf vs. decaf coffee), in two groups: (a) well-rested participants, tested after a normal night of sleep; and (b) sleep-deprived participants, tested between 4:00 and 6:30 a.m. Both groups were deprived of caffeine during the 12 hours preceding testing. Sleep-deprived participants reported lowest levels of vigor compared to the well-rested participants. All participants felt more energetic in the caffeine condition compared to placebo. Similarly, feelings of fatigue were decreased by caffeine, in particular for the fatigued participants. In the caffeine condition, participants also reported less anger. No changes in feelings of depression or tension were found. It was concluded that caffeine effects are more pronounced in fatigued participants than in well-rested ones (at similar levels of caffeine withdrawal).

Penetar et al. (1993) studied participants who were 49 hours sleep deprived and 72 hours caffeine deprived. They found that sleep deprivation lowered tense and energetic arousal, hedonic tone, confidence, and talkativeness, and increased "sleepiness," "irritability," and "confusion." Compared to placebo, subsequent caffeine administration (range: 150 to 600 mg/70 kg body weight) then reversed these effects of sleep deprivation by increasing energetic arousal, confidence, and talkativeness, and decreasing confusion for over 2 hours. Moreover, energetic arousal was reversed for over 12 hours. However, a side effect of caffeine was increased tense arousal, including an increase in "anxiety" lasting for 2 hours and a 12-hour increase in feelings of "nervousness/jitteriness." This confirms the effects of moderate to high doses of caffeine on anxiety observed in (many) other studies (e.g., Brauer et al., 1994; Hasenfratz & Bättig, 1994; Liguori, Hughes, & Oliveto, 1997; Silverman & Griffiths, 1992).

Brauer et al. (1994) found that when people were deprived of caffeine on Day 1, administration of 300 mg caffeine (equivalent to three cups of strong coffee) on Day 2 strongly increased perceived anxiety. On the other hand, Lader et al. (1996) deprived participants for 48 hours after overnight abstinence but found no direct effects on anxiety when subjects were then given caffeine. They did, however, conclude that a faster caffeine metabolism also meant a faster drop in anxiety during *withdrawal* and a slower return when resuming caffeine consumption.

Concluding, it appears that caffeine has positive effects on hedonic tone at lower doses and that effects on energetic and tense arousal increase with increasing caffeine dose. Additionally, it decreases sleep deprivation-related fatigue. Other effects (jitteriness, nervousness, stomach problems, headache, anxiety) seem to be related to higher amounts of caffeine. However, the research discussed earlier also endorses the view that the effects of caffeine can only be fully understood when the effects of caffeine deprivation are also examined.

EFFECTS OF CAFFEINE DEPRIVATION ON MOOD

The way in which mood is affected through caffeine deprivation in caffeine consumers is typically studied by comparing caffeine abstinence with caffeine administration, using a double-blind design. The results of studies addressing caffeine abstinence all point toward one typical symptom profile, which incorporates a deprivation duration factor. In a study comparing the effects of 250 mg caffeine with placebo, the latter condition (caffeine deprivation after overnight abstinence) was associated with increased sleepiness and yawning and decreased energetic arousal compared to caffeine administration (Phillips–Bute & Lane, 1998). Using a more naturalistic setting, Lane (1997) found that, compared to normal caffeine consumption, lunchtime measures after overnight abstinence showed a decrease in energetic arousal and hedonic tone, "desire to socialize/talkativeness," and "ability to concentrate" and increased levels of "light headed/dizzy," "headache," "flu-like feelings," and "heavy arms and legs."

Similarly, Schuh and Griffiths (1997) showed that after overnight abstinence, caffeine had a significant improving effect on "headache," "flu-like feelings," "worn out," "alert," and "helpful." In this study, headache relief seemed the most important caffeine deprivation symptom because it explained the most variance in the crossover point data from a choice of reward questionnaire (caffeine or money). Jones, Herning, Cadet, and Griffiths (2000) reported that prolonged overnight caffeine deprivation decreased energetic arousal, "ability to concentrate," and "friendliness" compared to caffeine administration and increased heavy feelings in arms and legs, possibly a more physical aspect of fatigue.

Also, Robelin and Rogers (1998) found that overnight caffeine deprivation decreased scores on the energetic mood dimension compared to caffeine administration in capsules; in line with other research, they found no effects on tense moods or any of the other mood adjectives used in the mood questionnaire administered. In another study, when cola (33 mg/serving) was replaced by placebo, 50% of participants reliably showed an increase in "headache," "drowsiness," and "fatigue." Only 25% of participants experienced identical symptoms when cola containing 17 mg/serving was replaced by placebo (Liguori, Hughes, & Oliveto, 1997).

Brauer et al. (1994) used two consecutive days of testing; on each of the days participants received 300 mg caffeine or placebo. Their data showed higher headache scores in the deprived condition compared to the nondeprived condition; headache ratings were highest at baseline on Day 2. Also, subjects reported significantly more disorientation following caffeine administration compared to placebo. Day 2 showed main effects (caffeine vs. placebo) and Dose × Time interactions for various adjectives related to energetic arousal. Perhaps surprisingly, when deprived on Day 1 and receiving a caffeine dose on Day 2, participants became more anxious. However, regardless of the condition on Day 1, caffeine administration on Day 2 significantly increased hedonic tone.

Compared to 4 days of 3 × 100 mg caffeine spread out over the day, two subsequent days of placebo administration increased "headache" ratings and decreased energetic arousal and feeling "anxious" and "self-confident" (Comer, Haney, Foltin, & Fischman, 1997). Compared to placebo, postplacebo caffeine increased hedonic tone and energetic arousal, as well as feeling "jittery" and "self-confident," and decreased feeling "unmotivated." Silverman, Evans, Strain, and Griffiths (1992) found that 52% of participants (mean daily caffeine intake = 235 mg) showed headaches, 8 to 11% experienced depression- and anxiety-related symptoms, and 13% used analgesic over-the-counter medication during the 2-day placebo (caffeine abstinence) period of their study. Anecdotal comments from these participants clearly characterized these effects as "severe and disruptive of their normal activities," as indicated by the key descriptors "headache," "flu-like," "vomiting," "fatigue," "glum," "lack of concentration," and "depressed."

Mitchell, de Wit, and Zacny (1995) found that consumers of high amounts of caffeine who abstained from caffeine for 33.5 hours showed increased scores on "headache" and lower energetic arousal. Lader et al. (1996) deprived 40 participants (users of moderate to high amounts) of caffeine overnight plus an additional 48 hours; they found that 27 reported tiredness and lethargy, followed by a feeling of "cerebral fullness," which then developed into a nonmigranous, diffuse throbbing headache in 18 participants. In five cases, this was accompanied by nausea and sickness. Although participants fell asleep faster and reported a higher quality of sleep (see also James, 1998), they felt more tired and less alert upon awakening.

Two-day caffeine deprivation also decreased energetic arousal. Furthermore, tiredness increased during the first day of abstinence, but subsequently decreased during the second day, and the ability to concentrate was rated lower only after 48 hours of caffeine deprivation. Heatherley, Hayward, Seers, and Rogers (2005) gave their participants a predose of 1.2 mg/kg caffeine, followed by the same dose or placebo after 4, 6, or 8 hours. Their results clearly showed that only after 8 hours of caffeine deprivation did caffeine improve energetic arousal and hedonic tone, whereas at 4 and 6 hours no effects on mood were observed.

Only one study has evaluated double-blind caffeine abstinence effects in users of moderate to very high caffeine amounts with a diagnosis of caffeine dependence (based on the criteria for substance dependence from the *DSM-IV*). It showed evidence of caffeine deprivation during the placebo period in 9 out of 11 participants, 8 of which reported functional impairment in normal daily activities, while 7 showed increased ratings of fatigue or depression with decreased ratings of vigor (Strain, Mumford, Silverman, & Griffiths, 1994).

Höfer and Bättig (1994) compared many of their post-test results (0 and 50 mg in decaf, ad lib access) with habitual intake as a baseline measure. Their findings indicate that acute caffeine deprivation causes a general decrease in energetic arousal and hedonic tone, along with an increase in headache and nausea scores. These deprivation symptoms had all disappeared after 3 days of caffeine abstinence. However, of all caffeine deprivation research, Evans and Griffiths' (1999) must be the most thorough and complete. Using a "maintenance dose" baseline where participants consumed a set amount of caffeine during the course of several days after which they received their experimental manipulations, the authors found no difference in withdrawal symptoms following multiday single daily doses of 300 and 3 × 100 mg caffeine (the latter spread out over the day).

On switching to placebo, headache and "flu-like symptoms" increased and energetic arousal and hedonic tone decreased. When they kept participants on maintenance doses (MDs) of 100 to 600 mg/day followed by a 2-day placebo course, clear Drug × Dose interactions for energetic arousal, hedonic tone, confusion, and headache were found. The actual effects of placebo substitution showed increased headaches and tiredness after all MDs. However, following the 600-mg MD, placebo also decreased energetic arousal and hedonic tone, whereas placebo after the 300-mg MD showed no decrease in hedonic tone. After the 100-mg MD, placebo only caused tiredness and headache, where the increase in headache was related to the MD caffeine level.

In a third experiment, using a baseline MD of 300 mg caffeine/day, the authors found dose substitution effects for energetic arousal and "total mood disturbance." Drug × Dose Substitution interaction effects were found for headache and energetic arousal. Only subsequent doses of 100 mg or lower showed some caffeine deprivation effects. Tiredness increased with the 100- and 50-mg follow-up dose, with added decreases in energetic arousal in the 25-mg follow-up dose and added headaches and decreased hedonic tone in the placebo condition.

Finally, their fourth experiment showed that more regular caffeine use gives rise to more profound withdrawal symptoms upon acute caffeine deprivation. After 1 day of 2 × 150 mg caffeine following a 7-day placebo period, no caffeine deprivation symptoms were found. After 3 days of caffeine use, placebo decreased energetic arousal and increased headache scores. Following 7 days of caffeine use, placebo increased headache symptoms even further. The authors concluded that daily consumption of caffeine can result in physical dependence and subsequent deprivation symptoms upon termination of caffeine intake, irrespective of the pattern of intake across the day, and even at habitual doses of 100 mg/day. The symptoms described in Evans and Griffiths' 1999 paper are fully consistent with the other research discussed in this section.

In conclusion, it appears that caffeine deprivation is mainly represented by a decrease in energetic arousal, where more severe deprivation (related to such factors as daily caffeine consumption, metabolic rate, time of day, etc.) also includes increased headaches and decreased hedonic tone. In particular, deprivation symptoms are less severe and less acute in users of lower and moderate amounts of caffeine (e.g., Green & Suls, 1996) than in those using higher amounts.

Effects on anxiety levels appear to be less reliable, but seem to be lowered during caffeine abstinence (e.g., Comer et al., 1997). This effect clearly draws parallels with the anxiogenic characteristics of caffeine at medium and higher doses (Brauer et al., 1994; Hasenfratz & Bättig, 1994; Liguori, Hughes, & Oliveto, 1997; Penetar et al., 1993; Silverman & Griffiths, 1992). Lader et al. (1996) concluded that a faster caffeine metabolism also meant a faster drop in anxiety during *withdrawal* and a slower return when resuming caffeine consumption. In general, their findings indicate marked individual differences in caffeine and caffeine-withdrawal effects and their severity, with faster caffeine metabolizers experiencing less strong acute caffeine effects, but with stronger caffeine deprivation effects.

OTHER ASPECTS OF THE EFFECTS OF CAFFEINE AND CAFFEINE DEPRIVATION ON MOOD

Time of Day

If overnight caffeine-deprived participants need caffeine to reverse their cognitive functioning back to baseline and consecutive caffeine doses appear to avoid deprivation rather than reverse them, it is clear that caffeine should have different effects dependent on the time of consumption. Indeed, in a self-administering study, Green and Suls (1996) provided coffee (decaf with 0 or 125 mg caffeine in capsule). Compared to placebo, caffeine increased tense arousal during midmorning and afternoon, but there were no early morning or evening effects of caffeine on tense arousal. Surprisingly, the authors also found no effects of caffeine on energetic arousal, but this might be more closely related to expectancy effects of the vehicle than to their explanation in terms of conditioning or tolerance to the alerting effects of caffeine.

In a slow-release caffeine study, Sicard et al. (1996) showed caffeine to be awakening at 5 hours and marginally after 2 and 10 hours after the test compared to placebo. Compared to baseline scores, however, it increased energetic arousal and tense arousal. No effects were found in the placebo group (but then, habitual caffeine intake is not mentioned here) or on hedonic tone.

A. P. Smith and colleagues have produced an ecologically valid range of studies looking at the effects of caffeinated coffee when consumed with the three main meals of the day, in overnight caffeine (and carbohydrate) deprived participants. Breakfast (vs. no breakfast) led to greater post-test calmness, whereas caffeinated coffee (2×100 mg vs. 0 [decaffeinated]) provided improved alertness at the same time. The results indicate two very distinct profiles of effects for breakfast cereal and coffee (Smith, Clark, & Gallagher, 1999). However, 1 hour after administering a 0- (placebo) versus 4-mg/kg dose in decaf coffee with breakfast, caffeine increased alertness.

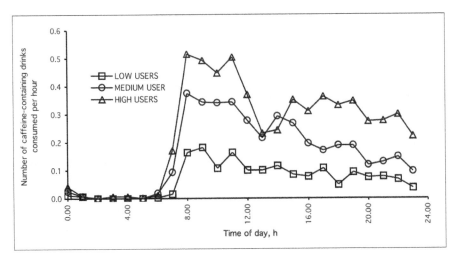

FIGURE 10.1 Caffeine intake as a function of time of day, measured in "low," "medium," and "high" caffeine consumers (Jas & Rogers, unpublished data). n_{low} = 448; n_{med} = 1,036; n_{high} = 1,575 (total number of caffeinated beverages consumed in each group).

Also, breakfast + caffeine made people feel more "friendly" compared to the breakfast + no caffeine condition, whereas caffeine showed no effects in the no-breakfast condition. Two hours after breakfast, caffeine increased scores for "alert," "attentive," "proficient," "happy," "friendly," "interested," "sociable," and "outward going" (Smith, Kendrick, Maben, & Salmon, 1994). When used in combination with an evening meal (vs. no meal), caffeine (vs. placebo) had little effect on how elated the no-meal group felt, but greatly increased elation in the meal group (Smith, Maben, & Brockman, 1994).

Evidence supportive of a link between habitual caffeine intake levels and the prevalence of caffeine withdrawal symptoms comes from Jas and Rogers (unpublished data). They found that users of high amounts of caffeine consume more caffeine in the early morning compared to low caffeine users of low amounts of caffeine, who use caffeine more regularly throughout the day (see Figure 10.1).

Age

Strikingly, Rapoport et al. (1981) found that despite similar salivary caffeine concentrations in children (mean age = 11 years) and adults (22 years) following 3 or 10 mg/kg caffeine administration, children did not experience any adverse side effects (e.g., headache and nausea) at the higher dose; however, adults consuming low and high amounts of caffeine did. Their results indicate a lower prevalence of caffeine-induced (negative) objective effects in children than in adults, which they then link to the possibility that "caffeine is activating some biological substrate which is not fully developed in children...." This suggests that children and adults differ in methylxanthine metabolism, as reviewed by Ginsberg, Hattis, Russ, and Sonawane (2004), and that children are experiencing exclusively *positive* effects of caffeine, regardless of the dose.

However, in a later study (average age of participants = 10 years), the same authors reported that children consuming low amounts of caffeine were perceived by their parents as more emotional, inattentive, and restless when given caffeine. Children consuming higher levels of caffeine did not show any changes in this respect. Rapoport, Berg, Ismond, Zahn, and Neims (1984) concluded that "these differences cannot be attributed to tolerance, withdrawal or subject selection, and suggest a possible physiological basis in children for dietary caffeine preference" (Rapoport et al., 1984).

Although a meta-analysis of nine caffeine studies in children showed little evidence for adverse caffeine effects in children (Stein, Krasowski, Leventhal, Phillips, & Bender, 1996), Bernstein et al. (1998) reported impaired cognitive performance (average age = 10 years). Consistent with findings elsewhere (e.g., Richardson, Rogers, Elliman, & O'Dell, 1995), these withdrawal effects persisted for 1 week after caffeine deprivation commenced.

In a study comparing effects of caffeine in participants in their early 20s and in 50- to 65-year-olds, participants were deprived of caffeine for only 1 to 2 hours prior to testing. Even so, caffeine (vs. placebo) improved ratings of hedonic tone in the older but not younger age group. Moreover, only the older age group rated themselves less amicable (post-test vs. pretest) after having received placebo (Rees, Allan, & Lader, 1999). The researchers concluded that the effects of caffeine tended to be greater in older than in younger people, producing subjective improvements in alertness, particularly in the elderly who showed a greater decline in alertness during the day. Rogers and Dernoncourt (1998), on the other hand, found no age-related differences in the effects of caffeine on simple reaction time performance (SRT is very sensitive to changes in levels of alertness; Smit & Rogers, 2000).

Concluding, although relatively little research has been conducted in this area, it appears that, compared to adults, children have little or no side effects of caffeine consumption, although caffeine withdrawal symptoms have been found. This might make children especially vulnerable to caffeine's reinforcing effects. Future research could determine to what extent preadolescent caffeine exposure is linked with adult adverse effects of caffeine in users and nonusers.

PRACTICAL IMPLICATIONS

Health Care

Caffeine has analgesic effects equivalent to acetaminophen (Ward, Whitney, Avery, & Dunner, 1991), and it increases the analgesic effects of many anesthetics—for example, ibuprofen (McQuay, Angell, Carroll, Moore, & Juniper, 1996). As indicated by Silverman et al. (1992), the adverse effects of any imposed caffeine abstinence could have a serious impact on pre- and post-surgical well-being of hospitalized patients and could be confounded with complaints that relate to the actual medical issue for which the patient is hospitalized. However, personal communication with various local hospital preadmission staff and nutrition advisors has revealed that, after almost 10 years, no hospital nutrition and dietetics guidelines seem to be in place currently to address this issue so relevant to patient care.

Furthermore, Hughes (1996) argues that "a question deserving of further study is whether caffeine use in various groups, such as alcohol/drug abusers, can be especially problematic or can interfere with recovery ..." It appears that the public health sector is not fully aware of the effects caffeine consumption may have on diagnosis, treatment and recovery.

Safety Issues

The fact that performance and mood can be seriously affected by caffeine abstinence raises some important questions regarding safety in everyday life situations. Many vehicle accidents are caused by falling asleep at the wheel, especially under monotonous driving conditions. Individual measures to combat sleepiness—for example, the use of a radio or cold air—are only effective for a short period of time. Much more effective in fighting sleep are taking a short nap (<15 minutes) or consuming a caffeine-containing drink (Horne & Reyner, 1996). Vehicle drivers curtailing their normal nighttime sleep can also reduce their sleepiness and accidental risk by consuming a strong cup of coffee (200 mg caffeine) 30 minutes before driving (Reyner & Horne, 2000). This is confirmed by Brice and Smith (2001), who used 3 mg/kg caffeine after overnight caffeine deprivation. Clearly, caffeine withdrawal may be a significant cause of driver sleepiness because caffeine intake is an effective countermeasure.

DISTINGUISHING BETWEEN WITHDRAWAL REVERSAL AND NET BENEFICIAL EFFECTS OF CAFFEINE

Because of the way in which the effects of caffeine are usually interpreted in the literature, conclusions tend to support the traditional view that caffeine is a psycho-stimulant. However, the overview in Table 10.1 also suggests that, typically, caffeine is tested against placebo using caffeine consumers who were caffeine deprived overnight—a deprivation time usually exceeding 8 hours and therefore long enough for caffeine to improve energetic arousal (Heatherley et al., 2005). Consequently these results may show no more than the reversal by caffeine of the negative effects of caffeine abstinence.

Goldstein, Kaizer, and Whitby (1969) noted this possibility over 30 years ago. They found that caffeine abstainers (i.e., caffeine nonusers) felt no effects after placebo administration, but responded to caffeine with negative effects (jittery, nervous, upset stomach, etc.). Habitual caffeine users, on the other hand, showed negative effects upon receiving placebo (acute deprivation), reporting sleepiness and irritability. When caffeine users received caffeine, however, they reported positive effects after deprivation overnight but only to the extent that, for example, their alertness was raised to the lame level as that of the caffeine nonusers (whose alertness was affected by caffeine).

Most subsequent studies that have claimed to test the net beneficial effects of caffeine, or net detrimental effects of caffeine deprivation for that matter, have in effect compared reversed caffeine abstinence with prolonged caffeine abstinence (RCA–PCA). Whereas this would be an appropriate way of investigating withdrawal reversal effects of caffeine, using this approach to test for caffeine or caffeine deprivation effects is highly inappropriate. Moreover, because of the severity of prolonged caffeine withdrawal and therefore also of withdrawal reversal, the RCA–PCA design is not only used to (wrongly) test the effects of caffeine *or* caffeine deprivation, it also fails to distinguish between two essentially different concepts.

An excellent example to illustrate these points is shown in the study published by Brauer et al. (1994). Their aim was to investigate effects of caffeine deprivation. "Abstinence effects" (Day 1) and "acute (caffeine) effects" (Day 2) data were obtained and analyzed comparing a caffeine condition to a placebo condition in overnight caffeine-deprived participants. Apart from the fact that the results of Day 2 are inevitably confounded with those of Day 1, their graphs clearly show an increase in headache after placebo and an increase in energetic arousal after caffeine.

However, the significance of those effects only exists by virtue of one extreme (prolonged deprivation) having been measured against the other extreme (caffeine). Their graphs help interpret the significant effects reported (e.g., they indicate a strong stimulating effect of caffeine, but no decrease in stimulation in the placebo condition). However, most papers in this area have not published such graphs and leave an inter- pretational "void" as to whether the effects mentioned are merely those of the caffeine (deprivation reversal) or the placebo (prolonged deprivation) condition, or both.

This leaves us to conclude that investigating the effects of caffeine on mood is more complex than previously thought and that it therefore requires a different approach from the one generally taken. Some researchers have dealt with this issue quite ingeniously, identifying different approaches that can be taken when investi- gating the effects of caffeine.

BASELINE APPROACH

Testing net beneficial effects requires a more neutral "baseline," or "0," against which to test the effects of caffeine (deprivation), but this also imposes a problem. In Lader et al. (1996), participants were already caffeine withdrawn at baseline, which shows this approach to be but a variation on the RCA–PCA approach. Other researchers have acknowledged this problem and have taken a different line of thought.

Rather than comparing caffeine with early morning pretest baseline in overnight deprived participants, Höfer and Bättig (1994) compared many of their post-test results (0 and 50 mg in decaf, ad lib access) with habitual intake as a baseline measure. Unfortunately, because the average coffee consumption was 5.3 cups per day, the active dose lies well below the baseline intake. Evans and Griffiths (1999) used a more sophisticated baseline measure. They investigated caffeine deprivation effects by creating an experimentally relevant baseline by, for example, administering 300 mg caffeine per day spread out over two doses, for 7 days. Likewise, researching the net beneficial effects of caffeine, one could keep participants on a baseline dose for 7 days (but see predosing approach that follows) or could abstain participants for 7 days (but see 'long-term withdrawn consumer approach' that follows) and use that as a benchmark against which to test the effects of caffeine.

PREDOSING APPROACH

Warburton (1995) let regular coffee drinkers (more than three cups/day) consume a cup of coffee containing 75 mg caffeine 1 hour before arriving at the laboratory for testing. Because consecutive caffeine dose (75 or 150 mg) increased clearheadedness, happiness, and calmness, and decreased tenseness compared to placebo, it was concluded that the effects found could not represent caffeine withdrawal reversal, but rather represented absolute (net beneficial) effects. However, although the design of Warburton's study appears to ensure that participants were not caffeine deprived, it is possible that the predose of caffeine had not fully reversed caffeine withdrawal (James, 1998) because the average habitual daily caffeine consumption well exceeded the caffeine dose of 75 mg.

This argument also stands for a similar approach taken by Rees et al. (1999), who found effects on "interested–bored" and "contented" with 250 mg caffeine compared to placebo, 1 to 2 hours after participants consumed a light breakfast with a cup of coffee or tea. Note that here also, as in the Warburton study, no overall caffeine effects were found on energetic arousal. Even though caffeine withdrawal effects do reliably occur from 8 hours after caffeine consumption (Robelin & Rogers, 1998; Heatherley et al., 2005), this is still no guarantee that the effects found are true net beneficial effects of caffeine. Again, it may very well be that the predose did not fully reverse the effects of overnight caffeine deprivation.

NONCONSUMER APPROACH

Although one could presume that the ideal participants for a study investigating the effects of caffeine would be nonconsumers, it remains a possibility that these people are in fact "self-selected" by virtue of experiencing negative effects of caffeine consumption—for example, they experience nervousness, jitteriness, and anxiety after caffeine consumption (thus, simply avoiding caffeine because they do not experience any benefit upon its consumption). Hawk (1929) reported that one to three cups of coffee in nonconsumers of coffee indeed induced nervousness, tremors, headache, and dizziness. It also decreased length and quality of sleep and ability to concentrate. The idea of self-selection in caffeine nonconsumers has been highlighted by Goldstein et al. (1969), who concluded that "it is therefore essential to find ways of investigating whether the demonstrated differences in response to caffeine are consequences of habitual caffeine use or whether they were present at the outset, before caffeine use began" (referring to intrinsic, possibly genetically determined factors).

Animal research has proven exactly that point by showing the development of taste aversions in caffeine-naïve rats given caffeine and in caffeine-deprived rats given "placebo" (Vitiello & Woods, 1977). Although this approach would certainly work if one could use people who have never been exposed to caffeine (e.g., those avoiding caffeine on religious grounds or possibly some groups of people in more remote parts of this world), this may be impractical; certainly, it could be regarded as "unethical" to expose these nonexposed people to a drug that is not part of their lives.

A small compromise that alleviates the ethical problem was employed by Rogers, Martin, Smith, Heatherley, and Smit (2003); their two studies used participants whose caffeine intake did not involve tea or coffee, but only cola drinks, no more frequently than one 330-ml can per week. They compared those with participants who exceeded an average caffeine consumption of 200 mg/day. At the outset, in both studies, overnight caffeine-deprived consumers rated lower alertness and higher tension scores than the nonconsumers. Not only does this confirm the caffeine withdrawal–reversal theory, it also shows that consumers of very low amounts of caffeine provide a good alternative to absolute nonconsumers.

LONG-TERM WITHDRAWN CONSUMER APPROACH

Because this is an ethically acceptable and powerful approach to the problem of investigating the "net" effects of caffeine consumption, it is surprising that it has not been used more often. The approach is to test the effects of caffeine in consumers who have abstained from caffeine long enough so as not to experience its deprivation effects anymore. Rogers et al. (1995) administered 0 (placebo) and 70 mg caffeine in novel juice drinks for 10 consecutive workdays and took several measures 1 hour after the test. They found that consumers of moderate but not low amounts of caffeine showed decreased levels of energetic arousal and feeling "cheerful" when given placebo compared to caffeine-containing juice during the first 5 days of the experiment. These effects were smaller on Day 6 through Day 10, suggesting that caffeine abstinence effects take several days to clear during a period of continuous caffeine deprivation.

This is in line with Richardson et al. (1995), who found that certain caffeine abstinence effects take more than 7 days to clear. They compared the deprivation effects of caffeine in three groups who consumed moderate to high amounts of caffeine: 90 minutes, overnight, or 7 days deprived. Acute withdrawal effects of caffeine were found in the overnight and week groups, showing increased levels of "headache" and decreased scores for aspects of energetic arousal and hedonic tone on the morning of the test session.

Overnight abstinence showed the highest levels of caffeine withdrawal symptoms and also resulted in marginally higher scores of "angry," "dejected," "tired," and "drowsy." Moreover, "headache" accounted for changes in "clearheaded" but not "cheerful" or "friendly," whereas "tired" ratings accounted for differences in "angry," "dejected," and "drowsy." Even participants in the longest deprivation condition (7 days) showed symptoms characteristic of caffeine withdrawal, although these symptoms were strongly reduced compared to the effects of overnight withdrawal.

These results clearly suggest a detrimental effect of chronic caffeine intake that is reversed by caffeine. Indeed, James (1998) found that during such a prolonged daily predosing phase (Day 1 to Day 6), caffeine decreased alertness compared to placebo. However, irrespective of the condition during this phase (0 or 3×1.75 mg/kg daily), James recorded increased energetic arousal[*] upon acute caffeine administration on the "challenge day" (Day 7), and no effects were reported for items relating to tense arousal and hedonic tone. Headaches were most frequent in

---

[*] Note that caffeine nonusers in this study (and in one of our recent studies, as yet unpublished) showed an increase in energetic arousal following caffeine that was inconsistent with the failure of caffeine to improve performance. Our interpretation of this result is that these participants have (mis)labeled caffeine-induced "jitteriness" as "alertness."

the chronic (6-day) caffeine exposure (C) followed by a placebo challenge (p). In agreement with the withdrawal reversal hypothesis, this was followed by Pc and Pp and, finally, Cc. Also, the first condition showed increased severity and duration of the headaches compared to the average of the other three.

Rogers, Stephens, and Day (1998) found that although overnight caffeine participants benefited from receiving an 85-mg dose of caffeine, their reaction time performance was only improved to the same level as that of chronically (10 days) caffeine-deprived participants who received placebo. Crucially, caffeine did not benefit performance in long-term deprived subjects. If anything, it impaired it. However, this idea is nothing new. Goldstein et al. (1969) already found that "users but not abstainers require caffeine in the morning to achieve a sufficient state of alertness and readiness to face the day's tasks."

Moreover, these long-term caffeine withdrawal studies clearly suggest that long-term users deprived of caffeine perform similarly and feel similar to users deprived of caffeine overnight when given caffeine. They also suggest that a caffeine withdrawal period longer than 7 days reverses deprivation effects sufficiently for testing net beneficial effects of caffeine and that such effects, if they exist at all, are very small in comparison to the effects of caffeine withdrawal reversal.

To complete the perspective on this issue, it is important to note that long-term abstinent (past) caffeine consumers are not necessarily equivalent to "never" consumers. This is because exposure to caffeine may produce long-lasting neuroadaptive effects (Debry, 1994), as occurs with other drugs such as cocaine (Keys & Ellison, 1999), alcohol (Hunt & Nixon, 1993) and nicotine (Carlson, Armstrong, Switzer, & Ellison, 2000). Some evidence also suggests that irregular or low consumption promotes tolerance to the deprivation effects of caffeine (Höfer & Bättig, 1994).

In conclusion, it appears that little research so far has provided an unequivocal test of the net effects of caffeine (or caffeine deprivation, for that matter) on mood. From a practical standpoint, the best approach to this problem is that of comparing the effects of caffeine in longer term abstaining consumers. Although the abstinence duration required to avoid confounding abstinence effects by creating caffeine nonconsumers is likely to exceed even a 7-day period, we propose this to be the only proper way of testing net beneficial effects of caffeine in man, even though caffeine exposure history may constitute a confounding factor.

CONCLUSIONS

Very little research has been published on net beneficial effects of caffeine in people not deprived of caffeine in comparison to a vast amount of literature reporting caffeine effects in participants deprived (usually overnight) of it. These studies are actually measuring the effects of caffeine withdrawal reversal against prolonged caffeine deprivation. The popularity of this method for testing the effects of caffeine is likely to be based upon the strength and reliability of the effects. More importantly, despite the claims of some researchers to have addressed this issue by testing the effects of caffeine in consumers not deprived of caffeine (e.g., Warburton, 1995), this method still leaves open the possibility that the effects observed are due to the reversal of some residual withdrawal effects.

In any case, other results (e.g., Rogers et al., 1998; James, 1998; Richardson et al., 1995; Goldstein, 1969) clearly indicate that deprivation reversal effects of caffeine are much stronger and more reliable than are any net beneficial effects. These publications suggest that caffeine has little or no net benefit effects. Because children who do not consume caffeine seem to experience fewer negative effects of caffeine compared to adults who do not consume it, it is not unlikely that the basis for caffeine-related flavor preference lies in childhood rather than in adulthood. More research in this area is definitely needed.

On top of the effects of caffeine deprivation, caffeine consumption is detrimental to sleep quality, thereby inevitably affecting mood (and performance) upon awakening and thereafter (Lader et al., 1996). This is probably partly what we recognize as overnight caffeine withdrawal and appears to be what drives caffeine users to have their first caffeine dose of the day (see Figure 10.1), adding strength to the argument that caffeine intake functions to reverse overnight deprivation symptoms. Clearly, caffeine intake also functions to prevent more severe abstinence symptoms that would occur after prolonged withdrawal (e.g., headaches and even nausea).

The observation that higher doses of caffeine in coffee make people drink less (Kozlowski, 1976) suggests that people balance their caffeine intake to a certain extent. Griffiths et al. (1986) confirmed and extended these findings by showing that a caffeine preload reduced consecutive coffee intake modestly, consistently, and in a dose-related fashion. Results by Lader et al. (1996) suggest that individuals metabolizing caffeine at a higher rate experience weaker acute effects of caffeine, but stronger effects of caffeine deprivation.

In summary, caffeine increases energetic arousal in a dose-dependent manner, and at low doses it improves hedonic tone and may reduce anxiety. Also, maintenance doses appear to improve hedonic tone rather than energetic arousal. At high doses, caffeine increases tense arousal, including such symptoms as anxiety, nervousness, and jitteriness. All of these effects are modified by a variety of contextual and other factors, but by far the most important modifying factor is the individual's level of habitual caffeine use. This is because the acute "positive" effects of caffeine felt by caffeine consumers (and measured in the typical caffeine experiment) may represent no more than the reversal of negative effects of short-term caffeine withdrawal. Consequently, it is doubtful that any net beneficial effects for mood can be gained from regular caffeine consumption. Future research should take this doubt seriously by at last adopting research designs that can distinguish between caffeine and caffeine-deprivation effects.

The review of recent literature presented in this chapter was preceded by a reference to tales and legends about the discovery of caffeine-containing plants. The symptoms reported in the case of Kaldi and his herd (see chapter 2) appear to be similar in nature to some of the adverse caffeine effects known to occur in caffeine-naïve adults (restlessness, jitteriness). The much lower dose of caffeine from the tea leaves fallen into the emperor's container of boiling water, however, appears to have affected hedonic tone and energetic arousal. These tales may well prove to be a very early understanding of the true effects of caffeine in caffeine-naïve individuals.

REFERENCES

Balogh, A., Harder, S., Vollandt, R., & Staib, A. H. (1992). Intraindividual variablility of caffeine elimination. *International Journal of Clinical Pharmacology, Therapy and Toxicology, 30*, 383–387.

Beaumont, M., Batejat, D., Pierard, C., Coste, O., Doireau, P., Beers, P. V., et al. (2001). Slow release caffeine on a prolonged (64-h) continuous wakefulness: effects on vigilance and congnitive performance. *Journal of Sleep Research, 10*, 265–276.

Benowitz, N. L., Hall, S. M., & Modin, G. (1989). Persistent increase in caffeine concentrations in people who stop smoking. *British Medical Journal, 298*, 1075–1076.

Bernstein, G. A., Carroll, M. E., Walters Dean, N., Crosby, R. D., Perwien, A. R., & Benowitz, N. L. (1998). Caffeine withdrawal in normal school-age children. *Journal of the American Academy of Child & Adolescent Psychiatry, 37*, 858–865.

Brauer, L. H., Buican, B., & de Wit, H. (1994). Effects of caffeine deprivation on taste and mood. *Behavioral Pharmacology, 5*, 111–118.

Brice, C., & Smith, A. (2001). The effects of caffeine on simulated driving, subjective alertness and sustained attention. *Human Psychopharmacology, 16*, 523–531.

Campbell, D. L. (1995). *The tea book.* Gretna, LA: Pelican Publishing Company, Inc.

Carlson, J. C., Armstrong, B., Switzer, R. C., & Ellison, G. (2000). Selective neurotoxic effects of nicotine on axons in fasciculus retroflexus further support evidence that this is a weak link in brain across multiple drugs of abuse. *Neuropharmacology, 39*, 2792–2798.

Chauchard, P., Mazoué, H., & Lecoq, R. (1945). Inhibition par les sucres de l'effet excitant qu'exercent les bases puriques sur le système nerveux (Inhibition by sugars of the excitatory effect methylxanthines exert on the nervous system). *Société de Biologie Séance, 13*, January, 12–13.

Chvasta, T. E., & Cooke, A. R. (1971). Emptying and absorption of caffeine from the human stomach. *Gastroenterology, 61*, 838–843.

Comer, S. D., Haney, M., Foltin, R. W., & Fischman, M. W. (1997). Effects of caffeine withdrawal on humans living in a residential laboratory. *Experimental and Clinical Psychopharmacology, 5*, 399–403.

Czok, G. (1974). Zur Frage der biologischen Wirksamkeit von Methylxanthinen in Kakao-produkten (Addressing the question of the biological activity of methylxanthines in cocoa products). *Zeitschrift für Ernährungswissenschaft, 13*, 165–171.

Debry, G. (1994). *Coffee and health.* Paris: John Libbey Eurotext.

Evans, S. M., & Griffiths, R. R. (1999). Caffeine withdrawal: A parametric analysis of caffeine dosing conditions. *The Journal of Pharmacology and Experimental Therapeutics, 289*, 285–294.

Flaten, M. A., & Blumenthal, T. D. (1999). Caffeine-associated stimuli elicit conditioned responses: An experimental model of the placebo effect. *Psychopharmacology, 145*, 105–112.

Fredholm, B. B., Bättig, K., Holmén, J., Nehlig, A., & Zvartau, E. E. (1999). Actions of caffeine in the brain with special reference to factors that contribute to its widespread use. *Pharmacological Reviews, 51*, 83–133.

Gilbert, R. M. (1984). Caffeine consumption. In G. A. Spiller (Ed.), *The methylxanthine beverages and foods: Chemistry, consumption and health effects* (pp. 185–214). New York: Alan R. Liss.

Ginsberg, G., Hattis, D., Russ, A., & Sonawane, B. (2004). Physiologically based pharmaco-kinetic (PBPK) modeling of caffeine and theophylline in neonates and adults: implications for assessing children's risks from environmental agents. *Journal of Toxicology and Environmental Health, 67*, 297–329.

Goldstein, A., Kaizer, S., & Whitby, O. (1969). Psychotropic effects of caffeine in man. IV. Quantitative and qualitative differences associated with habituation to coffee. *Clinical Pharmacology and Therapeutics, 10*, 489–497.

Green, P. J., & Suls, J. (1996). The effects of caffeine on ambulatory blood pressure, heart rate, and mood in coffee drinkers. *Journal of Behavioral Medicine, 19*, 111–128.

Griffiths, R. R., Bigelow, G. E., Liebson, I. A., O'Keeffe, M., O'Leary, D., & Russ, N. (1986). Human coffee drinking: Manipulation of concentration and caffeine dose. *Journal of the Experimental Analysis of Behavior, 45*, 133–148.

Hasenfratz, M., & Bättig, K. (1994). Acute dose–effect relationships of caffeine and mental performance, EEG, cardiovascular and subjective parameters. *Psychopharmacology, 114*, 281–287.

Hawk, P. B. (1929). A study of the physiological and psychological reactions of the human organism to coffee drinking. *American Journal of Physiology, 90*, 380–381.

Heatherley, S. V., Hayward, R. C., Seers, H. E., & Rogers, P. J. (2005). Cognitive and psychomotor performance, mood, and pressor effects of caffeine after 4, 6 and 8 h caffeine abstinence. *Psychopharmacology, 178*, 461–470.

Herz, R. S. (1999). Caffeine effects on mood and memory. *Behavior Research and Therapy, 37*, 869–879.

Hindmarch, I., Quinlan, P., Moore, K. L., & Parkin, C. (1998). The effects of black tea and other beverages on aspects of cognition and psychomotor performance. *Psychopharmacology, 139*, 230–238.

Hirsh, K. (1984). Central nervous system pharmacology of the dietary methylxanthines. In G. A. Spiller (Ed.), *The methylxanthine beverages and foods: Chemistry, consumption and health effects* (pp. 236–301). New York: Alan R. Liss.

Höfer, I., & Bättig, K. (1994). Cardiovascular, behavioral, and subjective effects of caffeine under field conditions. *Pharmacology, Biochemistry and Behavior, 48*, 899–908.

Horne, J. A., & Reyner, L. A. (1996). Counteracting driver sleepiness: Effects of napping, caffeine, and placebo. *Psychophysiology, 33*, 306–309.

Hughes, J. R. (1996). What alcohol/drug abuse clinicians need to know about caffeine. *The American Journal on Addictions, 5*, 49–57.

Hunt, J. N., & Knox, M. T. (1969). The slowing of gastric emptying by nine acids. *Journal of Physiology, 201*, 161–179.

Hunt, W. A., & Nixon, S. J. (Eds.) (1993). Alcohol-induced brain damage. *NIAAA Monograph, 22*, USA: Rockville.

James, A., & Rogers, P. (2005). Effects of caffeine on performance and mood: Withdrawal reversal is the most plausible explanation. *Psychopharmacology, 182*, 1–8.

James, J. E. (1991). *Caffeine and health*. London: Academic Press.

James, J. E. (1998). Acute and chronic effects of caffeine on performance, mood, headache, and sleep. *Neuropsychobiology, 38*, 32–41.

Jones, H. E., Herning, R. I., Cadet, J. L., & Griffiths, R. R. (2000). Caffeine withdrawal increases cerebral blood flow velocity and alters quantitative electroencephalography (EEG) activity. *Psychopharmacology, 147*, 371–377.

Keys, A., & Ellison, G. (1999). Autoradiographic analysis of enduring receptor and dopamine transporter alterations following continuous cocaine. *Pharmacology and Toxicology, 85*, 144–150.

Kozlowski, L. T. (1976). Effect of caffeine on coffee drinking. *Nature, 264*, 354–355.

Lader, M., Cardwell, C., Shine, P., & Scott, N. (1996). Caffeine withdrawal symptoms and rate of metabolism. *Journal of Psychopharmacology, 10*, 110–118.

Landolt, H. -P., Werth, E., Borbély, A. A., & Dijk, D. -J. (1995). Caffeine intake (200 mg) in the morning affects human sleep and EEG power spectra at night. *Brain Research, 675*, 67–74.

Lane, J. D. (1997). Effects of brief caffeinated-beverage deprivation on mood, symptoms, and psychomotor performance. *Pharmacology and Biochemical Behavior, 58*(1), 203–208.

Lieberman, H. R., Wurtman, R. J., Emde, G. G., Roberts, C., & Coviella, I. L. G. (1987). The effects of low doses of caffeine on human performance and mood. *Psychopharmacology, 92,* 302–312.

Liguori, A., & Hughes, A. H. (1997). Caffeine self-administration in humans: 2. A within-subjects comparison of coffee and cola vehicles. *Experimental and Clinical Psychopharmacology, 5,* 295–303.

Liguori, A., Hughes, A. H., & Grass, J. A. (1997). Absorption and subjective effects of caffeine from coffee, cola and capsules. *Pharmacology, Biochemistry and Behavior, 58,* 721–726.

Liguori, A., Hughes, J. R., & Oliveto, A. H. (1997). Caffeine self-administration in humans: 1. Efficacy of cola vehicle. *Experimental and Clinical Psychopharmacology, 5,* 286–294.

Lorist, M. M., Snel, J., & Kok, A. (1994). Influence of caffeine on information processing stages in well rested and fatigued subjects. *Psychopharmacology, 113,* 411–421.

Lorr, M., & McNair, D. M. (1988). *Profile of mood states bi-polar form.* San Diego: Educational and Industrial Testing Service.

Lotshaw, S. C., Bradley, J. R., & Brooks, L. R. (1996). Illustrating caffeine's pharmacological and expectancy effects utilizing a balanced placebo dosing. *Journal of Drug Education, 26,* 13–24.

McQuay, H. J., Angell, K., Carroll, D., Moore, R. A., & Juniper, R. P. (1996). Ibuprofen compared with ibuprofen plus caffeine after third molar surgery. *Pain, 66,* 247–251.

Miller, L. S., Lombardo, T. W., & Fowler, S. C. (1995). Caffeine and time of day effects on a force discrimination task in humans. *Physiology and Behavior, 57,* 1117–1125.

Mitchell, S. H., de Wit, H., & Zacny, J. P. (1995). Caffeine withdrawal symptoms and self-administration following caffeine deprivation. *Pharmacology, Biochemistry and Behavior, 51,* 941–945.

Mumford, G. K., Benowitz, N. L., Evans, S. M., Kaminski, B. J., Preston, K. L., Sannerud, C. A., et al. (1996). Absorption rate of methylxanthines following capsules, cola and chocolate. *European Journal of Clinical Pharmacology, 51,* 319–325.

Mumford, G. K., Evans, S. M., Kaminski, B. J., Preston, K. L., Sannerud, C. A., Silverman, K., et al. (1994). Discriminative stimulus and subjective effects of theobromine and caffeine in humans. *Psychopharmacology, 115,* 1–8.

Penetar, D., McCann, U., Thorne, D., Kamimori, G., Galinski, C., & Sing, H. (1993). Caffeine reversal of sleep deprivation effects on alertness and mood. *Psychopharmacology, 112,* 359–365.

Phillips–Bute, B. G., & Lane, J. D. (1998). Caffeine withdrawal symptoms following brief caffeine deprivation. *Physiology and Behavior, 63,* 35–39.

Quinlan, P., Lane, J., Moore, K. L., Aspen, J., Rycroft, J. A., & O'Brien, D. C. (2000). The acute physiological and mood effects of tea and coffee: The role of caffeine level. *Pharmacology and Biochemical Behavior, 66,* 19–28.

Rapoport, J. L., Berg, C. J., Ismond, D. R., Zahn, T. P., & Neims, A. (1984). Behavioral effects of caffeine in children. *Archives of General Psychiatry, 41,* 1073–1079.

Rapoport, J. L., Jensvold, M., Elkins, R., Buchsbaum, M. S., Weingartner, H., Ludlow, C., et al. (1981). Behavioral and cognitive effects of caffeine in boys and adult males. *Journal of Nervous and Mental Disease, 169,* 726–732.

Rees, K., Allan, D., & Lader, M. (1999). The influences of age and caffeine on psychomotor and cognitive function. *Psychopharmacology, 145,* 181–188.

Reyner, L. A., & Horne, J. A. (2000). Early morning driver sleepiness: Effectiveness of 200 mg caffeine. *Psychophysiology, 37*, 1–6.

Richardson, N. J., Rogers, P. J., Elliman, N. A., & O'Dell, R. J. (1995). Mood and performance effects of caffeine in relation to acute and chronic caffeine deprivation. *Pharmacology, Biochemistry and Behavior, 52*, 313–320.

Robelin, M., & Rogers, P. J. (1998). Mood and psychomotor performance effects of the first, but not of subsequent, cup-of-coffee equivalent doses of caffeine consumed after overnight caffeine abstinence. *Behavioral Pharmacology, 9*, 611–618.

Rogers, P.J., & Dernoncourt, C. (1998). Regular caffeine consumption: A balance of adverse and beneficial effects for mood and psychomotor performance. *Pharmacology, Biochemistry and Behavior, 59*, 1039–1045.

Rogers, P. J., Martin, J., Smith, C., Heatherley, S. V., & Smit, H. J. (2003). Absence of reinforcing, mood and psychomotor performance effects of caffeine in habitual non-consumers of caffeine. *Psychopharmacology, 167*, 54–62.

Rogers, P. J., Richardson, N. J., & Elliman, N. A. (1995). Overnight caffeine abstinence and negative reinforcement of preference for caffeine-containing drinks. *Psychopharmacology, 120*, 457–462.

Rogers, P. J., Stephens, S., & Day, J. E. L. (1998). Contrasting performance effects of caffeine after overnight and chronic caffeine withdrawal. *Journal of Psychopharmacology, 12* (suppl. A), PA13.

Rush, C. R., Sullivan, J. T., & Griffiths, R. R. (1995). Intravenous caffeine in stimulant drug abusers: Subjective reports and physiological effects. *The Journal of Pharmacology and Experimental Therapeutics, 273*, 351–358.

Schuh, K. J., & Griffiths, R. R. (1997). Caffeine reinforcement: the role of withdrawal. *Psychopharmacology, 130*, 320–326.

Segal, M. (1996). Tea: A story of serendipity. *FDA Consumer, 30* (2) as viewed at http://www.fda.gov/fdac/features/296_tea.html.

Sicard, B. A., Perault, M. C., Enslen, M., Chauffard, F., Vandel, B., & Tachon, P. (1996). The effects of 600 mg of slow release caffeine on mood and alertness. *Aviation, Space, and Environmental Medicine, 67*, 859–862.

Silverman, K., Evans, S. M., Strain, E. C., & Griffiths, R. R. (1992). Withdrawal syndrome after the double-blind cessation of caffeine consumption. *New England Journal of Medicine, 327*, 1109–1114.

Silverman, K., & Griffiths, R. R. (1992). Low-dose caffeine discrimination and self-reported mood effects in normal volunteers. *Journal of the Experimental Analysis of Behavior, 57*, 91–107.

Smit, H. J., Cotton, J. R., Hughes, S. C., & Rogers, P. J. (2004). Mood and cognitive performance effects of "energy" drink constituents: Caffeine, glucose and carbonation. *Nutritional Neuroscience, 7*, 127–139.

Smit, H. J., Gaffan, E. A., & Rogers, P. J. (2004). Methylxanthines are the psychopharmacologically active constituents of chocolate. *Psychopharmacology, 176*, 412–419.

Smit, H. J., & Rogers, P. J. (2000). Effects of low doses of caffeine on cognitive performance, mood and thirst in low and higher caffeine consumers. *Psychopharmacology, 152*, 167–173.

Smith, A. P., Clark, R., & Gallagher, J. (1999). Breakfast cereal and caffeinated coffee: Effects on working memory, attention, mood, and cardiovascular function. *Physiology and Behavior, 67*, 9–17.

Smith, A. P., Kendrick, A., Maben, A., & Salmon, J. (1994). Effects of breakfast and caffeine on cognitive performance, mood and cardiovascular functioning. *Appetite, 22*, 39–55.

Smith, A. P., Maben, A., & Brockman, P. (1994). Effects of evening meals and caffeine on cognitive performance, mood and cardiovascular functioning. *Appetite, 22*, 57–65.

Smith, A. P., Whitney, H., Thomas, M., Perry, K., & Brockman, P. (1997). Effects of caffeine and noise on mood, performance and cardiovascular functioning. *Human Psychopharmacology, 12*, 27–33.

Stein, M. A., Krasowski, M., Leventhal, B. L., Phillips, W., & Bender, B. G. (1996). Behavioral and cognitive effects of methylxanthines: A meta-analysis of theophylline and caffeine. *Archives of Pediatrics and Adolescent Medicine, 150*, 284–288.

Strain, E. C., Mumford, G. K., Silverman, K., & Griffiths, R. R. (1994). Caffeine dependence syndrome. *The Journal of the American Medical Association, 272*, 1043–1048.

Thayer, R. E. (1978). Toward a psychological theory of multidimensional activation (arousal). *Motivation and Emotion, 2*, 1–34.

Thayer, R. E. (1989). *The biopsychology of mood and arousal.* New York: Oxford University Press.

Vitiello, M. V., & Woods, S. C. (1977). Evidence for withdrawal from caffeine by rats. *Pharmacology, Biochemistry and Behavior, 6*, 553–555.

Warburton, D. (1995). Effects of caffeine on cognition and mood without caffeine abstinence. *Psychopharmacology, 119*, 66–70.

Ward, N., Whitney, C., Avery, D., & Dunner, D. (1991). The analgesic effects of caffeine in headache. *Pain, 44*, 151–155.

Wellman, F.L. (1961). *Coffee. Botany, cultivation and utilization.* London: Leonard Hill.

Yesair, D. W., Branfman, A. R., & Callahan, M. M. (1984). Human disposition and some biochemical aspects of methylxanthines. In G. A. Spiller (Ed.), *The methylxanthine beverages and foods. Chemistry, consumption and health effects* (pp. 215–233). New York: Alan R. Liss.

11 Caffeine, Mood, and Performance: A Selective Review

Lorenzo D. Stafford, Jennifer Rusted, and Martin R. Yeomans

CONTENTS

INTRODUCTION

The apparent potential of caffeine to enhance human performance has been widely exploited in selling caffeinated products. Accordingly, it is suggested that caffeine can promote vigilance, improve workplace performance (particularly for nightshift workers), sustain attention, reduce appetite, and stave off the adverse effects of fatigue or the common cold. In this review, we will consider whether the empirical evidence supports such assertions. We do not intend this chapter to be simply an exhaustive review of the literature; there are a number of other excellent examples of this (see the collected chapters in Gupta & Gupta, 1999). Rather, we consider some of the important questions that should direct a critical appraisal of the research to date, and we present those questions in relation to selected areas of the literature.

We ask whether we are observing absolute changes in performance or simply the withdrawal reinstatement in regular consumers. We consider the extent to which the reported effects are dose and/or age dependent. In addition, we examine whether the apparent effects can be accurately "sourced": Are we observing direct effects of caffeine on cognitive performance via selective neurotransmitter changes or indirect effects of its mood-enhancing properties? These questions will be considered in relation to the literature on the effects of caffeine on mood, psychomotor performance, and memory.

CAFFEINE AND MOOD

Defining "mood" as it has been operationalized in studies assessing effects of psychoactive compounds is less easy than one might expect. This is because researchers have been inconsistent in their allegiance to the most obvious measure of mood—subjective rating scales—and have incorporated into the broad definition of mood objective measures of change in arousal state including changes in alertness response, reaction time measures, and attentional parameters. We consider subjective ratings of mood change independently from objective changes in psychomotor performance tasks, and only the studies examining subjective ratings of change in arousal and alertness will be considered in this section.

Self-ratings of the effects of caffeine intake provide the most direct measure of mood change as it affects the caffeine consumer. Various methods have been used for these self-ratings, including multiple adjective check lists, digital scales, visual analogue scales, and normed questionnaires. Multiple adjective check lists do not have the sensitivity of the bipolar scales and have generally failed to detect mood changes resulting from caffeine intake (e.g., Loke & Meliska, 1984).

In contrast, numerous early studies using bipolar or analogue scales reported increased alertness following caffeine consumption in habitual caffeine consumers (e.g., Clubley, Bye, Henson, Peck, & Riddington, 1979; Leathwood & Pollet, 1983; Fagan, Swift, & Tiplady, 1988; Frewer & Lader, 1991; Flaten & Elden, 1999) and a dose-related improvement in subjective measures of calmness and interest in healthy young volunteers administered caffeine. This dose-related effect suggests that the experience of enhanced mood may depend upon baseline arousal. Consistent with this notion, Rees, Allen, and Lader (1999) reported that at a fixed dose of 250 mg caffeine, older adults were more sensitive than younger volunteers to the mood-enhancing effects of caffeine, with older but not younger volunteers feeling more interested and less bored during the test session. Similar, but nonsignificant improvements were recorded on measures of alertness and mental quick wittedness.

Time of day effects may influence the reported mood changes, however. Smith and colleagues (A. P. Smith, Rusted, Eaton–Williams, Savory, & Leathwood, 1990; A. P. Smith, Kendrick, & Maben, 1992) reported that volunteers who received 3 mg/kg caffeine gave higher ratings of alertness and mental acuity than did volunteers given a decaffeinated drink. However, they found that this effect was more pronounced in the late morning, when dips in the natural cycle of mental alertness might be anticipated.

In an extensive study, Johnson, Spinweber, and Gomez (1990) examined the effects of a morning dose of 250 mg caffeine on volunteers who received placebo or benzodiazepines the evening before. They asked volunteers to rate mood at 2-hour intervals throughout the day. All caffeine groups reported significant improvements in alertness relative to the placebo and BZ groups at all time points. Again, however, the greatest difference was observed in the early morning assessments. In this study, caffeine successfully counteracted the daytime drowsiness normally associated with BZ use. If older volunteers are indeed more sensitive to the mood-enhancing effects of caffeine, it would have been interesting to consider the possible impact of age on the BZ-induced sedation.

Work has also studied the effects of caffeine at separate day- and nighttime sessions. One might suppose caffeine would have a larger effect at night when levels of arousal would be at their lowest (A. P. Smith, Brockman, Flynn, Maben & Thomas, 1993). Though ratings of alertness were confirmed to be lower at night, caffeine acted to increase levels equally over day and night sessions with no interactive (Caffeine/Placebo × Day/Night) effect, therefore suggesting no additional benefit at nighttime periods of low arousal.

Considering the time course of caffeine-induced changes from a somewhat different perspective, Zwyghuizen–Doorenbos, Roehrs, Lipschutz, Timms, and Roth (1990) reported that a 250-mg dose of caffeine induced improvements in alertness that could be maintained over the course of the day in healthy young volunteers by one morning and one lunchtime dose. A further naturalistic study by Hindmarch et al. (2000) using 4-hour paced doses of 75 mg caffeine (chosen to be comparable to caffeine from a single cup of coffee) confirmed this pattern of sustained improvements in mood over the day.

An earlier study by Mumford et al. (1994) also reported positive effects of single low doses of caffeine (56 mg) on measures of well-being, alertness, and concentration. Reducing the dose further, to levels comparable to those delivered by tea or some caffeinated soft drinks, Smit & Rogers (2000) reported that doses of 12 to 50 mg caffeine failed to change perceived levels of "energetic arousal" or "tense arousal," though the former was increased in the same volunteers when they received caffeine doses of 100 mg.

A much earlier study by Lieberman, Wurtman, Emde, Roberts, and Coviella (1987a) had also failed to find mood-changing effects with low-dose regimes (32 to 256 mg caffeine) to healthy young males. These results are somewhat surprising given that the Smit and the Lieberman studies involved overnight caffeine abstinence and demonstrated significant behavioral changes on tests of reaction time and vigilance, at even the lower end of the dose ranges used.

Caffeine-related mood changes are not always perceived as positive effects. Negative effects such as increased anxiety and tenseness have also been reported in habitual caffeine consumers (Greden, 1974; Loke & Meliska, 1984; Loke, 1988; Loke, Hinrichs, & Ghoneim, 1985; Roache & Griffiths, 1987). Chait (1992) failed to demonstrate any differential sensitivity of light versus heavy caffeine consumers to the anxiogenic effects of caffeine, with only baseline level of arousal correlating significantly with the experienced subjective response. This is in contrast to earlier studies suggesting that nonclinical (Gilliland, 1980; Greden, Fontaine, Lubetsky, & Chamberlain, 1978) and clinical (Charney, Heninger, & Jatlow, 1985) populations who habitually consumed large quantities of coffee over the course of the day maintain above average anxiety scores, while decreased consumption of coffee can reduce reported anxiety and irritability, at least in clinical populations (Shisslak et al., 1985).

Some evidence also suggests that high caffeine consumption and dependent status (*DSM-IV*) can relate to personality characteristics such as sensation seeking and impulsivity in student populations (Jones & Lejuez, 2005). Though earlier work appeared to suggest that personality types such as extroversion/introversion can predict contrasts in response to caffeine (Gilliland, 1980), more recent work employing two different doses of caffeine and multiple mood measures postconsumption failed to replicate these findings (Liguori, Grass, & Hughes, 1999).

Several researchers have explored the possibility that caffeine-related effects on mood may be more marked in fatigued volunteers. This is based on the premise that the size of the observed effect may be limited under normal circumstances by a ceiling level of optimal arousal for volunteers in a nonfatigued state. That caffeine improves subjective alertness under extreme fatigue conditions is clearly indicated in studies looking at extended sleep deprivation and overnight working (e.g., Walsh et al., 1990; Penetar et al., 1993; Muehlbach & Walsh, 1995; Wright, Badia, Myers, & Plenzler, 1997). The same interaction in studies with moderately fatigued volunteers, however, is not indicated.

Rosenthal, Roehrs, Zwyghuizendoorenbos, Plath, and Roth (1991) reported enhancement by caffeine on measures of alertness but no additional advantage for volunteers in the sleep-restricted condition (5 vs. 8 hours). Lorist, Snel, and Kok (1994) similarly registered a significant but noninteractive effect of caffeine on measures of energetic arousal in fatigued versus nonfatigued volunteers.

Studies that examine the effects of age may also be considered in this context as an extension of this general principle, while age-related decrements in ability to sustain alertness indicate suboptimal arousal under "normal" circumstances for this population. In fact, once again, there is little evidence for the anticipated interaction in this volunteer group. Swift and Tiplady (1988) reported differential effects in young and elderly adults, suggesting that only the young group experienced enhanced alertness following caffeine. However, two research groups (Yu, Maskray, Jackson, Swift, & Tiplady, 1991; Rees et al., 1999) have since reported positive effects of caffeine on alertness measures in the healthy elderly; the size of these effects is generally comparable to those seen in younger volunteers.

In summary, studies that consider whether caffeine can induce the subjective experience of mood change in healthy volunteers indicate that, in general, small but robust increases in perceived alertness can be detected with subjective rating tools, such as visual analogue scales, in deprived and nondeprived consumers. Highly fatigued volunteers are likely to experience greater subjective mood changes than non- or moderately fatigued volunteers, who do not differ. No additional benefits are apparent for suboptimally aroused systems, but some evidence exists of negative mood consequences associated with overaroused systems.

Some evidence suggests that the size of the mood-related effects may be affected by caffeine usage and that tolerance effects to mood changes associated with caffeine intake do develop. This may effectively induce a baseline dependency effect whereby pharmacological sensitivity decreases in habitual consumers. Consideration of baseline differences may clarify individual differences and some of the situational differences reported in the caffeine literature. We will return to these points later in the chapter.

CAFFEINE AND PSYCHOMOTOR PERFORMANCE

By definition, a psychomotor function refers to any measure of performance that combines decision making with some form of motor activity. Thus, many cognitive tasks that combine decision making with, for example, a response measure could be interpreted as psychomotor tasks. However, for the purposes of this discussion, tasks in which the primary dependent variable is a measure of cognitive performance in terms of acquisition, recall, verbal production, etc. are discussed in the following section on cognitive performance. This section discusses only those tasks in which the dependent variable is based on a motor response and the cognitive element is less demanding.

Because caffeine is widely believed to have a mild psychostimulant effect, many studies of its effects have used measures of psychomotor performance such as tapping speed, simple and choice reaction time (RT), and other tasks requiring prolonged attention to stimuli but including a reaction time measure (often described as vigilance tasks). In most studies, these tasks are presented as part of a performance battery that includes additional cognitive tasks and mood evaluations. Caffeine has been reported to affect all psychomotor response measures tested to date. However, effects are often small, and the literature is complex and often contradictory. The aim of this section is to evaluate the extent to which various measures of psychomotor performance are altered by caffeine administration, starting with tasks with little cognitive load (e.g., tapping) and then examining tasks with increasing cognitive demand.

EFFECTS ON TAPPING AND OTHER MOTOR TASKS

Tapping tasks simply involve some form of repetitive motor response in the form of tapping alternate targets with a stylus (e.g., Lieberman, Wurtman, Emde, & Coviella, 1987b) or pressing a computer switch (e.g., Rees et al., 1999). This task has little cognitive load and is commonly included in performance batteries as a measure of motor speed. Because the task is simple, it was included in many early studies of the effects of caffeine, and several of these studies reported enhanced response rates following caffeine administration (e.g., Hollingworth, 1912; Horst, Buxton, & Robinson, 1934; Thornton, Holck, & Smith, 1939), although some early studies found no effects (e.g., Adler, Burkhardt, Ivy, & Atkinson, 1950; Flory & Gilbert, 1943).

More recently, several studies have reported an increase in tapping rate with caffeine (Fagan et al., 1988; Riedel et al., 1995; Kaplan et al., 1997; Rees, 1999; Rogers et al., 2005); however, a large number of studies have found no effect (Bruce, Scott, Lader, & Marks, 1986; Lieberman et al., 1987a; Rogers & Derncourt, 1998; Robelin & Rogers, 1998). Thus, it appears that caffeine can enhance motor response rate, but that the effect is small and therefore hard to detect. A number of factors could explain some of these differences in results and these are explored later.

In addition to standardized tapping measures, researchers have included a wide variety of simple motor tasks in performance batteries testing effects of caffeine. These include the pegboard task (e.g., Lieberman et al., 1987a; A. P. Smith, Whitney, Thomas, Perry, & Brockman, 1997), pursuit rotor task (e.g., Kuznicki & Turner, 1986), measures of fine finger movement (e.g., Lieberman et al., 1987a), and other standardized measures of hand steadiness (e.g., Bovim, Naess, Helle, & Sand, 1995; Jacobson & Thurmanlacey, 1992).

For tasks measuring primarily movement time, no effect of caffeine has been reported (e.g., Lieberman et al., 1987a; A. P. Smith et al., 1997). However, caffeine has been reported to reliably decrease hand steadiness (Bovim et al., 1995; Jacobson & Thurmanlacey, 1992; James, 1990; Loke et al., 1985), an effect also reported in many earlier studies of caffeine's effects (e.g., Gilliland & Nelson, 1939; Franks, Hagedorn, Hensley, Hensley, & Starmer, 1975). Thus, decreased hand steadiness is one of the more reliable effects of caffeine on psychomotor performance and perhaps needs to be included more widely in test batteries measuring effects of caffeine because this effect may confound some more cognitive measures such as effects on reaction time.

EFFECTS ON SIMPLE AND CHOICE REACTION TIME TASKS

Early reviews of the research evidence on the effects of caffeine on RT performance concluded that improved performance is generally not observed (Goldstein, Kaizer, & Warren, 1965; Dews, 1982). Since the last of these reviews, several studies have reported data suggesting faster RT performance after caffeine relative to placebo, and more recent reviews conclude that RT can be improved by caffeine, at least in the case of regular caffeine consumers tested after a period of caffeine abstinence (Rogers & Derncourt, 1998; Rogers, 2000). However, others contend that improvements in RT extend beyond the reversal of withdrawal effects (e.g., Warburton, 1995), and this review examines the literature on RT in light of these opposing views.

Some measurement of RT has been included in a large number of investigations into the effects of caffeine on performance, dating back to some of the earliest psychopharmacological investigations. For example, caffeine was reported to enhance typing speed in studies as early as 1912 (Hollingworth), and reports of improvements on more standard, if somewhat technologically limited, measures of reaction time followed soon afterward (e.g., Cheney, 1936; A. R. Gilliland &

Nelson, 1939). However, other studies from that period reported no effect of caffeine on reaction time or even a slowing of reaction time (e.g., Eddy & Downs, 1928; Hawk, 1929).

A detailed review of this early literature concluded that caffeine did not improve performance "except, perhaps, when performance had been degraded by fatigue or boredom" (Weiss & Laties, 1962). The following two decades saw further studies with disparate results, some reporting improvements in RT (e.g., Goldstein et al., 1965; Clubley et al., 1979), some no effect (e.g., Franks et al., 1975), and others reporting impairments (e.g., Childs, 1978).

A thorough review of this updated literature in 1982 concluded that caffeine had real effects on returning degraded human performance towards optimum, although Dews noted that the effects were small and were in the range of effects "produced by a variety of everyday arousing and alerting influences: changes of environment, noises," etc. (Dews, 1982). However, further improvements in technology since then have allowed more accurate measurement of RT and better control of stimuli, and several more recent studies have reported improved RT (e.g., Lieberman et al., 1987a; Swift & Tiplady, 1988; Rosenthal et al., 1991; A. P. Smith, Kendrick, Maben, & Salmon, 1994; A. P. Smith, Maben, & Brockman, 1994; Durlach, 1998), although a minority of more recent studies still failed to find measurable improvements (e.g., Kuznicki & Turner, 1986; Foreman, Barraclough, Moore, Mehta, & Madon, 1989; Richardson, Rogers, Elliman, & O'Dell, 1995; A. P. Smith et al., 1997). The remaining part of this section explores some of the experimental factors that led to these disparate results and tries to determine conditions under which improvements in psychomotor performance have been observed.

A wide range of methodological factors could account for the variable nature of published effects of caffeine on psychomotor performance—most notably, inadequate sample sizes, short duration tests, inadequate control for placebo effects, limited range of caffeine doses, and differences in testing conditions. Thus, some failures to find effects can be discounted on the grounds of inadequate methodology. However, other studies that found no effects appear to be well designed, and it may be instead that the small size of the effects means, inevitably, that even well designed studies will fail to find effects in some tests.

Thus, some laboratories have reported effects of caffeine on RT in several studies (e.g., A. P. Smith et al., 1992; A. P. Smith, Kendrick, et al., 1994; A. P. Smith, Maben, et al., 1994), but failed to find significant effects in others (e.g., A. P. Smith et al., 1997). Some of the factors that seem to influence the extent to which RT is altered by caffeine are informative about the nature of these effects, however, so these are discussed in greater length later in this review.

Although the discussion so far has treated RT as a single unified variable, in practice the context in which the response is made has a large effect on RT. Simple RT tasks require no more than a response whenever a target is presented and improved (faster) performance has been reported under certain circumstances (discussed later) with visual stimuli (e.g., Jarvis, 1993; Smit & Rogers, 2000; A. P. Smith et al., 1993) and auditory stimuli (e.g., Clubley et al., 1979; Lieberman et al., 1987a). However, even small changes in procedure alter cognitive demand. For example, some RT tasks include target stimuli that require a response and other more frequent stimuli that require no response (e.g., Rees et al., 1999). Thus, this task combines RT with response inhibition. Other choice RT tasks do not include any inhibition component, but instead include several alternative responses (usually three or more response keys) that relate to different target stimuli.

It is clear that caffeine can improve performance on all of these tasks, but there is no one task that produces truly consistent results. Thus, performance on simple RT has been reported to be improved (e.g., Jacobson & Edgley, 1987; Durlach, 1998; Robelin & Rogers, 1998; Smit & Rogers, 2000; Haskell, Kennedy, Wesnes, & Scholey, 2005), unaffected (e.g., Franks et al. 1975; Bruce, Scott, & Lader, 1986; Lieberman et al., 1987b; A. Smith, Sturgess, & Gallagher, 1999; Christopher, Sutherland, & Smith, 2005), or impaired (e.g., Childs, 1978) by caffeine. Performance on choice RT improved significantly in some studies (e.g., Lieberman et al., 1987b; Kerr, 1991; Durlach, 1998; van Duinen, Lorist, & Zijdewind, 2005) but not in others (e.g., Kuznicki & Turner, 1986; Fagan et al., 1988; Foreman et al., 1989; Judelson et al., 2005; Haskell et al., 2005). Indeed, many studies include two or more RT measures but rarely find effects of caffeine on all RT tasks (cf. Durlach, 1998). Factors such as task duration, size of test battery, dose of caffeine, level of habitual caffeine use of test subjects, and test conditions all appear to affect the likelihood of detecting an effect of caffeine on RT.

Effects on Sustained and Focused Attention

Tasks measuring sustained attention typically combine an RT measure over a long duration task where a failure to attend to the stimulus features can lead to impaired performance. Two commonly used tasks in this category include the rapid visual information processing (RVIP) task, in which subjects are presented with a rapid stream of digits and an RT measure is taken whenever three consecutive odd or even digits have been displayed, or the long-duration variable fore-period RT task, which measures simple RT over an extended period during which the appearance of the target stimuli is unpredictable. Although it is often difficult to detect effects of caffeine in short-duration tasks, caffeine does appear to have more reliable effects on tasks requiring sustained attention (see Koelega, 1993, 1998), especially when performance decreases as a function of task duration.

As with RT, not all studies find effects (e.g., Loke & Meliska, 1984; Linde, 1995) and, when multiple tests were used, not all were affected by caffeine (e.g., Lieberman et al., 1987a; A. P. Smith, Maben, et al., 1994, Christopher et al., 2005). However, the majority of reported studies using tasks measuring sustained attention in some way find improved performance, including studies using the RVIP task (e.g., A. P. Smith et al., 1990; Frewer & Lader, 1991; Hasenfratz & Battig, 1994; Warburton, 1995; Rees et al., 1999; Yeomans, Ripley, Davies, Rusted, & Rogers, 2002; Haskell et al., 2005), repeated digits vigilance task (A. P. Smith et al., 1992; A. P. Smith, Maben, et al., 1994), digit cancellation task (Rees et al., 1999), auditory vigilance task (Lieberman et al. 1987a; Fagan, et al. 1988; Zwyghuizen–Doorenbos et al., 1990; Rosenthal et al., 1991), and various visual vigilance tasks (e.g., Goldstein et al., 1965; Fine et al., 1994; Kenemans & Lorist, 1995; Kenemans

& Verbaten, 1998). Thus, there is clear evidence that caffeine can help sustain attention on these demanding tasks.

In tasks of focused attention, the evidence is less clear. In such tasks, subjects must direct attention toward one group of information while ignoring competing information groups. An example of this is the Stroop task (Stroop, 1935). Evidence has been found that a 250-mg dose of caffeine can impair (Foreman et al., 1989) and enhance (Hasenfratz & Battig, 1992) performance. When numeric and color versions of the Stroop task are compared, again evidence indicates no differences between caffeine and placebo at doses of 125 and 250 mg (Edwards, Brice, Craig, & Penri–Jones, 1996) and also offers support for benefits of 250 mg on reaction times on the color Stroop (Kenemans, Wieleman, M. Zeegers, & Verbaten, 1999).

To try to account for these divergent findings, one can observe a number of methodological differences. For instance, though matched closely on the Foreman et al. (1989) design, Hasenfratz and Battig (1992) used regular smokers in an abstinent state; therefore, because of the similar stimulating actions of nicotine and caffeine, this may have contributed to the differing results.

Similarly, studies by Edwards et al. (1996) and Kenemans et al. (1999) differed in a number of ways, including period of deprivation (2 and 12 hours, respectively). In the former, because the half-life of caffeine can last up to 5 hours, if subjects consumed a caffeinated drink before arriving, it seems likely the subjects were not equally deprived, hence reducing the effect of the experimental treatment. At larger doses, a recent sleep-deprivation study also failed to find an effect of 600 mg of caffeine versus placebo on a color Stroop task (Wesensten, Killgore, & Balkin, 2005). The evidence to date, then, appears to show rather ambiguous effects of caffeine on more demanding tasks such as the Stroop, though clearly further work using more rigorous methodology is needed.

SUMMARY

This brief overview of the extensive literature on the effects of caffeine on psycho-motor performance suggests that caffeine can improve psychomotor performance, particularly in tasks requiring sustained attention. However, as noted in several recent reviews (e.g., James, 1994; Rogers & Derncourt, 1998; Rogers, 2000; James & Rogers, 2005), the majority of studies have tested regular caffeine consumers following a period of caffeine abstinence (typically overnight). Consequently, the extent to which the effects of caffeine represented an absolute improvement in performance or a restoration of performance degraded by caffeine withdrawal remains unclear. We return to this issue later.

CAFFEINE AND MEMORY

Psychological models of memory incorporate multiple components. These are defined in terms of durability (short- vs. long-term storage) or material nature (autobiograph-ical, episodic, semantic) of the memorial trace, or by the accessibility of those memory traces (explicit, implicit memories). For the most part, experimental studies of the potential of caffeine to affect memory have been limited to simple assessments of newly established episodic memory—that is, measures of acquisition and short-term storage of verbal materials presented in the form of unrelated word lists.

Exceptions include occasional studies measuring paired associate learning in which the interest is in the rate of acquisition of an association between two unrelated items; spatial memory, where memory for location of items is the variable of interest; or semantic memory, where access to stored representations of factual or lexical information is assessed. Some studies have considered "working memory," assessing the ability to hold and manipulate information held in a transient "workspace"; an example of this might be the ability to solve mental arithmetic problems.

On such measures of memory, the noted effects of caffeine have been far from robust and are most frequently entangled in interactions with other variables. As stated earlier, test selection and sensitivity differences may make it difficult to determine whether the effects of caffeine on mnemonic processes are direct but ephemeral actions on the neurochemical pathways associated with memory acquisition or indirect consequences of action on other variables. For example, mood changes and changes in sustained attention may have a clear impact on the volunteer's ability to process the material effectively for acquisition and subsequent retrieval.

In the 1980s, many studies examined and failed to find effects of caffeine on measures of memory; acquisition measures of spatial learning (Battig, Buzzi, Martin, & Feierabend, 1984), short-term verbal memory (Clubley et al., 1979; File, Bond, & Lister, 1982), and immediate or delayed recall of word lists (Loke et al., 1985; Roache & Griffiths, 1987; Lieberman, 1988; Loke, 1988) were variously tested and proved to be insensitive to caffeine-induced changes. Recent work has confirmed these null effects on a range of memory tasks at a number of caffeine doses (free recall and verbal reasoning tasks, at doses of 40 mg [A. P. Smith, Sturgess, et al., 1999] or 80 mg [Warburton, Bersellini, & Sweeney, 2001]) and similarly in delayed/immediate recall at a dose of 75 mg (Smit & Rogers, 2002) or 1.2 mg/kg (Rogers et al., 2005; Heatherley, Hayward, Seers, & Rogers, 2005).

Two studies that used the same 100-mg dose of caffeine found no effects on a short-term memory task (Hindmarch, Quinlan, Moore, & Parkin, 1998) or on a range of working memory tasks (A. P. Smith, Clark, & Gallagher, 1999). Positive findings have been reported, however, though these are often based on one measure of a given task or a limited number of trials within a task. For example, in a measure of verbal memory, 75- and 150-mg doses of caffeine appeared to improve performance on the delayed but not immediate version of the task (Warburton, 1995). However, in a later study, the same group failed to find an effect of either measure at a dose of 80 mg (Warburton et al., 2001).

Studies reporting caffeine enhancements in memory also need to be viewed from the perspective of whether memory or peripheral processes are affected. For example, early work by Paroli (cited in Sawyer, Julia, and Turin, 1982) found increased speed of correct response in completing math problems, a task that loads heavily on working memory. The latter result could in fact be explained in terms of caffeine-related increases in the psychomotor components of the math task and does not require any effect of caffeine on the memory component.

In assessing the weight of null effects reported, some authors looked to the population selection as a possible source of differences. It appeared that caffeine effects on memory were more likely to be demonstrated in volunteers who were habitual caffeine consumers (Gilliland & Andress, 1981; Loke, 1988) or in volunteers who were high on the extroversion scale (Terry & Phifer, 1986). Research has also hinted at possible benefits to older populations; for instance, one study reported that caffeine enhanced short-term memory for a middle-aged group (46 to 54) compared to young (26 to 34) and old (66 to 74) groups (Hogervorst, Riedel, Schmitt, & Jolles, 1998). Nevertheless, this advantage was limited to only one of five trials in which performance was essentially poorer for the middle-aged individuals consuming placebo. Given the higher habitual caffeine consumption by this group, this effect could be explained by increased withdrawal.

A more recent study investigated how caffeine interacted with time of day in elderly subjects (>65 years) receiving caffeinated or decaffeinated coffee at separate morning and afternoon sessions (Ryan, Hatfield, & Hofstetter, 2002). Short-delay recall was enhanced for those in the caffeine group with additional interactions with time of day; long-delay recall and recognition declined from morning to afternoon for those receiving decaffeinated but not caffeinated coffee. However, without pre-treatment measures, one cannot rule out pre-existing differences in memory between the two groups.

In addition to age, a number of studies suggested sex differences in response to caffeine, which may limit the generalizability of effects reported in mixed or all-male samples. For example, Erikson et al. (1985) and Arnold, Petros, Beckwith, Coons, and Gorman (1987) reported that word list recall was impaired by caffeine for male volunteers, but was facilitated, though not always robustly, for females (Arnold et al., 1987). B. D. Smith, Tola, and Mann, (1999) have argued, conversely, that most positive reports of caffeine effects on cognition use exclusively male volunteers. They suggest that, because of females' greater arousability (as indicated in studies testing EEG responses to affective material, e.g., B. D. Smith, Meyers, Kline, & Bozmen, 1987; B. D. Smith et al., 1995) they should be more likely to show negative effects of caffeine because caffeine-related effects work on a tight inverted-U shape facilitation/impairment curve.

The inconsistent findings and the radically different interpretations highlight once again the complexity of the caffeine-induced changes; dose titration, task sensitivity, and volunteer sample all contribute to the nature and extent of the performance effects observed.

INTERACTIVE EFFECTS OF CAFFEINE, ESTROGEN, AND ACETYLCHOLINE

Arnold et al. (1987) first suggested that an additional confound for female samples is a possible caffeine–estrogen interaction. This suggestion was based on the fact that their female sample, who showed positive caffeine-related performance effects, were in fact tested only during the menstrual cycle to standardize hormonal influences. This is a particularly interesting result, then, in light of increased evidence for changes in cognitive competence as a consequence in estrogen depletion in older female populations (e.g., Paganinihill & Henderson, 1994; Williams, 1998; Gibbs & Aggarwal, 1998). If estrogen depletion is associated with memory impairment, the fact that young women only show benefits of caffeine at the point in their cycle when estrogen levels take a substantive dip is entirely consistent with the view that, for the most part, healthy adults are working with optimized systems whose efficiency, in terms of cognitive processes at least, cannot be boosted significantly by stimulants.

In fact, such potential interactions on memory measures between estrogen and caffeine do not appear to have been systematically considered in the published literature. As summarized earlier, there appear to be no Age × Caffeine interactions on subjective assessments of mood change, despite a main effect of caffeine on mood. Many of these studies, however, were run on male-only samples; when mixed-sex samples were used, sex differences were not anticipated and sex was rarely incorporated as a factor in the analyses.

Similarly, on measures of memory, sex differences have rarely been systematically explored as a possible source of differential effects. Rees et al. (1999) tested a mixed older age sample of 24 males and 24 females and reported no significant effects of caffeine on digit span (a measure of working memory) or on immediate or delayed free recall of a 20-item word list. Rogers and Derncourt (1998) tested 11 women and seven male volunteers aged between 55 and 84 years on an immediate free recall task; caffeine had no significant effects on recall scores. Yu et al. (1991) tested 20 elderly volunteers on a paired associate learning task. They did not specify the sex ratio of their sample, but again found no significant effects of caffeine on cognitive performance levels. It remains possible that these null results may mask sex differences in caffeine-related performance effects and that women may be substantially more sensitive to caffeine-induced performance benefits during the menstrual cycle.

Estrogen-related effects on memory have been associated with the modulatory effects of this hormone on the cholinergic neurotransmitter system—the neurotransmitter system most closely associated with effective acquisition and storage of new memories (see Everitt and Robbins, 1997, for an excellent review). One study by Riedel et al. (1995) explored the pharmacological basis of caffeine's cognitive-enhancing effects by testing its ability to reverse the robust impairments induced by the drug scopolamine. Scopolamine is a cholinergic antagonist that produces transient dose-dependent impairments in memory and attention when administered to healthy volunteers. It is commonly used as a model of age- and dementia-related changes in cognitive performance because changes in efficiency of the cholinergic system are robustly associated with age- and dementia-related cognitive decline.

Riedel and colleagues (1995) reported that moderate doses of caffeine (250 mg) reversed the scopolamine-induced deficit in immediate and delayed recall of unrelated word lists, while having no effect on memory scanning times, visual search, simple choice or incompatible choice RT measures. In a control condition, coadministration of nicotine (a cholinergic agonist) with scopolamine reversed the scopolamine-induced deficits in incompatible choice RT and in immediate but not delayed recall. The authors conclude that the cognitive-enhancing properties of caffeine and nicotine are therefore distinct and although nicotine may affect primarily speeded and sustained attentional processes, caffeine's effects appear to be more memorial than attentional in nature. They conclude that caffeine may have cognitive-enhancing effects via its cholinergic connections and not solely via its adenosine antagonism, as has generally been assumed (Yu et al., 1991; Nehlig, Daval, & Debry, 1992).

SPECIFICITY OF INTERACTIVE EFFECTS ON BRAIN NEUROTRANSMITTER SYSTEMS

This cholinergic connection provides a pharmacological basis for an estrogen–caffeine interaction. Indeed, the work by Riedel and colleagues clearly predicts an age-related increase in the effects of caffeine and an augmented effect in women during menstruation. This possibility and its implications clearly warrant exploration. In terms of pharmacological specificity, however, the results of the Riedel study must be interpreted cautiously. There are no other direct tests of this caffeine–cholinergic link in the human literature, although Myers, Johnson, and McVey (1999) report a series of animal studies that show the same synergistic relationship between caffeine and choline, the precursor of acetylcholine.

Earlier human studies, however, suggest that caffeine can reverse the mood impairments induced by the gaba-ergic agonists lorazepam (File et al., 1982) and diazepam (Mattila, Palva, & Savolainen, 1982). The latter result with diazepam was not confirmed by Loke et al. (1985). However, a more recent study by Rush, Higgins, Bickel, and Hughes (1994) presented evidence that doses of 250 mg/kg caffeine can offset psychomotor and mood changes induced by doses of 2.8 and 5.6 m/kg lorazepam to healthy young volunteers and can also reverse BZ-induced memory deficits. These reversals, then, must be taken to indicate the complex and interactive nature of neurotransmitter effects on cognitive function, rather than the specificity of neurochemical actions by the compounds in question.

More recently, noradrenaline has also been suggested to play a role in the effect of caffeine on behavior; one study administered clonidine (a drug that reduces noradrenaline activity and arousal) or placebo to individuals followed by caffeine or placebo (A. P. Smith, Brice, Nash, Rich, & Nutt, 2003). Results revealed significant Clonidine × Caffeine interactions on a range of mood and performance measures, thus appearing to suggest that caffeine was able to counteract clonidine-induced decreases in arousal. Unfortunately, the absence of post-hoc tests makes it difficult to see whether key group differences are significant.

Specificity of effects is a vital issue in the human psychopharmacology of psychoactive compounds. Although the source of any beneficial effects of caffeine may be of little importance to the healthy adult coffee drinker, it is critical to those interested in the potential of a given compound to improve cognitive function. Understanding caffeine's potential as a moderator of human mood and cognition, as well as the nature of the neurotransmitter interactions underlying those effects, has relevance not only for those interested in the cognitive-enhancing qualities of the compound, but also for those concerned with the mental and physical health consequences of caffeine usage.

FACTORS INFLUENCING EFFECTS OF CAFFEINE ON COGNITION AND PERFORMANCE

Considering the literature reviewed in this chapter, it is clear that recurrent themes emerge regarding factors that modulate the robustness of caffeine-related performance effects. We will consider each of these factors in turn in this final section.

Dose–Response Relationships

First, differences exist between studies on such basic design factors as dosage of caffeine employed. Reviewing the literature, we observe clear dose-dependent effects on performance measures. Thus, on measures of mood, dose-dependent increases in calmness and interested alertness were reported by Frewer and Lader (1991) and Lieberman et al. (1987a), but negative effects such as anxiety and irritability begin to emerge when high doses are administered (e.g., Loke et al., 1985; Roache & Griffiths, 1987; Loke, 1988). The same pattern—an inverted U-shaped curve—with improvements at lower doses and impairments at high doses is observed on psycho-motor and memory tasks (Foreman et al., 1989; Kaplan et al., 1997).

The boundaries of the dose ranges within which we observe positive versus negative effects are necessarily broad because they are determined directly by the individual differences in baseline arousal at test and indirectly by task factors affecting that baseline (i.e., complex tasks are more arousing than low-level tasks). We also need to know whether habitual patterns of intake among participants and baseline levels of caffeine are considered, and whether other conditions (such as diet) or habits (such as smoking) affecting metabolism of the compound are controlled in the pre-experimental period.

We can also explore dose–response effects within the historical change that we see in the size of the doses tested. Most recently, a clear shift has taken place toward the use of smaller doses and the existence of caffeine-induced performance changes at doses habitually encountered in hot and cold beverages. Interestingly, performance effects have emerged with some consistency with smaller than average doses of caffeine (Smit and Rogers, 2000). More intriguingly, some evidence suggests some dissociation between the effects of caffeine on mood and on performance measures, particularly at the lower dose range (Rogers, Richardson, & Demoncourt, 1995; Rusted, 1999).

Test Selection and Sensitivity

A significant contribution to the diverse range of results reported with caffeine can be accounted for by the diversity of test selection across studies. Although the choice of vigilance or mood tasks is less critical to the demonstration of caffeine's effects, the choice of tests for monitoring effects on tasks of learning, memory, and other complex cognitive function is more varied and more problematic. Apart from the fact that many of the tests employed necessarily involve multifaceted cognitive processes, it is also true to say that the relatively small benefits that might be anticipated may be difficult to demonstrate unless rigorous measures are taken on all other potential confounding factors.

Placebo Effects

Another potentially confounding factor in studies of the effects of caffeine is the response to the placebo condition. When caffeine is administered in capsule form, this is not a problem, although the pharmacokinetics of caffeine administered in this way differ markedly from that seen when caffeine is consumed as a drink (e.g., peak saliva/caffeine levels; Liguori, Hughes, & Grass, 1997). However, many studies have contrasted effects of drinks such as caffeinated coffee with decaffeinated coffee as a placebo control. The potential problem with this approach is that prior experience of the postingestive effects of coffee may lead to conditioned responses to coffee flavor that may be placebo-like (that is, the decaffeinated drink produces conditioned caffeine-like responses) or even, possibly, compensatory responses (where the conditioned response counteracts the anticipated effects of normal coffee).

The potential for placebo effects has been elegantly demonstrated. Subjects who consumed a placebo drink but were told that it contained caffeine and that caffeine would improve performance performed faster on a motor task, whereas those told that caffeine would impair performance performed worse (Fillmore & Vogel–Sprott, 1992). Thus, inadequate control of placebo effects can, potentially, have large effects on the likelihood of detecting an actual effect of caffeine on mood and performance.

Another important aspect pertaining to experimental vehicles is whether the other active compounds in tea and coffee may be responsible for any reported effects. For instance, there is evidence that flavonoids are capable of interacting with benzodiazepine receptors (Medina et al., 1997). Flavonoids are also present in black and green tea (Wang & Helliwell, 2001), so this raises the prospect that, presumably, the anxiolytic and related effects of tea might be modulated via this compound.

Therefore, studies finding a difference between decaffeinated and caffeinated tea are studying the effects not only of caffeine but also of other potentially active compounds. An alternative approach is to use drinks not known to contain any active compounds, such as various fruit teas and juices. Such beverages have the advantage of matching the pharmacokinetics of normally consumed caffeinated drinks more closely than capsules do. Also, they neatly disguise the nature of the study and hence expectancy effects are minimized.

THRESHOLD LEVELS OF AROUSAL

Under this heading, we include factors that determine the baseline level of arousal of an individual at the outset of the test session and therefore the strength and behavioral consequences of the stimulatory effects induced by a given dose of caffeine. Thus, age, fatigue, dependence, and withdrawal are factors that may appear to be quite disparate but act by inducing suboptimal cognitive operating systems upon which caffeine-induced performance change will be superimposed. Age and fatigue effects were considered in some detail in the mood and the memory sections of this chapter and will be summarized only briefly here. Issues of dependence and deprivation, which continue to feed theoretical controversies, will be considered in more detail.

EFFECTS OF AGE

Despite the anticipated interaction of age with caffeine-related improvements in mood and performance, little evidence is found in the literature for larger effects of a given dose of caffeine in an older adult volunteer than in a younger one. It is important to consider, however, that relatively few studies within the caffeine literature have compared young and older adults and that the range of tasks tested has been limited. Certainly, measures of performance particularly sensitive to age-related decrements—for example, measures of sustained attention—had been expected to be sensitive to such an interaction.

On the other hand, the more recent emphasis in cognitive psychology on the difficulties attached to dual task performance and selective inhibition in older volunteers (see Craik, 1994, for a review) have not yet been tested in psychopharmacological manipulations. Clearly, more studies examining a wider range of cognitive processes are needed before any definite conclusions can be drawn.

Effects of Fatigue

For the most part, researchers have focused their attention on the interactive effects of caffeine and fatigue on mood and psychomotor performance. The accumulated evidence clearly indicates that highly fatigued volunteers are likely to experience greater subjective mood change than volunteers who are only moderately or not fatigued. The evidence for differential effects in the latter two groups remains equivocal. In contrast, the results on tasks of psychomotor performance show a smoother and more sensitive fatigue-related change in caffeine effects. Caffeine-induced performance benefits can thus be identified within nonfatigued volunteers over, for example, a 5-minute test of sustained attention (e.g., Smit and Rogers, 2000) and appear to be reliable and robustly observed in even minimally deprived volunteers (e.g., Warburton, 1995).

In general, reviews of the literature have treated this short-term task-induced fatigue as distinct from sleep-induced fatigue (e.g., Snel & Lorist, 1999). One key consideration in assessing the size of the caffeine effects in studies employing longer term sleep deprivation, however, has been the potential confound between sleep deprivation and the concurrent caffeine deprivation imposed in the design of most of those studies. Some of the more recent studies have argued that the use of shorter sleep deprivations periods (e.g., Wright et al., 1997, used 48 hours only) ensures that caffeine withdrawal effects are minimal and therefore do not constitute a significant confound. This raises the obvious question as to what constitutes withdrawal and, once again, we can point to the need to consider short-term and longer term withdrawal effects.

Certainly, longer term withdrawal (3 days +) is associated with more chronic feelings of fatigue, poor motivation, and sometimes depression, but 24-hour withdrawal produces subjective reports of headache and irritability; both carry attendant performance decrements (e.g., Bruce et al., 1991; Juliano & Griffiths, 2004). Indeed, recent research has identified mood decrements, with perhaps less pronounced performance decrements, after the 12-hour or overnight abstinence commonly employed as a "washout" period in many of the early studies. The relative contribution to apparent performance enhancement of these short-term withdrawal reinstatement effects remains a source of contention (see James, 1994).

Effects of Withdrawal and Dependence

As highlighted throughout this review, an important issue is the extent to which effects of caffeine on mood and performance represent a real benefit from consuming caffeine or represent the normalization of mood and performance adversely affected by the effects of caffeine withdrawal. The vast majority of studies used caffeine consumers tested after a washout period, which is typically overnight drink abstinence. Under these circumstances, it is very difficult to determine whether any effects of caffeine on mood and performance represent reversal of withdrawal effects or absolute effects of caffeine (the "net benefit"; Rogers, Richardson, & Dernoncourt, 1995). This problem has been highlighted in several recent articles (James, 1994; Rogers, 2000; James & Rogers, 2005), but the issue remains unresolved.

The nature of withdrawal effects and behavioral consequences of abstinence are not fully discussed here because they are reviewed elsewhere in this volume and in the wider literature (e.g., Griffiths & Woodson, 1988; Rogers & Derncourt, 1998; Juliano & Griffiths, 2004). Instead, we consider only whether caffeine abstinence is a prerequisite for detecting reliable effects of caffeine on mood and performance. If caffeine abstinence is a necessary precondition, then two obvious premises follow: Caffeine-related changes will not be observed in volunteers who do not abstain, and people who do not habitually consume caffeine should not show caffeine-related performance benefits. We address each of these premises in turn.

Caffeine-Related Changes Will Not Be Observed in Nonabstinent Volunteers

As with so much of the caffeine literature, results that address this issue are conflicting. For example, Loke and Meliska (1984) contrasted the effects of placebo, 195, and 325 mg caffeine subjects who consumed high and low amounts of caffeine following 2 hours of caffeine abstinence. Neither reaction time nor hit-rate on a visual vigilance task was altered by either caffeine dose. In contrast, several recent studies suggest that caffeine can improve mood and performance in the absence of caffeine deprivation. Thus, subjects who had been asked to refrain from consuming caffeine for 1 hour prior to testing had faster RT and performed more accurately on a sustained attention task following caffeine (A. P. Smith, Maben, et al., 1994); subjects asked to drink their normal morning drink were reported to have improved mood and attention in response to caffeine administered 1 (Warburton, 1995) or 2 (Rees et al., 1999) hours later. All three studies relied on self-dosing, and a criticism is that no measure was taken to confirm compliance.

Also using a self-administration method but checking compliance via analysis of caffeine/saliva levels, a more recent study reported some enhancements in mood and performance after caffeinated tea/coffee (2 mg/kg) versus placebo (Christopher et al., 2005). Importantly, however, the key measure of reaction time was unaffected by caffeine in three of the four tasks (focused attention, categoric search, simple reaction time), and elevations in alertness were seen only at the first time point following consumption. Interestingly, no significant differences were found after completion of the test battery, approximately 20 minutes later, though one might have predicted stronger differences in mood after a (presumably) mildly fatiguing set of cognitive tasks. Together with methodological problems discussed elsewhere (James & Rogers, 2005), these results cannot be taken as firm evidence of consistent benefits of caffeine in nonabstinent individuals.

In studies in which caffeine administration has been controlled by the experimenter, one study found that RVIP performance and alertness were enhanced by caffeine, but only for those individuals preloaded 1 hour before with placebo but not caffeine (Yeomans et al., 2002). This demonstrated that the beneficial effects of caffeine are evident only in individuals previously deprived of caffeine ($\approx$11 hours) and presumably in some state of withdrawal. No equivalent enhancement was observed in the caffeine-sated volunteers. More recent work manipulated the duration of caffeine abstinence (4, 6, or 8 hours) and found the strongest effects of caffeine on performance—and particularly mood—emerging after 8 hours (Heatherley et al., 2005), implying that caffeine offered few benefits when individuals were minimally withdrawn.

The findings of these two studies suggest that caffeine has the clearest benefit when the period of deprivation is in excess of 8 hours, which is around the same duration as an individual's routine overnight abstinence. Though this would tend to support the argument for few beneficial effects of caffeine beyond the reversal of caffeine withdrawal, this is based upon only a few studies and clearly more research is needed. Furthermore, because these two studies tested participants in the morning and early evening, it is unclear whether shorter periods of deprivation in combination with natural decreases in arousal (e.g., postlunch "dip") could possibly reveal some enhancement from caffeine as previous work has suggested (A. P. Smith et al., 1990).

People Who Do Not Habitually Consume Caffeine Should Not Show Caffeine-Related Performance Benefits

If caffeine simply reverses the adverse effects of caffeine withdrawal, then it would be expected that people who do not habitually consume caffeine should not see any improvement in performance or mood when given caffeine. There have been several studies of the effects of caffeine on mood and performance in nonconsumers, many of which failed to find effects of caffeine in nonconsumers but reporting effects in caffeine-deprived moderate or high consumers (Loke & Meliska, 1984; Kuznicki & Turner, 1986; Zahn & Rapoport, 1987; B. D. Smith, Rafferty, Lindgren, Smith, & Nespor, 1992). The only studies showing no difference in response to caffeine between low and high consumers (Lieberman et al., 1987a; Richardson et al., 1995) did not include any independent tests showing an actual improvement in nonconsumers and failed to find an interaction between habitual use and change in mood or performance.

More recently, however, it was shown that caffeine consumers' and nonconsumers' alertness was enhanced in response to caffeine (Rogers, Martin, Smith, Heatherley, & Smit, 2003). Although no separate analyses were completed to confirm this, the mean values suggest similar benefits to consumers and nonconsumers. Still more recently, a study found benefits in consumers and nonconsumers from caffeine in certain measures of mood and performance (Haskell et al., 2005). However, separate analysis for each group revealed a rather complex pattern—for instance, caffeine acted to improve aspects of mood (alertness) and performance (RVIP) for consumers but not for nonconsumers. Hence, although the findings provide evidence for some advantages for non- or low consumers of caffeine, they do not show a consistent effect for both groups on key measures known to be sensitive to the effects of caffeine.

In summary then, although the majority of studies to date have shown no consistent effects from caffeine in nonconsumers, further research that also analyzes effects of caffeine separately for consumers and nonconsumers is required. Interestingly when this has been completed (e.g., Haskell et al., 2005), the results suggest differential effects of caffeine in consumers and nonconsumers. The existence of such effects highlights one of the problems in using nonconsumers: There are marked individual responses to caffeine and nonconsumers may represent a subpopulation who do not find the effects of these drinks beneficial.

This idea is supported in studies of liking for caffeinated drinks, which has been shown to develop through conditioned associations between drink flavor and the postingestive effects of caffeine. Although regular caffeine consumers who experience caffeinated drinks when they are caffeine deprived develop a liking for novel drinks containing caffeine (Rogers, Richardson, & Elliman, 1995; Yeomans, Spetch, & Rogers, 1998; Yeomans, Jackson, Lee, Nesic, & Durlach, 2000), subjects who habitually drink little or no caffeine tend to develop a dislike for novel caffeinated drinks (Rogers et al., 1995).

If nonconsumers represent a subpopulation that does not find caffeine beneficial, then the finding that these subjects do not show improved performance following caffeine administration cannot be taken as strong evidence that the effects of caffeine on mood and performance can be explained through caffeine dependence. A more stringent test would be to take a group of regular caffeine consumers (who presumably do find the effects of caffeine beneficial) and then test them following a period of caffeine abstinence longer than the time taken for the effects of physical dependence to be reversed. If these fully abstinent consumers were found to show beneficial effects of caffeine, this would demonstrate that withdrawal reversal was an inadequate explanation for the effects of caffeine on mood and performance.

To date, only four such studies have been reported, three of which provide evidence that abstinent consumers do not show improved mood and performance when caffeine is administered (James, 1998; Rogers, Stephens, & Day, 1998; Rogers et al., 2005). The fourth study found that energetic ratings were increased by caffeine for those individuals maintained and withdrawn from caffeine (Tinley, Yeomans, & Durlach, 2003). However, though mean values imply a benefit to both groups (maintained caffeine and placebo), no separate analyses were carried out to answer this question decisively. In summary, although more studies of this sort are needed, the balance of evidence to date points toward no positive effects of caffeine for regular consumers who are withdrawn long term from caffeine.

CONCLUSIONS

This selective review of the effects of caffeine on mood and performance has highlighted the disparate nature of the findings reported in the literature over the years. We have attempted to draw attention to the confounding variables that make comparative evaluation of research reports difficult, but that equally have driven the recent resurgence in interest in the effects of caffeine on human information processing and produced increasingly sophisticated attempts to untangle the complexities of the psychoactive effects of this compound. The combination of individual differences, pharmacokinetic factors, dependency issues, and task and process sensitivities provides sufficient challenge indeed to the most innovative and determined of researchers.

REFERENCES

Adler, H. F., Burkhardt, W. L., Ivy, A. C., & Atkinson, A. J. (1950). Effect of various drugs on psychomotor performance at ground level and at simulated altitudes of 18,000 feet in a low pressure chamber. *Journal of Aviation Medicine, 21,* 221–236.

Arnold, M. E., Petros, T. V., Beckwith, B. E., Coons, G., & Gorman, N. (1987). The effects of caffeine, impulsivity, and sex on memory for word lists. *Physiology & Behavior, 41*(1), 25–30.

Battig, K., Buzzi, R., Martin, J. R., & Feierabend, J. M. (1984). The effects of caffeine on physiological functions and mental performance. *Experientia, 40*(11), 1218–1223.

Bovim, G., Naess, P., Helle, J., & Sand, T. (1995). Caffeine influence on the motor steadiness battery in neuropsychological tests. *Journal of Clinical and Experimental Neuropsychology, 17*(3), 472–476.

Bruce, M., Scott, N., Lader, M., & Marks, V. (1986). The psychopharmacological and electrophysiological effects of single doses of caffeine in healthy human subjects. *British Journal of Clinical Pharmacology, 22,* 81–87.

Bruce, M., Scott, N., & Lader, M. (1991). Caffeine withdrawal: A contrast of withdrawal symptoms in normal subjects who have abstained from caffeine for 24 hours and for 7 days. *Journal of Psychopharmacology, 5*(2), 129–134.

Chait, L. D. (1992). Factors influencing the subjective response to caffeine. *Behavioral Pharmacology, 3*(3), 219–228.

Charney, D. S., Heninger, G. R., & Jatlow, P. I. (1985). Increased anxiogenic effects of caffeine in panic disorders. *Archives of General Psychiatry, 42*(3), 233–243.

Cheney, R. H. (1936). Reaction time behavior after caffeine and coffee consumption. *Journal of Experimental Psychology, 19,* 357–369.

Childs, J. M. (1978). Caffeine consumption and target scanning performance. *Human Factors, 20*(1), 91–96.

Christopher, G., Sutherland, D., & Smith, A. (2005). Effects of caffeine in non-withdrawn volunteers. *Human Psychopharmacology—Clinical and Experimental, 20*(1), 47–53.

Clubley, M., Bye, C. E., Henson, T. A., Peck, A. W., & Riddington, C. J. (1979). Effects of caffeine and cyclizine alone and in combination on human performance, subjective effects and EEG activity. *British Journal of Clinical Pharmacology, 7*(2), 157–163.

Craik, F. I. M. (1994). Memory changes in normal aging. *Current Directions in Psychological Science, 3,* 155–158.

Dews, P. B. (1982). Caffeine. *Annual Review of Nutrition, 2,* 323–341.

Durlach, P. J. (1998). The effects of low dose of caffeine on cognitive performance. *Psychopharmacology, 140,* 116–119.

Eddy, N. B., & Downs, A. W. (1928). Tolerance and cross-tolerance in the human subject to the diuretic effect of caffeine, theobromine and theophylline. *Journal of Pharmacology and Experimental Therapeutics, 33,* 167–174.

Edwards, S., Brice, C., Craig, C., & Penri–Jones, R. (1996). Effects of caffeine, practice, and mode of presentation on Stroop task performance. *Pharmacology Biochemistry & Behavior, 54*(2), 309–315.

Erikson, G. C., Hager, L. B., Houseworth, C., Dungan, J., Petros, T., & Beckwith, B. E. (1985). The effects of caffeine on memory for word lists. *Physiology & Behavior*, *35*(1), 47–51.

Everitt, B. J., & Robbins, T. W. (1997). Central cholinergic systems and cognition. *Annual Review of Psychology*, 48, 649–684.

Fagan, D., Swift, C. G., & Tiplady, B. (1988). Effects of caffeine on vigilance and other performance tests in normal subjects. *Journal of Psychopharmacology*, *2*(1), 19–25.

File, S. E., Bond, A. J., & Lister, R. G. (1982). Interaction between effects of caffeine and lorazepam in performance tests and self-ratings. *Journal of Clinical Psychopharmacology*, *2*(2), 102–106.

Fillmore, M. T., & Vogel–Sprott, M. (1992). Expected effect of caffeine on motor performance predicts the type of response to placebo. *Psychopharmacology*, *106*(2), 209–214.

Fine, B. J., Kobrick, J. L., Lieberman, H. R., Marlowe, B., Riley, R. H., & Tharion, W. J. (1994). Effects of caffeine or diphenhydramine on visual vigilance. *Psychopharmacology*, *114*(2), 233–238.

Flaten, M. A., & Elden, A. (1999). Caffeine and prepulse inhibition of the acoustic startle reflex. *Psychopharmacology*, *147*(3), 322–330.

Flory, C. D., & Gilbert, J. (1943). The effects of benzedrine sulphate and caffeine citrate on the efficiency of college students. *Journal of Applied Psychology*, 27, 121–134.

Foreman, N., Barraclough, S., Moore, C., Mehta, A., & Madon, M. (1989). High doses of caffeine impair performance of a numerical version of the Stroop task in men. *Pharmacology Biochemistry & Behavior*, *32*, 399–403.

Franks, H. M., Hagedorn, H., Hensley, V. R., Hensley, W. J., & Starmer, G. A. (1975). Effect of caffeine on human performance, alone and in combination with ethanol. *Psychopharmacologia*, *45*(2), 177–181.

Frewer, L. J., & Lader, M. (1991). The effects of caffeine on two computerized tests of attention and vigilance. *Human Psychopharmacology—Clinical and Experimental*, *6*(2), 119–128.

Gibbs, R. B., & Aggarwal, P. (1998). Estrogen and basal forebrain cholinergic neurons: Implications for brain aging and Alzheimer's disease-related cognitive decline. *Hormones and Behavior*, *34*(2), 98–111.

Gilliland, A. R., & Nelson, D. (1939). The effects of coffee on certain mental and physiological functions. *Journal of General Psychology*, *21*, 339–348.

Gilliland, K. (1980). The interactive effect of introversion-extraversion with caffeine induced arousal on verbal performance. *Journal of Research in Personality*, *14*(4), 482–492.

Gilliland, K., & Andress, D. (1981). Ad-lib caffeine consumption, symptoms of caffeinism, and academic performance. *American Journal of Psychiatry*, *138*(4), 512–514.

Goldstein, A., Kaizer, S., & Warren, R. (1965). Psychotropic effects of caffeine in man. II. Alertness, psychomotor coordination and mood. *Journal of Pharmacology and Experimental Therapeutics*, *150*(1), 146–151.

Greden, J. F. (1974). Anxiety or caffeinism—Diagnostic dilemma. *American Journal of Psychiatry*, *131*(10), 1089–1092.

Greden, J. F., Fontaine, P., Lubetsky, M., & Chamberlin, K. (1978). Anxiety and depression associated with caffeinism among psychiatric-inpatients. *American Journal of Psychiatry*, 135, 963–966.

Griffiths, R. R., & Woodson, P. P. (1988). Caffeine physical dependence: A review of human and laboratory animal studies. *Psychopharmacology*, 94, 437–451.

Gupta, B. S., & Gupta, U. (1999). *Caffeine and behavior: Current views and research trends.* Boca Raton, FL: CRC Press.

Hasenfratz, M., & Battig, K. (1992). Action profiles of smoking and caffeine: Stroop effect, EEG, and peripheral physiology. *Pharmacology Biochemistry & Behavior, 42,* 155–161.

Hasenfratz, M., & Battig, K. (1994). Acute dose–effect relationships of caffeine and mental performance, EEG, cardiovascular and subjective parameters. *Psychopharmacology, 114,* 281–287.

Haskell, C. F., Kennedy, D. O., Wesnes, K. A., & Scholey, A. B. (2005). Cognitive and mood improvements of caffeine in habitual consumers and habitual nonconsumers of caffeine. *Psychopharmacology, 179*(4), 813–825.

Hawk, O. G. (1929). A study of the physiological and psychological reactions of the human organism to coffee drinking. *American Journal of Physiology, 90,* 380–381.

Heatherley, S. V., Hayward, R. C., Seers, H. E., & Rogers, P. J. (2005). Cognitive and psychomotor performance, mood, and pressor effects of caffeine after 4-, 6-, and 8-h caffeine abstinence. *Psychopharmacology, 178*(4), 461–470.

Hindmarch, I., Quinlan, P. T., Moore, K. L., & Parkin, C. (1998). The effects of black tea and other beverages on aspects of cognition and psychomotor performance. *Psychopharmacology, 139,* 230–238.

Hindmarch, I., Rigney, U., Stanley, N., Quinlan, P., Rycroft, J., & Lane, J. (2000). A naturalistic investigation of the effects of day-long consumption of tea, coffee and water on alertness, sleep onset and sleep quality. *Psychopharmacology, 149*(3), 203–216.

Hogervorst, E., Riedel W. J., Schmitt J. A. J., & Jolles, J. (1998). Caffeine improves memory performance during distraction in middle aged, but not in young or old subjects. *Human Psychopharmacology, 13,* 277–284.

Hollingworth, H. (1912). The influence of caffeine on mental and motor efficiency. *Archives of Psychology (New York), 3,* 1–166.

Horst, K., Buxton, R. E., & Robinson, W. D. (1934). The effect of habitual use of coffee or decaffeinated coffee upon blood pressure and certain motor reactions in normal young men. *Journal of Pharmacology and Experimental Therapeutics, 52,* 322–337.

Jacobson, B. H., & Edgley, B. M. (1987). Effects of caffeine on simple reaction time and movement time. *Aviation Space and Environmental Medicine, 58*(12), 1153–1156.

Jacobson, B. H., & Thurmanlacey, S. R. (1992). Effect of caffeine on motor performance by caffeine-naive and caffeine-familiar subjects. *Perceptual and Motor Skills, 74*(1), 151–157.

James, J. E. (1990). The influence of user status and anxious disposition on the hypertensive effects of caffeine. *International Journal of Psychophysiology, 10*(2), 171–179.

James, J. E. (1994). Does caffeine enhance or merely restore degraded psychomotor performance? *Neuropsychobiology, 30*(2–3), 124–125.

James, J. E. (1998). Acute and chronic effects of caffeine on performance, mood, headache, and sleep. *Neuropsychobiology, 38,* 32–41.

James, J. E., & Rogers, P. J. (2005). Effects of caffeine on performance and mood: Withdrawal reversal is the most plausible explanation. *Psychopharmacology, 182*(1), 1–8.

Jarvis, M. J. (1993). Does caffeine intake enhance absolute levels of cognitive performance? *Psychopharmacology, 110*(1–2), 45–52.

Johnson, L. C., Spinweber, C. L., & Gomez, S. A. (1990). Benzodiazepines and caffeine— Effect on daytime sleepiness, performance, and mood. *Psychopharmacology, 101*(2), 160–167.

Jones, H. A., & Lejuez, C. W. (2005). Personality correlates of caffeine dependence: The role of sensation seeking, impulsivity, and risk taking. *Experimental and Clinical Psychopharmacology, 13*(3), 259–266.

Judelson, D. A., Armstrong, L. E., Sokmen, B., Roti, M. W., Casa, D. J., & Kellogg, M. D. (2005). Effect of chronic caffeine intake on choice reaction time, mood, and visual vigilance. *Physiology & Behavior, 85*(5), 629–634.

Juliano, L. M., & Griffiths, R. R. (2004). A critical review of caffeine withdrawal: Empirical validation of symptoms and signs, incidence, severity, and associated features. *Psychopharmacology, 176*(1), 1–29.

Kaplan, G. B., Greenblatt, D. J., Ehrenberg, B. L., Goddard, J. E., Cotreau, M. M., Harmatz, J. S., et al. (1997). Dose-dependent pharmacokinetics and psychomotor effects of caffeine in humans. *Journal of Clinical Pharmacology, 37*(8), 693–703.

Kenemans, J. L., & Lorist, M. M. (1995). Caffeine and selective visual processing. *Pharmacology Biochemistry and Behavior, 52*(3), 461–471.

Kenemans, J. L., & Verbaten, M. N. (1998). Caffeine and visuospatial attention. *Psychopharmacology, 135*(4), 353–360.

Kenemans, J. L., Wieleman J. S. T., Zeegers, M., & Verbaten, M. N. (1999). Caffeine and Stroop interference. *Pharmacology Biochemistry & Behavior, 63*(4), 589–598.

Kerr, J. S., Sherwood, N., & Hindmarch, I. (1991). Separate and combined effects of the social drugs on psychomotor performance. *Psychopharmacology, 104*, 113–119.

Koelega, H. S. (1993). Stimulant drugs and vigilance performance—A review. *Psychopharmacology, 111*(1), 1–16.

Koelega, H. S. (1998). Effects of caffeine, nicotine and alcohol on vigilance performance. In J. Snel, & M. M. Lorist (Ed.), *Nicotine, caffeine and social drinking*. Harwood.

Kuznicki, J. T., & Turner, L. S. (1986). The effects of caffeine on caffeine users and nonusers. *Physiology and Behavior, 37*, 397–408.

Leathwood, P. D., & Pollet, P. (1983). Diet-induced mood changes in normal populations. *Journal of Psychiatric Research, 17*(2), 147–154.

Lieberman, H. R. (1988). Beneficial effects of caffeine. Paper presented at the Twelfth international Scientific Colloquium on Coffee, Paris.

Lieberman, H. R., Wurtman, R. J., Emde, G. G., & Coviella, I. L. G. (1987b). The effects of caffeine and aspirin on mood and performance. *Journal of Clinical Psychopharmacology, 7*(5), 315–320.

Lieberman, H. R., Wurtman, R. J., Emde, G. G., Roberts, C., & Coviella, I. L. G. (1987a). The effects of low doses of caffeine on human performance and mood. *Psychopharmacology, 92*(3), 308–312.

Liguori, A., Grass, J. A., & Hughes, J. R. (1999). Subjective effects of caffeine among introverts and extraverts in the morning and evening. *Experimental and Clinical Psychopharmacology, 7*(3), 244–249.

Liguori, A., Hughes, J. R., & Grass, J. A. (1997). Absorption and subjective effects of caffeine from coffee, cola and capsules. *Pharmacological Biochemistry and Behavior, 58*(3), 721–726.

Linde, L. (1995). Mental effects of caffeine in fatigued and nonfatigued female and male subjects. *Ergonomics, 38*(5), 864–885.

Loke, W. H. (1988). Effects of caffeine on mood and memory. *Physiology and Behavior, 44*, 367–372.

Loke, W. H., Hinrichs, J. V., & Ghoneim, M. M. (1985). Caffeine and diazepam—Separate and combined effects on mood, memory, and psychomotor performance. *Psychopharmacology, 87*(3), 344–350.

Loke, W. H., & Meliska, C. J. (1984). Effects of caffeine use and ingestion on a protracted visual vigilance task. *Psychopharmacology, 84*(1), 54–57.

Lorist, M. M., Snel, J., & Kok, A. (1994). Influence of caffeine on information processing stages in well rested and fatigued subjects. *Psychopharmacology, 113*, 411–421.

Mattila, M. J., Palva, E., & Savolainen, K. (1982). Caffeine antagonizes diazepam effects in man. *Medical Biology, 60*(2), 121–123.

Medina, J. H., Viola, H., Wolfman, C., Marder, M., Wasowski, C. D. C., et al. (1997). Overview—Flavonoids: A new family of benzodiazepine receptor ligands. *Neurochemical Research, 22*(4), 419–425.

Muehlbach, M. J., & Walsh, J. K. (1995). The effects of caffeine on simulated night-shift work and subsequent daytime sleep. *Sleep, 18*(1), 22–29.

Mumford, G. K., Evan, S. M., Kaminski, B. J., Preston, K. L., Sannerud, C. A., Silverman, K., et al. (1994). Discriminative stimulus and subjective effects of theobromine and caffeine in humans. *Psychopharmacology, 115*(1–2), 1–8.

Myers, J. P., Johnson, D. A., & McVey, D. E. (1999). Caffeine in the modulation of brain function. In B. S. Gupta and U. Gupta (Eds.), *Caffeine and behavior: Current views and research trends* (pp. 1–16). Boca Raton, FL: CRC Press.

Nehlig, A., Daval, J. L., & Debry, G. (1992). Caffeine and the central nervous system—Mechanisms of action, biochemical, metabolic and psychostimulant effects. *Brain Research Reviews, 17*(2), 139–169.

Paganinihill, A., & Henderson, V. W. (1994). Estrogen deficiency and risk of Alzheimer's disease in women. *American Journal of Epidemiology, 140*(3), 256–261.

Penetar, D., McCann, U., Thorne, D., Kamimori, G., Galinski, C., Sing, H., et al. (1993). Caffeine reversal of sleep-deprivation effects on alertness and mood. *Psychopharmacology, 112*(2–3), 359–365.

Rees, K., Allen, D., & Lader, M. (1999). The influences of age and caffeine on psychomotor and cognitive function. *Psychopharmacology, 145*(2), 181–188.

Richardson, N. J., Rogers, P. J., Elliman, N. A., & O'Dell, R. J. (1995). Mood and performance effects of caffeine in relation to acute and chronic caffeine deprivation. *Pharmacology Biochemistry & Behavior, 52*(2), 313–320.

Riedel, W., Hogervorst, E., Leboux, R., Verhey, F., Vanpraag, H., & Jolles, J. (1995). Caffeine attenuates scopolamine-induced memory impairment in humans. *Psychopharmacology, 122*(2), 158–168.

Roache, J. D., & Griffiths, R. R. (1987). Interactions of diazepam and caffeine—Behavioral and subjective dose effects in humans. *Pharmacology Biochemistry and Behavior, 26*(4), 801–812.

Robelin, M., & Rogers, P. J. (1998). Mood and psychomotor performance effects of the first, but not of subsequent, cup of coffee equivalent doses of caffeine consumed after overnight caffeine abstinence. *Behavioral Pharmacology, 9*(3), 1–8.

Rogers, P. J. (2000). Why we drink caffeine-containing beverages, and the equivocal benefits of regular caffeine intake for mood and cognitive performance. In T. H. Parliament, C.T. Ho, & P. Schieberle (Eds.), *Caffeinated beverages: Health benefits, physiological effects and chemistry* (Vol. 754, pp. 37–45). Washington, D.C.: ACS symposium series, American Chemical Society.

Rogers, P. J., & Derncourt, C. (1998). Regular caffeine consumption: A balance of adverse and beneficial effects for mood and psychomotor performance. *Pharmacology Biochemistry & Behavior, 59*(4), 1039–1045.

Rogers, P. J., Heatherley, S. V., Hayward, R. C., Seers, H. E., Hill, J., & Kane, M. (2005). Effects of caffeine and caffeine withdrawal on mood and cognitive performance degraded by sleep restriction. *Psychopharmacology, 179*(4), 742–752.

Rogers, P. J., Martin, J., Smith, C., Heatherley, S. V., & Smit, H. (2003). Absence of reinforcing, mood and psychomotor performance effects of caffeine in habitual nonconsumers of caffeine. *Psychopharmacology, 167,* 54–62.

Rogers, P. J., Richardson, N. J., & Dernoncourt, C. (1995). Caffeine use—Is there a net benefit for mood and psychomotor performance? *Neuropsychobiology, 31*(4), 195–199.

Rogers, P. J., Richardson, N. J., & Elliman, N. A. (1995). Overnight caffeine abstinence and negative reinforcement of preference for caffeine-containing drinks. *Psychopharmacology, 120,* 457–462.

Rogers, P. J., Stephens, S., & Day, J. E. L. (1998). Contrasting performance effects of caffeine after overnight and chronic caffeine withdrawal. *Journal of Psychopharmacology, 12*(Supp A), A13.

Rosenthal, L., Roehrs, T., Zwyghuizendoorenbos, A., Plath, D., & Roth, T. (1991). Alerting effects of caffeine after normal and restricted sleep. *Neuropsychopharmacology, 4*(2), 103–108.

Rush, C. R., Higgins, S. T., Bickel, W. K., & Hughes, J. R. (1994). Acute behavioral effects of lorazepam and caffeine, alone and in combination, in humans. *Behavioral Pharmacology, 5*(3), 245–254.

Rusted, J. M. (1999). Caffeine and cognitive performance: Effects on mood or mental processing. In B. S. Gupta & U. Gupta (Eds.), *Caffeine and behavior: Current views and research trends* (pp. 221–230). Boca Raton, FL: CRC Press.

Ryan, L., Hatfield, C., & Hofstetter, M. (2002). Caffeine reduces time-of-day effects on memory performance in older adults. *Psychological Science, 13*(1), 68–71.

Sawyer, D. A., Julia, H. L., & Turin, A. C. (1982). Caffeine and human behavior—Arousal, anxiety, and performance effects. *Journal of Behavioral Medicine, 5*(4), 415–439.

Shisslak, C. M., Beutler, L. E., Scheiber, S., Gaines, J. A., Wall, J. L., & Crago, M. (1985). Patterns of caffeine use and prescribed medications in psychiatric inpatients. *Psychological Reports, 57*(1), 39–42.

Smit, H., & Rogers, P. J. (2000). Effects of low doses of caffeine on cognitive performance, mood and thirst in low and higher caffeine consumers. *Psychopharmacology, 152,* 167–173.

Smit, H., & Rogers, P. J. (2002). Effects of energy drinks on mood and mental performance: critical methodology. *Food Quality and Preference,* 13, 317–326.

Smith, A., Sturgess, W., & Gallagher, J. (1999). Effects of a low dose of caffeine given in different drinks on mood and performance. *Human Psychopharmacology—Clinical and Experimental,* 14, 473–482.

Smith, A. P., Brice, C., Nash, J., Rich, N., & Nutt, D. J. (2003). Caffeine and central noradrenaline: Effects on mood, cognitive performance, eye movements and cardiovascular function. *Journal of Psychopharmacology, 17*(3), 283–292.

Smith, A. P., Brockman, P., Flynn, R., Maben, A., & Thomas, M. (1993). Investigation of the effects of coffee on alertness and performance during the day and night. *Neuropsychobiology,* 27, 217–223.

Smith, A. P., Clark, R., & Gallagher, J. (1999). Breakfast cereal and caffeinated coffee: Effects on working memory, attention, mood and cardiovascular function. *Physiology & Behavior, 67*(1), 9–17.

Smith, A. P., Kendrick, A. M., & Maben, A. L. (1992). Effects of breakfast and caffeine on performance and mood in the late morning and after lunch. *Neuropsychobiology, 26*(4), 198–204.

Smith, A. P., Kendrick, A., Maben, A., & Salmon, J. (1994). Effects of breakfast and caffeine on cognitive performance, mood and cardiovascular functioning. *Appetite, 22*(1), 39–55.

Smith, A. P., Maben, A., & Brockman, P. I. P. (1994). Effects of evening meals and caffeine on cognitive performance, mood and cardiovascular functioning. *Appetite, 22*(1), 57–65.

Smith, A. P., Rusted, J. M., Eaton–Williams, P., Savory, M., & Leathwood, P. (1990). Effects of caffeine given before and after lunch on sustained attention. *Neuropsychobiology, 23*(3), 160–163.

Smith, A. P., Whitney, H., Thomas, M., Perry, K., & Brockman, P. (1997). Effects of caffeine and noise on mood, performance and cardiovascular functioning. *Human Psychopharmacology—Clinical and Experimental, 12*(1), 27–33.

Smith, B. D., Meyers, M. Kline, R., & Bozman, A. (1987). Hemispheric-asymmetry and emotion-lateralized parietal processing of affect and cognition. *Biological Psychology, 25*, 247–260.

Smith, B. D., Kline, R., Lindgren, K., Ferro, M., Smith, D. A., & Nespor, A. (1995). The lateralized processing of affect in emotionally labile extroverts and introverts—Central and autonomic effects. *Biological Psychology, 39*(2–3), 143–157.

Smith, B. D., Rafferty, J., Lindgren, K., Smith, D. A., & Nespor, A. (1992). Effects of habitual caffeine use and acute ingestion—Testing a biobehavioral model. *Physiology & Behavior, 51*(1), 131–137.

Smith, B. D., Tola, K., & Mann, M. (1999). Caffeine and arousal: A biobehavioral theory of physiological, behavioral and emotional effects. In B. S. Gupta & U. Gupta (Eds.), *Caffeine and behavior: Current views and research trends* (pp. 87–135). Boca Raton, FL: CRC Press.

Snel, J., & Lorist, M. M. (1999). Caffeine and fatigue. In B. S. Gupta & U. Gupta (Eds.), *Caffeine and behavior: Current views and research trends* (pp. 151–159). Boca Raton, FL: CRC Press.

Stroop, J. R. (1935). Studies of interference in serial verbal reactions. *Journal of Experimental Psychology, 18*, 643–662.

Swift, C. G., & Tiplady, B. (1988). The effect of age on the response to caffeine. *Psychopharmacology, 94*, 29–31.

Terry, W. S., & Phifer, B. (1986). Caffeine and memory performance on the AVLT. *Journal of Clinical Psychology, 42*(6), 860–863.

Thornton, G. R., Holck, H. G. O., & Smith, E. L. (1939). The effect of benzedrine and caffeine upon performance in certain psychomotor tasks. *Journal of Abnormal Psychology, 34*, 96–113.

Tinley, E. M., Yeomans, M. R., & Durlach, P. J. (2003). Caffeine reinforces flavor preference in caffeine-dependent, but not long-term withdrawn, caffeine consumers. *Psychopharmacology, 166*, 416–423.

van Duinen, H., Lorist, M. M., & Zijdewind, I. (2005). The effect of caffeine on cognitive task performance and motor fatigue. *Psychopharmacology, 180*(3), 539–547.

Walsh, J. K., Muehlbach, M. J., Humm, T. M., Dickins, Q. S., Sugerman, J. L., & Schweitzer, P. K. (1990). Effect of caffeine on physiological sleep tendency and ability to sustain wakefulness at night. *Psychopharmacology, 101*(2), 271–273.

Wang, H. F., & Helliwell, K. (2001). Determination of flavonols in green and black tea leaves and green tea infusions by high-performance liquid chromatography. *Food Research International, 34*(2–3), 223–227.

Warburton, D. M. (1995). Effects of caffeine on cognition and mood without caffeine abstinence. *Psychopharmacology, 119*(1), 66–70.

Warburton, D. M., Bersellini, E., & Sweeney, E. (2001). An evaluation of a caffeinated taurine drink on mood, memory and information processing in healthy volunteers without caffeine abstinence. *Psychopharmacology, 158*, 322–328.

Weiss, B., & Laties, V. G. (1962). Enhancement of human performance by caffeine and the amphetamines. *Pharmacological Review, 14,* 1–36.

Wesensten, N. J., Killgore, W. D. S., & Balkin, T. J. (2005). Performance and alertness effects of caffeine, dextro amphetamine, and modafinil during sleep deprivation. *Journal of Sleep Research, 14*(3), 255–266.

Williams, C. L. (1998). Estrogen effects on cognition across the life span. *Hormones and Behavior, 34*(2), 80–84.

Wright, K. P., Badia, P., Myers, B. L., & Plenzler, S. C. (1997). Combination of bright light and caffeine as a countermeasure for impaired alertness and performance during extended sleep deprivation. *Journal of Sleep Research, 6*(1), 26–35.

Yeomans, M. R., Jackson, A., Lee, M. D., Nesic, J., & Durlach, P. J. (2000). Expression of flavor preferences conditioned by caffeine is dependent on caffeine deprivation state. *Psychopharmacology, 150,* 208–215.

Yeomans, M. R., Ripley, T., Davies, L. H., Rusted, J. M., & Rogers, P. J. (2002). Effects of caffeine on performance and mood depend on the level of caffeine abstinence. *Psychopharmacology, 164*(3), 241–249.

Yeomans, M. R., Spetch, H., & Rogers, P. J. (1998). Conditioned flavor preference negatively reinforced by caffeine in human volunteers. *Psychopharmacology, 137*(4), 401–409.

Yu, G., Maskray, V., Jackson, S. H. D., Swift, C. G., & Tiplady, B. (1991). A comparison of the central nervous system effects of caffeine and theophylline in elderly subjects. *British Journal of Clinical Pharmacology, 32*(3), 341–345.

Zahn, T. P., & Rapoport, J. L. (1987). Autonomic nervous system effects of acute doses of caffeine in caffeine users and abstainers. *International Journal of Psychophysiology, 5*(1), 33–41.

Zwyghuizen–Doorenbos, A., Roehrs, T. A., Lipschutz, L., Timms, V., & Roth, T. (1990). Effects of caffeine on alertness. *Psychopharmacology, 100,* 36–39.

12 Caffeine and Multicomponent Task Performance

Uma Gupta and B. S. Gupta

CONTENTS

INTRODUCTION: REVIEW OF THE LITERATURE

Caffeine is a widely consumed (D'Amicis & Viani, 1993; Debry, 1994; Barone & Roberts, 1996; Lundsberg, 1998; B. D. Smith, Kinder, Osborne, & Trotman, 2002), stimulating (Boulenger & Uhde, 1982; Zahn & Rapoport, 1987a, b; Rall, 1990; Nehlig, Daval, & Debry, 1992; Nehlig and Debry, 1994) substance. Its effects upon human performance depend upon a variety of factors, such as habituation to caffeine, basal arousal and initial response level, adequacy of experimental design, caffeine dosage, and several other factors related particularly to task demands determined by the nature of task and its level of difficulty and complexity (Estler, 1982; Dews,

311

1984; Bättig & Welzel, 1993; B. D. Smith & Tola, 1998; B. D. Smith, Tola, & Mann, 1999; Snel, Lorist, & Tieges, 2004).

Caffeine effects, therefore, may vary not only from situation to situation but also from task to task. For instance, caffeine has been reported to enhance performance on tasks involving

visual vigilance (Baker & Theologus, 1972; Regina, Smith, Keiper, & McKelvey, 1974; Fagan, Swift, & Tiplady, 1988; Fine et al., 1994; Kenemans & Lorist, 1995; Kenemans & Verbaten, 1998)

auditory vigilance (Lieberman, Wurtman, Emde, & Coviella, 1987, Lieberman, Wurtman, Emde, Roberts, & Coviella, 1987; Fagan et al., 1988; Pons, Trenque, Bielecki, Moulin, & Potier, 1988; Zwyghuizen–Doorenbos, Roehrs, Lipschutz, Timms, & Roth, 1990; Rosenthal, Roehrs, Zwyghuizen–Doorenbos, Plath, & Roth, 1991; Linde, 1995)

prolonged vigilance task (Loke & Meliska, 1984; Lieberman, Emde, Roberts, et al., 1987; Linde, 1994; Stein, Bender, Phillips, Leventhal, & Karsowski, 1996; Lin, McCann, Slate, & Uhde, 1997; Rogers & Dernoncourt, 1998; Rees, Allen, & Lader, 1999; Gilbert, Dibb, Plath, & Hiyane, 2000; Van Dongen et al., 2001)

endurance (Ivy, Costill, Fink, & Lower, 1979)

verbal reasoning or decision making (9 out of 12 studies demonstrated positive results: Borland, Rogers, Nicholson, Pascoe, & Spencer, 1986; Rogers, Spencer, Stone, & Nicholson, 1989; A. P. Smith, Rusted, Savory, Eaton–Williams, & Hall, 1991; A. P. Smith, Kendrick, & Maben, 1992; A. P. Smith, Brockman, Flynn, Maben, & Thomas, 1993; A. P. Smith, Kendrick, Maben, & Salmon, 1994; A. P. Smith, Maben, & Brockman, 1994; Mitchell & Redman, 1992; Bonnet & Arand, 1994; Linde, 1994; A. Smith, 1994; Warburton, 1995)

verbal abilities and intelligence (Gupta, 1988a, b; Anderson, 1994)

incidental learning (Gupta, 1991, 1993; Jarvis, 1993)

attention (Pons et al., 1988; Zwyghuizen–Doorenbos et al., 1990; Frewer & Lader, 1991; Kenemans & Lorist, 1995; Lorist, Snel, Mulder, & Kok, 1995; Warburton, 1995; Debrah, Kerr, Murphy, & Sherwin, 1996; Wijers, Lange, Mulder, & Mulder, 1997)

information processing (Bättig & Buzzi, 1986; Lorist, Snel, & Kok, 1994; Lorist, Snel, Kok, & Mulder, 1994; Lorist et al., 1995; Ruijter, De Ruiter, & Snel, 2000; Ruijter, De Ruiter, Snel, & Lorist, 2000)

rapid information processing (Hasenfratz, Jacquet, Aeschbach, & Bättig, 1991; Hasenfratz, Buzzini, Cheda, & Bättig, 1994; Hasenfratz & Bättig, 1993, 1994)

However, caffeine leads to a decrement in hand steadiness (Weiss & Laties, 1962; Nash, 1966; Ghoneim, Hinrichs, Chiang, & Loke, 1986) and has inconsistent effects on reaction time (see reviews by Estler, 1982, and Kerr, Sherwood, & Hindmarch, 1991; Bryant et al., 1998; Durlach, 1998; Rogers & Dernoncourt, 1998; Smit & Rogers, 2000; Ruijter, Lorist, Snel, & De Ruiter, 2001) and memory (Erikson et al.,

1985; Terry & Phifer, 1986; Landrum, Meliska, & Loke, 1988; Loke, 1988; Foreman, Barraclough, Moore, Mehta, & Madon, 1989; Loke, 1992; Jarvis, 1993; Turner, 1993; Barraclough & Foreman, 1994; A. Smith, 1994; Linde, 1995; Riedel et al., 1995; Warburton, 1995; Wright, Badia, Myers, & Plenzer, 1997; Hindmarch, Quinlan, Moore, & Parkin, 1998; Rogers & Dernoncourt, 1998; B. D. Smith & Tola, 1998; Herz, 1999; Hogervorst, Riedel, Kovacs, Brouns, & Jolles, 1999; Rees et al., 1999; B. D. Smith et al., 1999; Warburton, Bersellini, & Sweeney, 2001; Ryan, Hatfield, & Hofstetter, 2002; B. D. Smith, Osborne, Mann, Jones, & White, 2004).

The studies cited here, however, do not suggest that contradictory evidence is not available. This variability in outcomes may be interpreted in terms of caffeine effects being highly specific to task and situation (Rall, 1990). Moreover, the differences in results across studies perhaps also reflect differences in groups and tasks: Some tasks may not be sensitive in detecting subtle effects produced by caffeine administration, dosage level, and many subjective variables like habituation to caffeine and nicotine, sleep deprivation, fatigue, and withdrawal symptoms.

Another major difficulty in assessing and interpreting the effects of caffeine on human performance is that caffeine interacts with the characteristics of the person to whom the drug is administered. Personality characteristics reported to interact with caffeine in their effects on behavior include extraversion (Gilliland, 1980; B. D. Smith, Rypma, & Wilson, 1981; B. D. Smith, Wilson, & Jones, 1983; B. D. Smith, Wilson, & Davidson, 1984; Gupta, 1988b; Gupta & Gupta, 1994), impulsivity (Revelle, Humphreys, Simon, & Gilliland, 1980; Anderson & Revelle, 1982, 1983; Bowyer, Humphreys, & Revelle, 1983; Erikson et al., 1985; Arnold, Petros, Beckwith, Coons, & Gorman, 1987; Gupta, 1988a, 1991, 1993; Anderson, Revelle, & Lynch, 1989; Gupta & Gupta, 1990, 1999; A. P. Smith et al., 1991; A. P. Smith, Kendrick, et al., 1992; Gupta, Dubey, & Gupta, 1994; Gupta, Singh, & Gupta, 1999), and sensation seeking (Andrucci, Archer, Pancoast, & Gordon, 1989; Davidson & Smith, 1989). However, studies are also available in which the observed effects of caffeine were not influenced by individual differences.

The effects of caffeine are likely to reflect on several components of human performance, such as attentional dispositions, information transformation rate, primary memory capacity, capacity to access information in long-term storage, and response bias in a choice task. Kahneman (1973) also states that manipulations of activation yield effects on long- and short-term memory, attention distribution, stimulus discrimination and speed–accuracy trade-off. Broadbent's (1971) warning that the effects of such a manipulation manifested in terms of increase/decrease of errors, benefit/loss of speed, and so on are likely to vary from arouser to arouser seems pertinent in this context. The performance efficiency would therefore depend upon the functional level of various processing mechanisms set by the state induced by an arouser and the extent to which each of these is deployed in accordance with the task demands while performing a particular task. Thus, the interaction of the quality of a particular state with the quality of task demands put forth by a particular task will determine performance (Hamilton, Hockey, & Rejman, 1977; Eysenck, 1982).

The emphasis in most of the studies referred to in the above paragraphs of this chapter was on individual components observed mostly under "passive-machine"

(Kahneman, 1973) types of functional settings. However, the investigations of caffeine effects would be more revealing if studies are carried out on tasks that involve multicomponent skills ensuring active and effortful participation of the subject throughout while performing a task. For instance, in a letter transformation task, the subject is required to work through the alphabet a specified distance (usually between one to four letters) from a given letter or groups of letters; for example, the answer to "DN + 2" is "FP" and the answer to "KCHS + 4" is "OGLW."

Varying the number of letters requiring transformation between one and four and also the transformation requirement between one and four, a matrix of 16 (4 × 4) tasks that demand varying emphasis on processing of new input and holding capacity can be devised. Response (output) is not permitted until all letters are transformed. At least three major factors are involved in the performance of this task (Eysenck, 1982):

     access to long-term memory and locating the appropriate part of the alphabet
     performance of the transformation
     rehearsal and storage of accumulating answers

The letter transformation task outlined here creates a range of tasks that vary from having pure processing power to striking a balance between maintaining storage and processing new input. Moreover, the subject's active and effortful participation throughout is ensured while this task is performed. Investigation of caffeine effects on a task that requires active and effortful participation of the organism, on the one hand, and depends heavily upon more than one component of performance on the other would certainly be more useful and helpful in understanding the subtleties of caffeine effects on behavior. Hence, a study reported in the succeeding section was planned to use the letter transformation task for exploration of caffeine effects. The central objective was to investigate the dose–response relationship in caffeine effects.

EXPERIMENT 1

METHODS

The effects of four doses of caffeine citrate (1, 2, 3, or 4 mg/kg body weight) or placebo (citric acid) dissolved in a glass of orange-flavored drink were examined on a letter transformation task that involved multicomponent skills. Similar drug doses were also used in our earlier studies (Gupta & Gupta, 1990, 1994; Gupta, 1991, 1993; Gupta et al., 1994). Citric acid has also been used in investigations devoted to studying caffeine effects (White, Lincoln, Pearce, Reeb, & Vaida, 1980; Gupta, 1991, 1993; Gupta et al., 1994; Gupta & Gupta, 1999).

Subjects

Fifty postgraduate, right-handed male students aged 19 to 24 years volunteered as subjects. They were assigned randomly in equal numbers to five treatments (four doses of caffeine and a placebo). They were subsequently randomly assigned serial numbers from 1 to 10 in each treatment group.

Students who did not take coffee at all or were only casual coffee drinkers (taking not more than one cup of coffee a day for only 3 to 4 days a week) and who were nonsmokers and only casual cola and tea consumers were accepted as subjects. This was done because it is well known that the habitual level of caffeine or nicotine consumption influences response to challenge doses and consequently affects performance (Loke & Meliska, 1984; Loke, 1988; Fine & McCord, 1991; B. D. Smith, Rafferty, Lindgren, Smith, & Nespor, 1992; Herz, 1999; A. P. Smith, Clark, & Gallagher, 1999; Smit & Rogers, 2000). In addition, only persons who did not use any kind of drug, such as opioid analgesics, CNS depressants, CNS sympathomimetics, tranquilizers, cannabinoids, or psychedelics, qualified as subjects.

Materials

The stimulus material was patterned after the letter transformation task employed by Hamilton et al. (1977; Experiment V) as a test for closed-system thinking. In the simplest version of the task, the subjects are simply required to indicate the letter following a given letter (e.g., D + 1 = E). The task was changed in two ways: (a) by varying the number of letters requiring transformation between one and four (e.g., D + 1 = E; MTEK + 1 = NUFL); and (b) by varying the size of the required transformation between one and four (e.g., D + 1, 2, 3, or 4). The storage load (number of letters requiring transformation) and transition length (size of the required transformation) were varied in a 4 × 4 matrix shown in Table 12.1. In this way, 16 tasks were constructed. Letters of the alphabet were arranged on sheets of paper as columns of single letters and groups of two, three, or four letters; there were 16 such sheets, one for each task.

Experimental Design

A factorial design involving five treatments (four caffeine doses and a placebo), four storage loads (zero, one, two, and three letters), and four process levels (+1, +2, +3, +4 letters from a given letter) with repeated measures on the last two factors was used. Ten subjects were randomly assigned to each of the five treatments.

TABLE 12.1
Storage and Processing Conditions for Letter Transformation Task with Examples of Task Performed

Storage Level	Process Level						
	Add 1		Add 2	Add 3	Add 4		
	Stimulus	Response			Stimulus	Response	
Storage 0	D	E	—	—	D	H	
Storage 1	—	—	—	—	—	—	
Storage 2	—	—	—	—	—	—	
Storage 3	GBRE	HCSF	—	—	GBRE	KFVI	

Procedure

Prior to the day of testing, subjects were advised to fast overnight, to have their normal night's sleep, and to abstain from caffeinated/nicotinic beverages, alcohol, and drugs, as mentioned earlier, 10 h prior to the experiment.

To control for diurnal variations in arousal (Blake, 1967; Folkard, Knauth, Monk, & Rutenfranz, 1976; Eysenck & Folkard, 1980; Revelle et al., 1980), all experimental sessions began at the fixed time, i.e., 9.00 A.M. (Gupta & Gupta, 1990, 1994; Gupta, 1991). All subjects, tested individually, were weighed and a saliva sample was taken to determine the caffeine level at baseline. After giving written consent for administration of caffeine, the subject was given the orange-flavored cold drink that contained caffeine citrate or placebo, using a double-blind procedure.

Caffeine was administered in orange-flavored cold drinks because the subjects who provided data for the study were almost nonusers of coffee who might not much like the taste and smell of caffeinated/decaffeinated coffee. Subjects then completed a questionnaire about their previous night's sleep, food consumption, smoking, and alcohol or drug consumption. Following a 30-min absorption period to allow caffeine to reach peak plasma levels (Gilbert, 1976; B. D. Smith et al., 1981), a second saliva sample was taken. This was subsequently followed by the performance session, which began 45 min after the drink was ingested.

For the experiment, the procedure employed by Hamilton et al. (1977; Experiment V) was followed. The subject was instructed to make forward transition of variable length from a given letter in the alphabet and to give his response as a single unit rather than transform and output each letter separately when the letters were presented in groups. The subject was required to work down the columns on the sheets, performing a prearranged transformation. All the tasks were performed by all subjects in a balanced design. Work on each sheet was terminated before all items had been transformed, and time at task was recorded. Time at work for each subject was converted to time per letter output for each work sheet (Hamilton et al.).

RESULTS

The time per letter output of each subject for each of the four caffeine conditions (1, 2, 3, or 4 mg/kg body weight) in respect of each work sheet was divided by the corresponding placebo time. That is, the time figure obtained by the subject at Sr. No. 1 under each of the four caffeine conditions in respect of all Storage Load × Process Level conditions was divided by the corresponding time figure obtained by the subject at Sr. No. 1 in placebo condition. The scores thus derived served as units for all statistical analyses.

The data were treated by three-way (four caffeine treatments × four storage loads × four process levels) analysis of variance with repeated measures on the last two factors (Winer, 1971). The analysis showed that caffeine interacted significantly with storage load as well as with process level: Caffeine × Storage Load ($F = 26.48$; $df = 9, 108$; $p < .001$), Caffeine × Process Level ($F = 75.74$; $df = 9, 108$; $p < .001$), and Caffeine × Storage Load × Process Level ($F = 7.04$, $df = 27, 324$; $p < 0.001$). In light of these significant interactions, the main effect of caffeine, though statistically significant ($F = 275.48$; $df = 3, 36$; $p < .001$), was not considered important.

To obtain more detailed information, trend analysis was carried out to examine the variation accounted for by various trend components in caffeine effects for each of these interactions.

Caffeine × Storage Load

The trend analysis revealed that when storage load was zero (i.e., the letters were presented singly), the cubic trend in caffeine effects accounted for most of the variation (68.94%), the quadratic trend accounted for 29.88% variation, and the linear trend accounted for only negligible variation (1.18%). The linear trend accounted for most of the variation when the letters were presented in groups of two (61.52%), three (71.87%), or four (64.80%) letters. The corresponding figures for the quadratic component were 35.37, 28.13, and 30.72%, respectively. The cubic trend accounted for a negligible amount of variation.

The Caffeine × Storage Load interaction is illustrated in Figure 12.1. The figure indicates that when storage load is nil, a slight benefit can be had from caffeine administration in various doses. This benefit is also observed for all other storage conditions up to the dose of 3 mg/kg; however, with a 4-mg/kg dose, the performance seems to be worse than that under placebo conditions. Moreover, the rate of change in performance efficiency appears to be higher for a 4-mg/kg dose than that under lower doses of caffeine.

Caffeine × Process Level

The trend analysis showed that when the process level was minimal (+1 processing condition)—that is, the subject was simply required to give the next letter from the given letter—the quadratic trend in caffeine effects accounted for most of the variation (85.94%), the cubic trend accounted for 13.73% variation, and the linear trend

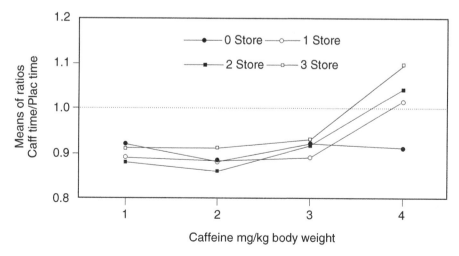

FIGURE 12.1 Effects of caffeine on letter transformation performance in various memory load conditions.

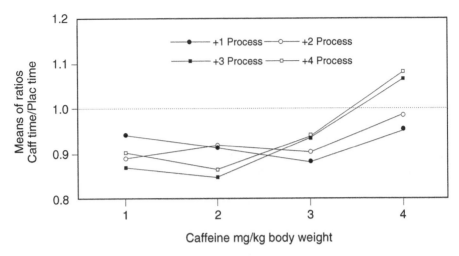

FIGURE 12.2 Effects of caffeine on letter transformation performance in various processing conditions.

accounted for negligible variation (0.33%). The linear trend accounted for most of the variation when the process level was increased: +2 (67.23%), +3 (77.78%), and +4 (69.83%). The corresponding figures for quadratic components were 15.53%, 21.76%, and 29.53% respectively. The cubic trend accounted for negligible amounts of variation except for the +2 level (17.24%). Thus, caffeine effects were more or less similar to those observed for conditions with higher storage load.

The Caffeine × Process Level interaction is shown in Figure 12.2. The figure indicates that the slight benefit observed under caffeine administration for all four doses of caffeine disappears with higher processing requirements (i.e., +3 and +4 processing levels) under the influence of 4 mg/kg of caffeine as compared with that of placebo. The rate of change in performance efficiency also seems to be higher for a 4-mg/kg dose than that under lower doses of caffeine.

Caffeine × Storage Load × Process Level

The results of trend analysis for this interaction (reported in Table 12.2) present quite a massive array of caffeine effects. However, in Figure 12.3, a discernible trend is quite obvious. With an increase in task demands caused by increased storage and processing requirements, the benefit derived from caffeine administration disappears, the performance turns worse with the increasing caffeine dose, and the dose–response trends become essentially linear.

Discussion

The results illustrated in Figure 12.1 for the statistically significant interaction between caffeine and storage load indicate quite clearly that caffeine improves performance (i.e., decreases processing time) on the simpler version of the letter

TABLE 12.2
Results of Trend Analysis in Caffeine Effects

Storage Level	Process Level	Percentage of Contributed Variation		
		Linear	Quadratic	Cubic
Storage 0	+1	65.36	0.11	34.52
	+2	26.72	73.10	0.18
	+3	53.34	25.80	20.86
	+4	31.90	68.09	0.01
Storage 1	+1	0.06	76.49	23.45
	+2	21.25	63.68	15.07
	+3	91.11	6.51	2.38
	+4	74.68	24.41	0.91
Storage 2	+1	8.70	73.91	17.39
	+2	94.25	5.74	0.01
	+3	74.14	25.45	0.41
	+4	74.34	20.63	5.03
Storage 3	+1	17.14	28.12	54.74
	+2	56.51	16.49	27.00
	+3	71.87	27.76	0.37
	+4	72.96	27.04	0

transformation task (i.e., one-letter task); on the more difficult versions (i.e., two-, three-, or four-letter tasks), caffeine improves performance when administered in doses up to 3 mg/kg. However, performance worsens (processing time is enhanced, i.e., performance is slowed down) with a 4-mg/kg dose.

Caffeine in the highest dose (4 mg/kg) perhaps works like a stressor and slows the letter transformation performance on two-, three-, and four-letter tasks. Moreover, caffeine effects are curvilinear (cubic trend accounts for 68.94% variation) when the memory load is zero (one-letter task), but such effects become essentially linear with increase in memory load—that is, when the subjects are required to transform letters presented in groups of two, three, or four letters (response was not permitted until all letters were transformed). The rate of change in performance efficiency across various doses of caffeine seems comparable for the simpler version of the task. Similar effects were also observed for the more difficult versions under the influence of caffeine administered in doses up to 3 mg/kg, but the rate of such change was higher when caffeine was administered in a 4-mg/kg dose.

Caffeine in all doses facilitates letter transformation performance with smaller process levels (i.e., +1 and +2 processing conditions); for higher process levels (i.e., +3 and +4 processing conditions), the facilitating effects have been observed with doses up to 3 mg/kg of caffeine. Contrarily, the highest dose (i.e., 4 mg/kg) affects the performance adversely. Caffeine effects are curvilinear (quadratic trend accounted for 85.94% variation) when subjects are required to provide the letter following the given letter (i.e., +1 processing condition).

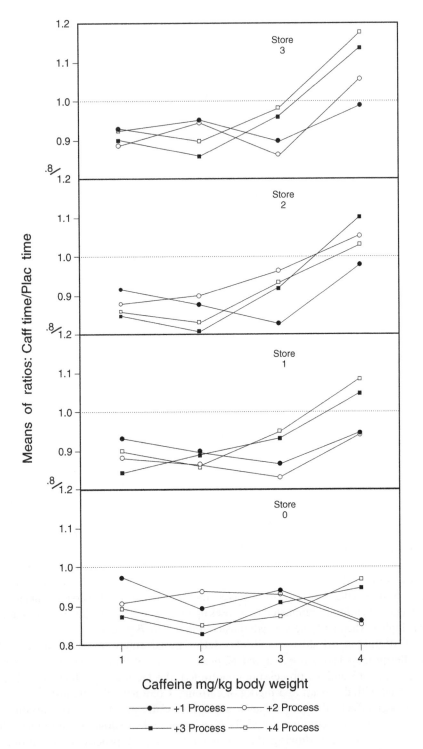

FIGURE 12.3 Effects of caffeine on letter transformation performance in various Memory Load × Processing Conditions.

The effects are primarily linear when the subjects work at higher (+2, +3, or +4) process levels (variation in caffeine effects accounted for by the linear trend ranges from 67.23 to 77.78%). The rate of change in response efficiency also appears to be higher with a 4-mg/kg dose for higher process levels (i.e., +3 and +4 processing conditions).

The higher order significant interaction, illustrated in Figure 12.3, indicates that when the letters are presented singly (one-letter task)—that is, where the primary emphasis is on processing speed, caffeine produces a facilitating influence on performance in all the transition length conditions used for letter transformation. Similarly, caffeine facilities performance with +1 process level in all memory load conditions (one- to four-letter tasks). This facilitating influence of caffeine has also been observed for doses up to 3 mg/kg with increasing memory storage and processing requirements; the 4-mg/kg dose, however, affects the performance adversely. With the increase in task demands caused by increased storage and processing requirements, the dose–response trends turn essentially linear (Table 12.2 and Figure 12.3).

EXPERIMENT 2

When administered in doses up to 3 mg/kg, caffeine produces beneficial effects on letter transformation performance (total solution time per letter output) in all Storage Load × Process Level conditions. The 4-mg/kg dose, however, not only produces differential effects but also worsens performance in certain conditions. This finding is potentially interesting, but it seems limited in that it is not clear which processing component or components of more complex problems were adversely affected by the 4-mg/kg dose of caffeine. At least three processing components can be identified for each letter:

access to long-term storage
letter transformation performance
rehearsal and storage

The aim of the experiment reported in this section was to analyze performance at the level of individual processing components as outlined here.

METHODS

The effects of 4 mg/kg of caffeine citrate and a placebo (citric acid) dissolved in a glass of orange-flavored drink were examined on letter transformation performance using a four-letter task and +4 process level.

Twenty postgraduate, right-handed male students aged 19 to 24 years volunteered as subjects. They were assigned randomly to two treatments (caffeine and a placebo) in equal numbers. Students fulfilled the qualifying criteria as specified in Experiment 1 for being accepted as subjects.

The letters in the four-letter task were presented sequentially and the subject was required to press a key after he had processed a letter to see the next letter on the screen; the processing time for each letter was inferred from the time between successive key presses. In addition, the subject performed transformation out loud. The time elapsing between key presses and the length of the speech phase were timed by computer. The total processing time for each letter could therefore be divided into three successive stages corresponding to the three processing components mentioned earlier. Thus, a four-letter task would have 12 processing components and caffeine might affect any or all of them.

RESULTS AND DISCUSSION

The data were analyzed by three-way (two treatments × four letters × three processing components) analysis of variance with repeated measures on the last two factors. The results revealed that the three main effects were statistically significant: treatments (F = 5.84; df = 1, 18; $p < 0.05$), letters (F = 4.47; df = 3, 54; $p < 0.01$), and processing components (F = 4.91; df = 2, 36, $p < 0.02$).

The mean solution times for the components of the letter transformation task in respect of the treatment groups (caffeine and placebo) are shown diagrammatically in Figure 12.4. The figure clearly indicates that the adverse effects of the 4-mg/kg dose of caffeine, expressed in terms of increase in processing time (indicative of slowing down the speed of processing), occur primarily during rehearsal and storage stages of processing. Thus, the primary locus of slowing down observed under the influence of 4 mg/kg of caffeine was the task component concerned with storage and updating operations.

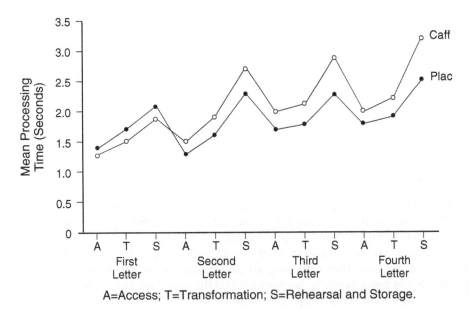

A=Access; T=Transformation; S=Rehearsal and Storage.

FIGURE 12.4 Effects of caffeine on components of the letter transformation task.

GENERAL DISCUSSION

The findings obtained in Experiment 1 make it quite clear that caffeine in relatively smaller doses (up to 3 mg/kg body weight) facilitates letter transformation performance but worsens it with a higher dose (4 mg/kg body weight)—especially in conditions with increasing task demands caused by increased storage and processing requirements. Humphreys and Revelle (1984) and Weiss and Laties (1962) also report that caffeine produces no effect or impairs performance on complex tasks (i.e., when task demands are high). This finding appears to be in line with the observations of Lieberman (1992), who suggests that the positive effects of caffeine are likely to occur up to about 300 mg and contrarily negative effects may occur with doses above 300 mg.

However, the authors are aware that great individual variability exists in sensitivity to caffeine. It is obvious from the results of Experiment 2 that the 4-mg/kg dose of caffeine does not produce uniform effects on various components of the letter transformation task. It is also obvious that the component most affected (though adversely) is the component concerned with storage, rehearsal, and updating operations.

Caffeine is well known for its stimulating properties; however, the arousal state induced by caffeine is relatively general and undifferentiated, whereas the arousal state produced by task demands as a by-product of active processing is fairly specific. Broadbent (1971) suggests that arousal's consequences for information processing involve activity in two types of mechanisms: the lower and the upper mechanisms. According to Broadbent, the activity in the lower mechanism is increased by stimulating drugs (amphetamine, caffeine, etc.) and decreased by depressing drugs (barbiturates, alcohol, etc.); the activity in the upper mechanism is enhanced while short and simple tasks (with fewer task demands) are performed and decreased when long and complex tasks (with more task demands) are performed.

Eysenck (1982) has also proposed that arousal involves two different kinds of systems: (a) a passive arousal system; and (b) an active cognitive control system. According to Eysenck, the first simply determines whether the induced arousal state is appropriate for satisfactory performance on a certain task and the other actively monitors the operations of the first system and initiates compensatory efforts whenever they are needed for satisfactory performance. Because of the close interdependent functioning of the two systems, people can cope with the stress caused by arousing or de-arousing conditions in a more active and flexible manner.

The fundamental effect of substances, like caffeine, that change the organism's state is to alter the tendency to action within a task. Caffeine therefore might lead to an alteration in the function of a central selective process that governs various ongoing cognitive operations (Hockey, 1986, 1993; Pribram & McGuinness, 1975). The results of Experiment 2 in this chapter uphold the veracity of this assumption by clearly demonstrating that the central process of storage and rehearsal is most affected by caffeine, rather than the other two processes of access to the relevant part of the alphabet and the transformation performance.

The implication of this finding is that the effects of caffeine on task performance can be better understood if we can identify more precisely the ways in which tasks affect processing activities. Interaction between the induced arousal state and task demands determines specific processing strategies a person must adopt for optimal performance on a task. More research is still needed to understand the exact nature of such interactions, especially in tasks in which subjects' active and effortful participation is ensured throughout the experimental session.

SUMMARY

The present study addressed an important issue in that caffeine research may be more revealing if studies are carried out on tasks involving multicomponent skills and employing functional settings in which the subject's active and effortful participation is ensured throughout the testing session. As a test for this speculation, a letter transformation task that creates a range of tasks varying from pure processing power to striking a balance between maintaining storage and processing new input was used for studying caffeine effects; subjects remained active and effortful participants throughout. Two experiments were run. The findings have been discussed and interpreted in terms of processing of information as a function of interaction between an induced arousal state and task demands and have demonstrated that this speculation is valid.

REFERENCES

Anderson, K. J. (1994). Impulsivity, caffeine and task difficulty: A within-subject test of the Yerkes–Dodson law. *Personality and Individual Differences, 16*, 813–829.

Anderson, K. J., and Revelle, W. (1982). Impulsivity, caffeine and proofreading: A test of the Easterbrook hypothesis. *Journal of Experimental Psychology: Human Perception and Performance, 8*, 614–624.

Anderson, K. J., & Revelle, W. (1983). The interactive effects of caffeine, impulsivity and task demands on visual search task. *Personality and Individual Differences, 4*, 127–132.

Anderson, K. J., Revelle, W., & Lynch, M. J. (1989). Caffeine, impulsivity, and memory scanning: A comparison of two explanations for the Yerkes–Dodson effect. *Motivation and Emotion, 13*, 1–20.

Andrucci, G. L., Archer, R. P., Pancoast, D. L., & Gordon, R. A. (1989). The relationship of MMPI and sensation seeking scales to adolescent drug use. *Journal of Personality Assessment, 53*, 253–266.

Arnold, M. E., Petros, T. V., Beckwith, B. F., Coons, G., & Gorman, N. (1987). The effect of caffeine, impulsivity, and sex on memory for word lists. *Physiology and Behavior, 41*, 25–30.

Baker, W. J., & Theologus, G. C. (1972). Effects of caffeine on visual monitoring. *Journal of Applied Psychology, 56*, 422–427.

Barone, J. J., & Roberts, H. R. (1996). Caffeine consumption. *Food and Chemical Toxicology, 34*, 119–126.

Barraclough, S., & Foreman, N. (1994). Factors influencing recall of supraspan word lists: Caffeine dose and introversion. *Pharmacopsychoecologia, 7*, 229–237.

Bättig, K., & Buzzi, R. (1986). Effect of coffee on the speed of subject-paced information processing. *Neuropsychobiology, 16*, 126–130.

Bättig, K., & Welzl, H. (1993). Psychopharmacological profile of caffeine. In S. Garattini (Ed.), *Caffeine, coffee and health* (pp. 213–253). New York: Raven Press.

Blake, M. J. F. (1967). Relationship between circadian rhythm of body temperature and introversion–extraversion. *Nature, 215,* 896–897.

Bonnet, M. H., & Arand, D. L. (1994). The use of prophylactic naps and caffeine to maintain performance during a continuous operation. *Ergonomics, 37,* 1009–1020.

Borland, R. G., Rogers, A. S., Nicholson, A. N., Pascoe, P. A., & Spencer, M. B. (1986). Performance overnight in shift workers operating a day-night schedule. *Aviation, Space and Environmental Medicine, 57,* 241–249.

Boulenger, J. P., and Uhde, T. W. (1982). Caffeine consumption and anxiety: Preliminary results of a survey comparing patients with anxiety disorders and normal controls. *Psychopharmacology Bulletin, 18,* 53–57.

Bowyer, P. A., Humphreys, M. S., & Revelle, W. (1983). Arousal and recognition memory: The effects of impulsivity, caffeine and time on task. *Personality and Individual Differences, 4,* 41, 49.

Broadbent, D. E. (1971). *Decision and stress.* London: Academic Press.

Bryant, C. A., Farmer, A., Tiplady, B., Keating, J., Sherwood, R., Swift, C. G., & Jackson, S. H. (1998). Psychomotor performance: Investigating the dose–response relationship for caffeine and theophylline in elderly volunteers. *European Journal of Clinical Pharmacology, 54,* 309–313.

D'Amicis, A., & Viani, R. (1993). The consumption of coffee. In S. Garattini (Ed.), *Caffeine, coffee and health* (pp. 1–16). New York: Raven Press.

Davidson, R. A., & Smith, B. D. (1989). Arousal and habituation: Differential effects of caffeine, sensation seeking and task difficulty. *Personality and Individual Differences, 10,* 111–119.

Debrah, K., Kerr, D., Murphy, J., & Sherwin, R. S. (1996). Effect of caffeine on recognition and physiological responses to hypoglycemia in insulin-dependent diabetes. *Lancet, 347,* 19–24.

Debry, G. (Ed.) (1994). *Coffee and health.* Paris: John Libbey.

Dews, P. B. (Ed.) (1984). *Caffeine.* Berlin: Springer–Verlag.

Durlach, P. J. (1998). The effects of a low dose of caffeine on cognitive performance. *Psychopharmacology, 140,* 116–119.

Erikson, G. C., Hager, L. B., Houseworth, C., Dungan, J., Petros, T., & Beckwith, B. E. (1985). The effects of caffeine on memory for word lists. *Physiology and Behavior, 35,* 47–51.

Estler, C. J. (1982). Caffeine. In F. Hoffmeister & G. Stille (Eds.), *Psychotropic agents. Part III. Alcohol and psychotomimetics, psychotropic effects of central acting drugs* (pp. 369–389). Berlin: Springer–Verlag.

Eysenck, M. W. (1982). *Attention and arousal.* Berlin: Springer–Verlag.

Eysenck, M. W., & Folkard, S. (1980). Personality, time of day and caffeine: Some theoretical and conceptual problems in Revelle et al. *Journal of Experimental Psychology: General, 109,* 32–41.

Fagan, D., Swift, C. G., & Tiplady, B. (1988). Effects of caffeine on vigilance and other performance tests in normal subjects. *Journal of Psychopharmacology, 2,* 19–25.

Fine, B. J., Kobrick, J. L., Lieberman, H. R., Marlowe, B., Riley, R. H., & Tharion, W. J. (1994). Effects of caffeine or diphenhydramine on visual vigilance. *Psychopharmacology, 114,* 233–238.

Fine, B. J., & McCord, L. (1991). Oral contraceptives use, caffeine consumption, field dependence and the discrimination of colors. *Perceptual and Motor Skills, 73,* 931–941.

Folkard, S., Knauth, P., Monk, T. H., & Rutenfranz, J. (1976). The effect of memory load on the circadian variation in performance efficiency under a rapidly rotating shift system. *Ergonomics, 19*, 479–488.

Foreman, N., Barraclough, S., Moore, C., Mehta, A., & Madon, M. (1989). High doses of caffeine impair performance of a numerical version of the Stroop task in men. *Pharmacology, Biochemistry and Behavior, 32*, 399–403.

Frewer, L. J., & Lader, M. (1991). The effects of caffeine on two computerized tests of attention and vigilance. *Human Psychopharmacology, 6*, 119–128.

Ghoneim, M. M., Hinrichs, J. V., Chiang, C. K., & Loke, W. H. (1986). Pharmacokinetic and pharmacodynamic interactions between caffeine and diazepam. *Journal of Clinical Pharmacology, 6*, 75–80.

Gilbert, D. G., Dibb, W. D., Plath, L. C., & Hiyane, S. G. (2000). Effects of nicotine and caffeine, separately and in combination, on EEG topography, mood, heart rate, cortisol, and vigilance. *Psychophysiology, 37*, 583–595.

Gilbert, R. M. (1976). Caffeine as a drug of abuse. In R. J. Gibbins, Y. Israel, H. Kalant, R. E. Popham, W. Schmidt, & R. G. Smart (Eds.), *Research advances in alcohol and drug problems* (Vol. 3., pp. 49–176). New York: John Wiley & Sons.

Gilliland, K. (1980). The interactive effect of introversion–extraversion with caffeine induced arousal on verbal performance. *Journal of Research in Personality, 14*, 482–492.

Gupta, B. S., Singh, S., & Gupta, U. (1999). Effects of impulsivity, caffeine and time of day on cognitive performance. *Psychological Studies, 44*, 77–85.

Gupta, U. (1988a). Effects of impulsivity and caffeine on human cognitive performance. *Pharmacopsychoecologia, 1*, 33–41.

Gupta, U. (1988b). Personality, caffeine and human cognitive performance. *Pharmacopsychoecologia, 1*, 79–84.

Gupta, U. (1991). Differential effects of caffeine on free recall after semantic and rhyming tasks in high and low impulsives. *Psychopharmacology, 105*, 137–140.

Gupta, U. (1993). Effects of caffeine on recognition. *Pharmacology, Biochemistry and Behavior, 44*, 393–396.

Gupta, U., Dubey, G. P., & Gupta, B. S. (1994). Effects of caffeine on perceptual judgment. *Neuropsychobiology, 30*, 185–188.

Gupta, U., & Gupta, B. S. (1990). Caffeine differentially affects kinesthetic aftereffect in high and low impulsives. *Psychopharmacology, 102*, 102–105.

Gupta, U., & Gupta, B. S. (1994). Effects of caffeine on perceptual judgment: A dose–response study. *Pharmacopsychoecologia, 7*, 215–219.

Gupta, U., and Gupta, B. S. (1999). Caffeine, impulsivity and performance. In B. S. Gupta and U. Gupta (Eds.), *Caffeine and behavior: Current views and research trends* (pp. 191–205). Boca Raton, FL: CRC Press LLC.

Hamilton, P., Hockey, G. R. J., & Rejman, M. (1977). The place of the concept of activation in human information processing theory: An integrative approach. In S. Dornic (Ed.), *Attention and performance* (Vol. VI, pp. 463–486). New York: Academic Press.

Hasenfratz, M., & Bättig, K. (1993). Dose–effect relationships between caffeine and various psychophysiological parameters. In *Proceedings of the 15th International Scientific Colloquium on Coffee* (Vol. II, pp. 476–482).

Hasenfratz, M., & Bättig, K. (1994). Acute dose–effect relationships of caffeine and mental performance, EEG, cardiovascular and subjective parameters. *Psychopharmacology, 114*, 281–287.

Hasenfratz, M., Buzzini, P., Cheda, P., & Bättig, K. (1994). Temporal relationships of the effects of caffeine and alcohol on rapid information processing. *Pharmacopsychoecologia, 7*, 87–97.

Hasenfratz, M., Jacquet, F., Aeschbach, D., & Bättig, K. (1991). Interactions of smoking and lunch with the effects of caffeine on cardiovascular functions and information processing. *Human Psychopharmacology, 6,* 277–284.

Herz, R. S. (1999). Caffeine effects on mood and memory. *Behavior Research and Therapy, 37,* 869–879.

Hindmarch, I., Quinlan, P. T., Moore, K. L. & Parkin, C. (1998). The effects of black tea and other beverages on aspects of cognition and psychomotor performance. *Psychopharmacology, 139,* 230–238.

Hockey, G. R. J. (1986). A state control theory of adaptation and individual differences in stress management. In G. R. J. Hockey, A. W. K. Gaillard, & M. G. H. Coles (Eds.), *Energetics and human information processing* (pp. 285–298). Dordrech, The Netherlands: Nijhoff.

Hockey, G. R. J. (1993). Cognitive-energetical control mechanisms in the management of work demands and psychological health. In A. Baddley & L. Weiskrantz (Eds.), *Attention: Selection, awareness, and control: A tribute to Donald Broadbent* (pp. 328–345). Oxford: Clarendon Press.

Hogervorst, E., Riedel, W. J., Kovacs, E., Brouns, F., & Jolles, J. (1999). Caffeine improves cognitive performance after strenuous physical exercise. *International Journal of Sports Medicine, 20,* 354–361.

Humphreys, M. S., & Revelle, W. (1984). Personality, motivation, and performance: A theory of the relationship between individual differences and information processing. *Psychological Review, 91,* 153–184.

Ivy, J. L., Costill, D. L., Fink, W. J., & Lower, R. W. (1979). Influence of caffeine and carbohydrate feeding on endurance performance. *Medical Science Sports, 11,* 6–11.

Jarvis, M. J. (1993). Does caffeine intake enhance absolute levels of cognitive performance? *Psychopharmacology, 110,* 45–52.

Kahneman, D. (1973). *Attention and effort.* Englewood Cliffs, NJ: Prentice Hall.

Kenemans, J. L., & Lorist, M. M. (1995). Caffeine and selective visual processing. *Pharmacology, Biochemistry and Behavior, 52,* 461–471.

Kenemans, J. L., & Verbaten, M. N. (1998). Caffeine and visuospatial attention. *Psychopharmacology, 135,* 353–360.

Kerr, J. S., Sherwood, N., & Hindmarch, I. (1991). Separate and combined effects of the social drugs on psychomotor performance. *Psychopharmacology, 104,* 113–119.

Landrum, R. E., Meliska, C. J., & Loke, W. H. (1988). Effects of caffeine and task experience on task performance. *Psychologia, 31,* 91–97.

Lieberman, H. R. (1992). Caffeine. In A. P. Smith and D. M. Jones (Eds.), *Handbook of human performance* (Vol. 2, pp. 49–72). London: Academic Press.

Lieberman, H. R., Wurtman, R. J., Emde, G. G., & Coviella, I. L. G. (1987). The effects of caffeine and aspirin on mood and performance. *Journal of Clinical Psychopharmacology, 7,* 315–320.

Lieberman, H. R., Wurtman, R. J., Emde, G. G., Roberts, C., & Coviella, I. L. G. (1987). The effects of low doses of caffeine on human performance and mood. *Psychopharmacology, 92,* 308–312.

Lin, A. S., McCann, U. D., Slate, S. O., & Uhde, T. W. (1997). Effects of intravenous caffeine administered to healthy males during sleep. *Depression and Anxiety, 5,* 21–28.

Linde, L. (1994). An auditory attention task: A note on the processing of verbal information. *Perceptual and Motor Skills, 78,* 563–570.

Linde, L. (1995). Mental effects of caffeine in fatigued and non-fatigued female and male subjects. *Ergonomics, 38,* 864–885.

Loke, W. H. (1988). Effects of caffeine on mood and memory. *Physiology and Behavior, 44,* 367–372.

Loke, W. H. (1992). The effects of caffeine and automaticity on a visual information processing task. *Human Psychopharmacology, 7*, 379–388.

Loke, W. H., & Meliska, C. J. (1984). Effects of caffeine use and ingestion on a protracted visual vigilance task. *Psychopharmacology, 84*, 54–57.

Lorist, M. M., Snel, J., & Kok, A. (1994). Influence of caffeine on information processing stages in well rested and fatigued subjects. *Psychopharmacology, 113*, 411–421.

Lorist, M. M., Snel, J., Kok, A., & Mulder, G. (1994). Influence of caffeine on selective attention in well rested and fatigued subjects. *Psychophysiology, 31*, 525–534.

Lorist, M. M., Snel, J., Mulder, G., & Kok, A. (1995). Aging, caffeine, and information processing: An event-related potential analysis. *Electroencephalography and Clinical Neurophysiology, 96*, 453–467.

Lundsberg, L. S. (1998). Caffeine consumption. In G. A. Spiller (Ed.), *Caffeine* (pp. 199–224). Boca Raton, FL: CRC Press LCC.

Mitchell, P. J., & Redman, J. R. (1992). Effects of caffeine, time of day and user history on study-related performance. *Psychopharmacology, 109*, 121–126.

Nash, H. (1966). Psychological effects and alcohol-antagonizing properties of caffeine. *Quarterly Journal of Studies in Alcohol, 27*, 727–734.

Nehlig, A., Daval, J. L., & Debry, G. (1992). Caffeine and the central nervous system: Mechanisms of action, biochemical, metabolic and psychostimulant effects. *Brain Research Reviews, 17*, 139–170.

Nehlig, A., & Debry, G. (1994). Effects of coffee on the central nervous system. In G. Debry (Ed.), *Coffee and health* (pp. 157–249). Paris: John Libbey.

Pons, L., Trenque, T., Bielecki, M., Moulin, M., & Potier, J. C. (1988). Attentional effects of caffeine in man: Comparison with drugs acting upon performance. *Psychiatry Research, 23*, 329–333.

Pribram, K. H., & McGuinness, D. (1975). Arousal, activation, and effort in the control of attention. *Psychological Review, 82*, 116–149.

Rall, T. W. (1990). Drugs used in the treatment of asthma. The methylxanthines, cromolyn sodium, and other agents. In A. G. Gilman, T. W. Rall, A. S. Nies, & P. Taylor (Eds.), *The pharmacological basis of therapeutics*, 8th ed. (pp. 618–637). London: Pergamon Press.

Rees, K., Allen, D., & Lader, M. (1999). The influences of age and caffeine on psychomotor and cognitive function. *Psychopharmacology, 145*, 181–188.

Regina, E. G., Smith, G. M., Keiper, C. G., & McKelvey, R. K. (1974). Effects of caffeine on alertness in simulated driving. *Journal of Applied Psychology, 59*, 483–489.

Revelle, W., Humphreys, M. S., Simon, L., & Gilliland, K. (1980). The interactive effects of personality, time of day, and caffeine: A test of arousal model. *Journal of Experimental Psychology: General, 109*, 1–31.

Riedel, W. J., Jolles, J., Van Praag, H., Verhey, F., Leboux, R., & Hogervorst, E. (1995). Caffeine attenuates scopolamine-induced memory impairment in humans. *Psychopharmacology, 122*, 158–165.

Rogers, A. S., Spencer, M. B., Stone, B. M., & Nicholson, A. N. (1989). The influence of a 1-h nap on performance overnight. *Ergonomics, 32*, 1193–1205.

Rogers, P. J., & Dernoncourt, C. (1998). Regular caffeine consumption: A balance of adverse and beneficial effects for mood and psychomotor performance. *Pharmacology, Biochemistry and Behavior, 59*, 1039–1045.

Rosenthal, L., Roehrs, T., Zwyghuizen–Doorenbos, A., Plath, D., & Roth, T. (1991). Alerting effects of caffeine after normal and restricted sleep. *Neuropsychopharmacology, 4*, 103–108.

Ruijter, J., De Ruiter, M. B., & Snel, J. (2000). The effects of caffeine on visual selective attention to color: An ERP study. *Psychophysiology, 37*, 427–439.

Ruijter, J., De Ruiter, M. B., Snel, J., & Lorist, M. M., (2000). The influence of caffeine on spatial-selective attention: An ERP study. *Clinical Neurophysiology, 111*, 2223–2233.

Ruijter, J., Lorist, M. M., Snel, J., & De Ruiter, M. B. (2001). The influence of caffeine on sustained attention: An ERP study. *Pharmacology, Biochemistry and Behavior, 66*, 29–38.

Ryan, L., Hatfield, C., & Hofstetter, M. (2002). Caffeine reduces time-of-day effects on memory performance. *Psychological Science, 13*, 68–71.

Smit, H. J., & Rogers, P. J. (2000). Effects of low doses of caffeine on cognitive performance, mood and thirst in low and higher caffeine consumers. *Psychopharmacology, 152*, 167–173.

Smith, A. P. (1994). Caffeine, performance, mood and states of reduced alertness. Special issue: Caffeine research. *Pharmacopsychoecologia, 7*, 75–86.

Smith, A. P., Brockman, P., Flynn, R., Maben, A., & Thomas, M. (1993). Investigation of the effects of coffee on alertness and performance during the day and night. *Neuropsychobiology, 27*, 217–223.

Smith, A. P., Clark, R., & Gallagher, J. (1999). Breakfast cereal and caffeinated coffee: Effects on working memory, attention, mood, and cardiovascular function. *Physiology and Behavior, 67*, 9–17.

Smith, A. P., Kendrick, A., Maben, A., & Salmon, J. (1994). Effects of breakfast and caffeine on cognitive performance, mood and cardiovascular functioning. *Appetite, 22*, 39–55.

Smith, A. P., Kendrick, A. M., & Maben, A. L. (1992). Effects of breakfast and caffeine on performance and mood in the late morning and after lunch. *Neuropsychobiology, 26*, 198–204.

Smith, A. P., Maben, A., & Brockman, P. (1994). Effects of evening meals and caffeine on cognitive performance, mood, and cardiovascular functioning. *Appetite, 22*, 57–65.

Smith, A. P., Rusted, J. M., Savory, M., Eaton–Williams, P., & Hall, S. R. (1991). The effects of caffeine, impulsivity and time of day on performance, mood and cardiovascular function. *Journal of Psychopharmacology, 5*, 120–128.

Smith, B. D., Kinder, N., Osborne, A., & Trotman, A. (2002). The arousal drug of choice: Major sources of caffeine. *Pharmacopsychoecologia, 15*, 1–34.

Smith, B. D., Osborne, A., Mann, M., Jones, H., & White, T. (2004). Arousal and behavior: Biopsychological effects of caffeine. In A. Nehlig (Ed.), *Coffee, tea, chocolate, and the brain* (pp. 35–52). Boca Raton, FL: CRC Press.

Smith, B. D., Rafferty, J., Lindgren, K., Smith, D. A., & Nespor, A. (1992). Effects of habitual caffeine use and acute ingestion: Testing a biobehavioral model. *Physiology and Behavior, 51*, 131–137.

Smith, B. D., Rypma, C. B., & Wilson, R. J. (1981). Dishabituation and spontaneous recovery of the electrodermal orienting response: Effects of extraversion, impulsivity, sociability and caffeine. *Journal of Research in Personality, 15*, 475–487.

Smith, B. D., & Tola, K. (1998). Caffeine: Effects on psychological functioning and performance. In G. A. Spiller (Ed.), *Caffeine* (pp. 251–299). Boca Raton, FL: CRC Press.

Smith, B. D., Tola, K., & Mann, M. (1999). Caffeine and arousal: A biobehavioral theory of physiological, behavioral, and emotional effects. In B. S. Gupta and U. Gupta (Eds.), *Caffeine and behavior: Current views and research trends* (pp. 87–135). Boca Raton, FL: CRC Press.

Smith, B. D., Wilson, R. D., & Davidson, R. A. (1984). Electrodermal activity and extraversion: Caffeine, preparatory signal and stimulus intensity effects. *Personality and Individual Differences, 5*, 59–65.

Smith, B. D., Wilson, R. J., & Jones, B. E. (1983). Extraversion and multiple levels of caffeine-induced arousal: Effects on overhabituation and dishabituation. *Psychophysiology, 20,* 29–34.

Snel, J., Lorist, M. M., & Tieges, Z. (2004). Coffee, caffeine and cognitive performance. In A. Nehlig (Ed.), *Coffee, tea, chocolate, and the brain* (pp. 53–71). Boca Raton, FL: CRC Press.

Stein. M. A., Bender, G. B., Phillips, W., Leventhal, B. L., & Karsowski, M. (1996). Behavioral and cognitive effects of methylxanthines: A meta-analysis of theophylline and caffeine. *Archives of Pediatric and Adolescent Medicine, 21,* 176–182.

Terry, W. S., & Phifer, B. (1986). Caffeine and memory performance on the AVLT. *Journal of Clinical Psychology, 42,* 860–863.

Turner, J. (1993). Incidental information processing: Effects of mood, sex and caffeine. *International Journal of Neuroscience, 72,* 1–14.

Van Dongen, H. P., Prince, N. J., Mullington, J. M. Szuba, M. P., Kapoor, S. C., & Kinges, D. F. (2001). Caffeine eliminates psychomotor vigilance deficits from sleeping inertia. *Sleep, 24,* 813–819.

Warburton, D. M. (1995). Effects of caffeine on cognition and mood without caffeine abstinence. *Psychopharmacology, 119,* 66–70.

Warburton, D. M., Bersellini, E., & Sweeney, E. (2001). An evaluation of a caffeinated taurine drink on mood, memory and information processing in healthy volunteers without caffeine abstinence. *Psychopharmacology, 158,* 322–328.

Weiss, B., & Laties, V. G. (1962). Enhancement of human performance by caffeine and the amphetamines. *Pharmacology Reviews, 14,* 1–36.

White, B. C., Lincoln, C. A., Pearce, N. W., Reeb, R., & Vaida, C. (1980). Anxiety and muscle tension as consequences of caffeine withdrawal. *Science, 209,* 1547–1548.

Wijers, A. A., Lange, J. J., Mulder, G., & Mulder, L. J. (1997). An ERP study of visual spatial attention and letter target detection for isoluminant and nonisoluminant stimuli. *Psychophysiology, 34,* 553–565.

Winer, B. J. (1971). *Statistical principles in experimental design,* 2nd ed. New York: McGraw Hill.

Wright, K. P., Badia, P., Myers, B. L., & Plenzer, S. C. (1997). Combination of bright light and caffeine as a countermeasure for impaired alertness and performance during extended sleep deprivation. *Journal of Sleep Research, 6,* 26–35.

Zahn, T. P., & Rapoport, J. L. (1987a). Acute autonomic nervous system and effects of caffeine in prepubertal boys. *Psychopharmacology, 91,* 40–44.

Zahn, T. P., & Rapoport, J. L. (1987b). Autonomic nervous system effects of acute doses of caffeine in caffeine users and abstainers. *International Journal of Psychophysiology, 5,* 33–41.

Zwyghuizen–Doorenbos, A., Roehrs, T. A., Lipschutz, L., Timms, V., & Roth, T. (1990). Effects of caffeine on alertness. *Psychopharmacology, 100,* 36–39.

13 Caffeinism: History, Clinical Features, Diagnosis, and Treatment

Iulian Iancu, Ahikam Olmer, and Rael D. Strous

CONTENTS

INTRODUCTION

Caffeine is considered to be the most commonly used psychoactive drug in the world. It is a powerful stimulant and its popularity results from this quality. It has been claimed that coffee promotes rapid, clear thinking, improves intellectual ability, enhances mental acuity, and decreases drowsiness, fatigue, and reaction time. Although these are all valued phenomena in an achievement-oriented society (Greden, 1974), caffeine also has deleterious effects and can cause a wide range of adverse effects due to abuse or abrupt interruption of its use. In this chapter we will summarize the data available concerning the syndrome of intoxication (caffeinism) and consider the clinical importance of the phenomenon.

EARLY REPORTS OF BEHAVIORAL EFFECTS

Historically, the use of caffeine-containing foods and beverages dates back 4,700 years. Use of these products has spread worldwide despite recurring efforts, motivated on moral, economic, medical, or political grounds, to restrict or eliminate their use (Griffiths & Mumford, 1995). The syndrome of excessive coffee drinking has long been reported. In Victorian England, the typical coffee drinker was characterized by members of the medical profession as: "tremulous, loses his self-command, is subject to fits of agitation and depression, and has a haggard appearance." It was further observed that a renewed dose of the "poison" gave temporary relief, but at the cost of "future misery" (Siegerist, 1943).

In America coffee became popular during the 18th century despite agitation by certain medical circles against its use (Mueller, 1967). Eighteenth-century physicians suggested that coffee and tea consumption promoted later use of alcohol, opium, and other stimulants (Greden, 1976). Medical case reports of caffeine toxicity, referred to as the "syndrome of coffee" (see Greden, 1974), appeared intermittently as early as the beginning of the 20th century. It is interesting that, following various observations of the effects of caffeine in soft beverages, several lawsuits (with subsequent research projects) were leveled at the beginning that century against the Coca-Cola company for marketing a beverage with a "deleterious ingredient": caffeine (Benjamin, Rogers, & Rosenbaum, 1991).

EPIDEMIOLOGY

No sound epidemiologic data on the prevalence of caffeine abuse and intoxication are available. Although the entity is well known, it remains underdiagnosed due to clinicians' omission of questioning about caffeine use in everyday practice. It remains unknown whether age, sex, race, or personality type has any effect on the rates of intoxication (Strain & Griffiths, 2000). Few studies have examined the prevalence of caffeine intoxication; most have examined selected populations (e.g., inpatients, college students) and used ambiguous criteria. One random-digit telephone survey of caffeine use in the general community found that 12% of respondents had met the *DSM-III-R* criteria for caffeine intoxication in the year previous to the investigation (Strain & Griffiths, 2000).

Bradley and Petree (1990) reported in a survey of university students that 18.9% out of 797 subjects endorsed the *DSM-III* caffeinism syndrome (presence of at least five signs). Students who consumed caffeine to obtain an enhanced performance used more coffee and had more caffeinism symptoms. Thus, it is plausible that students, physicians working long shifts, and high-tech employees would use large quantities of caffeine to obtain increased alertness and thus be at a higher risk of caffeine intoxication.

In a survey of 36,689 adult men and women (age range of 25 to 64 years) participating in population surveys in Finland between 1972 and 1992, Tanskanen et al. (2000a) reported that heavy use of coffee (seven cups or more per day) was found in 18.8% of men and 15.9% of women. Klatsky, Armstrong, and Friedman (1993) studied data of health examinations of 128,934 persons from northern California and reported that 16.3% of them reported daily intake of four or more cups of coffee. These studies suggest that up to a fifth of the population is at risk for caffeinism; however, more studies are required to define the extent of caffeine intoxication.

GENETICS

It has been suggested that the use of caffeine is influenced by the reinforcing properties of taste, hedonic psychoactive effects, and the desire to avoid withdrawal. However, preferences for caffeine and sensitivity to withdrawal vary widely between individuals (Kendler & Prescott, 1999). Twin studies have found heritable influences on coffee consumption. For example, in a study of female twins from a large population-based twin registry, Kendler and Prescott found greater concordance in monozygotic twin pairs for total caffeine consumption, heavy caffeine use, caffeine intoxication, and tolerance and withdrawal than in dizygotic twin pairs.

This study supports the findings of other studies suggesting that genetic differences may contribute to caffeine-related complications. Genetic risk factors may operate at several levels, including personality, vulnerability to psychopathology, caffeine metabolism (e.g., acetylation), and variations in adenosine receptors that may mediate the psychoactive effects of caffeine (see Kendler & Prescott, 1999).

PHARMACOLOGY

Caffeine is a naturally occurring xanthine derivative and is considerably more potent than another commonly known methylxanthine, theophylline. It is quickly absorbed in the oral, rectal, and subcutaneous routes and is distributed throughout all organ systems in proportion to body water (Haddad & Winchester, 1983). Approximately 90% of the caffeine in a cup of coffee is absorbed from the stomach within 20 minutes, with peak plasma concentrations occurring approximately 40 to 60 minutes later (O'Connell & Zurzola, 1984). It readily passes the blood–brain barrier as well as the placental barrier.

Caffeine is rapidly metabolized in the liver and excreted in the urine in almost equal parts as 1-methyluric acid and 1-methylxanthine. The half-life of caffeine is about 3.5 hours (Haddad & Winchester, 1983) and is shorter in cigarette smokers and prolonged in women, newborns, the elderly, patients with cirrhosis, and patients taking cimetidine (Tagamet) or oral contraceptives.

Caffeine undergoes hepatic metabolism via N-demethylation, acetylation, and oxidation. The CYP450-1A2 isoenzyme is largely responsible for the N-demethylation of caffeine to paraxanthine, the major metabolite. However, more than 25 metabolites have been identified and many are pharmacologically active. Caffeine's acetylation is under genetic control, and rapid acetylation is caused by an autosomal dominant gene. Slow acetylation leads to slow clearance and higher blood levels (Shils, Olson, Shike, & Ross, 1999). During elimination, approximately 85% of a dose is excreted in the urine within 48 hours, with approximately 1% as unchanged drug (Moffat, Osselton, Widdop, & Galichet, 2004).

Caffeine stimulates the medullary, respiratory, vasomotor, and vagal centers. At high doses, the spinal cord is stimulated. Whether regular consumption diminishes these stimulant effects remains unknown. The physiological effects of caffeine include stimulation of cardiac muscle and the central nervous system, a diuretic effect, elevation of plasma free fatty acid and glucose, smooth muscle relaxation, and stimulation of gastric acid secretion. Caffeine appears to stimulate synthesis and release of catecholamines, especially noradrenaline. The mild decrease in glucose tolerance following caffeine ingestion may be due to the catecholamine and subsequent cyclic adenosine monophosphate (cAMP) increase.

Caffeine's primary central mechanism of action appears to be its antagonism of adenosine receptors (Williams, 1995). This has several consequential effects because adenosine is well known as an important neuromodulator of several neurophysiologic processes. Activation of adenosine receptors activates an inhibitory G protein (Gi), thus inhibiting the formation of the second-messenger cAMP. Caffeine intake, therefore, results in an increase in intraneuronal cAMP concentrations in neurons that have adenosine receptors.

It has been estimated that as little as three cups of coffee may result in approximately 50% of the adenosine receptors being occupied by caffeine. Adenosine and adenosine triphosphate (ATP) are considered to be the primary cellular components involved in almost all stages of cellular function. They function as the endogenous agonists active at purinoreceptors.

Two classes of purinoreceptors have been described based on pharmacological criteria, P1 and P2 receptors. Adenosine and its analogs exhibit their agonistic action at P1 receptors, which may be blocked by various xanthines such as caffeine. P2 receptors are activated by ATP and no agents demonstrating clear antagonistic activity have been identified (Williams, 1995). P1 purinorecptors have further been subdivided into A1, A2a, A2b, A3, and A4 subclasses; the A prefix designates adenosine agonistic activity. Only A1, A2a, and A2b receptors are blocked by xanthines.

A1 receptors are found widely in the CNS with highest concentrations in the hippocampus, striatum, and the neocortex (Jacobson, van Gallen, & Williams, 1992). In contrast, A2a receptors are more limited to the substantia nigra, nucleus accumbens, globus pallidus, and olfactory tubercle. A2b receptors appear similarly, but are more widely distributed than those of A2a receptors. These distributions become important when effects of adenosine antagonism in these areas by caffeine activity are considered. Reflecting its important homeostatic role, adenosine is found in most areas of the CNS; thus, significant doses of caffeine have multiple and wide-ranging effects.

Adenosine is known to express potent inhibition of dopamine, GABA, glutamate, acetylcholine, serotonin, and norepinephrine release via presynaptic A1 receptors (Williams, 1995). Caffeine may be expected to produce an opposing effect at these receptors; thus, for example, it appears to stimulate synthesis and release of catecholamines, particularly noradrenaline, as well as enhance the actions of L-dopa and other dopamine agonists (Ferre, Fuxe, Von Euler, Johansson, & Fredholm, 1992).

It is well described that adenosine receptor agonists perform as functional dopamine antagonists (presumably at the A2a receptor site), so caffeine would demonstrate a considerably opposing effect—for example, observed as an exacerbation in psychosis in some cases. This interaction between A2a and D2 receptors has also been suggested to explain the stimulant effects of caffeine, and perhaps even to clarify some aspects of self-mutilation behavior such as is found in Lesch–Nyhan syndrome (Williams, 1995) and the lower incidence of Parkinson's disease related to caffeine use (Ross et al., 2000).

It has been suggested that P1 purinoreceptors might have a role in the mechanism of action of antipsychotic, antidepressant, and anxiolytic drugs (Ford, Delaney, Ling, Rose, & Erickson, 2001). It is interesting that knockout mice of P1 purinoreceptors have been found to be more aggressive (Ford et al., 2001). Postsynaptically, adenosine hyperpolarizes the postsynaptic membrane through A1 and A2 receptor modulation. As observed in decreased locomotor behavior, decreased schedule-controlled behavior, and high doses inducing ataxia and even cataplexy, adenosine demonstrates potent CNS depressant effects (hypothesized via A2 receptors). Therefore, it is not surprising that caffeine as an adenosine antagonist exhibits motor stimulant activity at these A2 receptors (Williams, 1995).

Interestingly, one of the hypothesized mechanisms of benzodiazepine action involves that of adenosine reuptake inhibition, thus potentiating its effects postsynaptically (Williams, 1995). Inosine, the deamination product of adenosine, was identified as a potential ligand for the central benzodiazepine receptor complex. It should be noted that, in contrast to adenosine, caffeine suppresses REM sleep and decreases total sleep time.

This has been further observed in the increase in total sleep following adenosine brain administration, as well as a resultant characteristic EEG sleep profile. Moreover, activation of central A1 and A2A receptors contributes to the ability of adenosine to produce sedation or sleep (Porkka–Heiskanen, T. et al., 1997; Radulovacki, Virus, Djuricic–Nedelson, & Green, 1984; Satoh, Matsumura, Suzuki, & Hayaishi, 1996). Caffeine was also shown to reduce ethanol-induced hypnotic effects in mammals caused by activation of A2A receptors (El Yacoubi, Ledent, Parmentier, Costentin, & Vaugeois, 2003).

It has been demonstrated that adenosine brain levels rise following ischemia and seizure activity and appear subsequently to result in an increased cerebral blood flow. Furthermore, it has been suggested that adenosine acts as an endogenous anticonvulsant, with adenosine acting as an endogenous anticonvulsant. This hypothesis is further substantiated by the observed proconvulsant and convulsant activity of caffeine in higher doses. Adenosine in this manner appears to exhibit neuroprotective effects with caffeine conversely displaying an opposing global cerebral vasoconstriction,

However, caffeine is also known to be a cognitive enhancer. This effect most likely results from a disinhibition of adenosine's inihibitory action on excitatory neurotransmission (Williams, 1995). Incidentally, some scientists have suggested that tolerance does not form to these vasoconstrictive effects and a rebound increase in cerebral flow is observed following caffeine withdrawal (Strain & Griffiths, 2000).

Interestingly, another important central effect potentially affected by methylxanthines such as caffeine is that of adenosine's proposed antinociceptive activity.

Such effects have been proposed to occur via A2 receptors, the activity of which may be antagonized by caffeine. Incidentally, although adenosine antagonists (with similar properties to caffeine) have been proposed as potential antidepressants due to their neurotransmitter release profile, evidence for their efficacy remains inconclusive and as yet unproven (Williams, 1995).

Tolerance may develop to several caffeine effects; however, in many cases it will be overcome by the nonlinear accumulation of caffeine with saturation of its metabolic pathway. This saturation may result from excessive caffeine ingestion or from pharmacokinetic interactions such as with over-the-counter or prescription medications. A particularly important stage of metabolism in this respect is that of the polycyclic aromatic hydrocarbon-inducible cytochrome P450 (CYP) 1A2.

Several medications, including certain selective serotonin reuptake inhibitors (particularly fluvoxamine), antiarrhytmics (mexiletine), antipsychotic medications (clozapine), psoralens, idrocilamide and phenylpropanolamine, bronchodilators (furafylline and theophylline), and quinolones (enoxacin), have been reported to be potent inhibitors of this isoenzyme. Fluvoxamine, for example, causes large reductions in the clearance of 1A2 substrates such as caffeine (Jeppensen, Loft, Poulsen, & Brosen, 1996; Rasmussen, Nielsen, & Brosen, 1998).

Pharmacokinetic interactions at the CYP1A2 enzyme level may induce toxic effects during concomitant administration of caffeine and these medications. It has therefore been suggested that dietary caffeine intake should be examined when considering or assuming response to drug therapy. One interesting possibility, for example, is that athletes might inadvertently exceed the urinary caffeine concentration limit set by sports authorities at 12 mg/L due to caffeine competing with other substances in the metabolic process (Carillo & Benitez, 2000). Caffeine metabolism is increased by smoking, and it is not uncommon to find higher rates of caffeine consumption in people who smoke tobacco.

Patients with schizophrenia receiving clozapine may complain of severe sedation and may drink large quantities of coffee. High doses of caffeine may lead to decreased metabolism of clozapine and increased clozapine levels, with increased sedation. The interruption of caffeine intake, on the other hand, may lead to decreased clozapine levels (Carillo, Hervaiz, Ramos, & Benitez, 1998; Hagg, Spigset, Mjorndal, & Dahlquist, 2000). It has therefore been recommended that individuals administered these drugs refrain from caffeine-containing foods and beverages or at least maintain their intake at a constant level (Shils et al., 1999).

While on the subject of caffeine metabolism, in neonates it is known that the pharmacokinetics of caffeine differs markedly from that in normal adults. The half-life of caffeine in infants is considerably longer. This may be a contributing factor to some of the reported cases of caffeine toxicity in neonates (Haddad & Winchester, 1983; Jokela & Vartiainen, 1959).

CLINICAL FEATURES OF CAFFEINE INTOXICATION

In contrast to the low level of importance assigned to caffeine dependence, there is a consensus that caffeinism (acute or chronic overuse of caffeine with resultant toxicity) is a syndrome of clinical significance. The mass media have described the

TABLE 13.1
Diagnostic Criteria for Caffeine Intoxication

Recent consumption of caffeine, usually in excess of 250 mg

At least five of the following signs developing during, or shortly after, caffeine use: restlessness, nervousness, excitement, insomnia, flushed face, diuresis, gastrointestinal disturbance, muscle twitching, rambling flow of thought and speech, tachycardia or cardiac arrhythmia, periods of inexhaustibility, and psychomotor agitation

Symptoms in preceding criterion cause clinically significant distress or impairment in social, occupational, or other important areas of functioning

Symptoms not due to any physical or other mental disorder, such as an anxiety disorder

Source: Adapted from American Psychiatric Association (2000). Diagnostic and statistical manual of mental disorders, 4th ed. Text Rev. Washington, D.C.: American Psychiatric Association.

constellation of symptoms characteristic of excessive caffeine use as "coffee nerves" (Greden, 1974), but in the medical profession, the syndrome is known as caffeinism.

Caffeinism can mimic or aggravate a number of physical and psychiatric disorders. The DSM classification has included caffeine intoxication since 1980. The *DSM-IV* diagnostic criteria for caffeine intoxication are provided in Table 13.1. The ICD-10 (World Health Organization, 1992) contains criteria for caffeine intoxication—"acute intoxication due to the use of other stimulants, including caffeine"—and appears to provide a more inclusive set of conditions regarding caffeine use compared to the *DSM-IV*.

In addition to the *DSM-IV* criteria, the literature on caffeinism also describes abdominal pain; aggravation of anxiety, panic disorder, or depression; and possible exacerbation of schizophrenia as possible consequences of excess caffeine intake. As discussed earlier, individuals vary considerably with respect to caffeine sensitivity, and considerable tolerance develops to its effects. However, loss of tolerance to varying degrees also occurs. When this happens, the user, who may not have altered his or her caffeine intake, may not recognize that symptoms are due to caffeine.

Caffeine intoxication is not commonly seen when daily intake is less than 250 mg. This amount of caffeine is found in three to five cups of coffee (depending on the coffee type), three to eight cups of tea, and 10 glasses of cola. The average cup of coffee or tea in the United States is reported to contain between 40 and 150 mg caffeine, although specialty coffees may contain much higher doses (McCusker, Goldberger, & Cone, 2003).

Diagnosis of caffeine intoxication is based on recent consumption of caffeine, usually in excess of 250 mg, excluding other causes and the presence of at least 5 of the 12 caffeine-induced signs and symptoms of caffeinism mentioned in Table 13.1. The amount of caffeine in cocoa, chocolate, and soft drinks can be enough to cause some symptoms of caffeine intoxication in small children when they ingest a candy bar and a 12-oz cola drink.

Initial effects may include insomnia, dyspnea, and excitement, progressing to a mild delirium. Alternating states of consciousness and muscle twitching may occur. Toxic sensory disturbances may include hyperesthesia, ringing in the ears, and visual flashes of light (Greden, 1974). Subsequent signs and symptoms may include diuresis, palpitations, arrhythmias (tachycardia, extrasystoles), hypotension, photo-phobia, and, in rare cases, rhabdomyolysis that can lead to renal failure. The terminal event in severe cases is seizures, although these have also been reported as the initial presentation (Haddad & Winchester, 1983).

Children demonstrate differing symptoms by age. Neonates show irritability, ophistothonos, muscular hypertonicity alternating with hypotonicity, upward ocular deviation, rigidity, and purposeless lip movements. Older children show alternating levels of consciousness, with intermittent agitation, muscle fasciculations, hyperten-sion, tachycardia, irritability with tonic posturing, hyperglycemia and ketonuria, and emesis or hematemesis. In children, the most characteristic finding is hyperirritability (Haddad & Winchester, 1983).

Several cases have been reported of subacute or chronic toxicity; however, the association still remains inconclusive. Cases of caffeine-induced manic depression and coffee-induced exacerbations of schizophrenic processes have been reported, but it is possible that the caffeine intake was coincidental with the beginning of the episode or may even have resulted from it. The psychoses appeared to relate to previous underlying psychiatric disease. In some cases, the reduction or discontin-uation of caffeine in the diet may lead to improvement or to greater efficacy of antipsychotic or antidepressant agents. In acute states, discontinuation of caffeine relieved the psychiatric symptoms. An association with an increase in anxiety and depressive symptoms in the population has also been reported. These symptoms, though, will respond to the simple elimination of caffeine.

Despite the fact that caffeine is widely used, few deaths have been reported (Haddad & Winchester, 1983). However, several deaths have been reported following ingestion of high-strength coffee-like preparation of coffee beans containing up to 5 g of caffeine. The acute oral lethal dose of caffeine in adults is considered to be greater than 10 g, or more than 1750 mg/kg. This dose is much lower in children.

The cause of death in acute toxicity is not clear, but it has been suggested that death may be due to seizures, pulmonary edema, or perhaps arrhythmias. Fatalities have been reported from 15 months to 61 years of age. These fatalities usually follow oral overdose, but also intravenous administration, with overall doses ranging from 3 to 50 g (Haddad & Winchester, 1983). In general, toxic and fatal reactions have been associated with blood concentrations in excess of 15 and 80 mg/L, respectively (Ford et al., 2001).

CAFFEINE AND ANXIETY DISORDERS

The observation of elevated anxiety symptoms among consumers of large amounts of caffeine may be expected because caffeine has pharmacological effects of central nervous stimulation and also increases catecholamine output as discussed previously. Furthermore, Cobb (1974) investigated unemployed auto workers and determined that, upon consumption of coffee with a stressful condition (after losing their jobs), their increase in norepinephrine output was greater than when they consumed it at nonstressful times and greater than that of controls.

Shanahan and Hughes (1986) confronted 46 students with a stressful or non-stressful task following ingestion of coffee that was heavily caffeinated or relatively caffeine free. State anxiety was found to be increased by exposure to the stressful situation. This trend was greater in subjects who had consumed caffeinated coffee. These findings support the anxiogenic role of caffeine.

Lane, Adcock, Williams, and Kuhn (1990) examined the effects of a moderate dose of caffeine on cardiovascular and neuroendocrine stress reactivity in 25 healthy males. Caffeine elevated blood pressure and plasma norepinephrine at rest, which contributed significantly to the effects of stress. Caffeine potentiated stress-related increases in plasma epinephrine and cortisol, more than double the responses observed in the control conditions. These effects were present in habitual and light consumers. The authors concluded that caffeine can potentiate cardiovascular and neuroendocrine stress reactivity and that habitual use of caffeine is not necessarily associated with development of tolerance to these effects.

We have previously proposed that caffeine may be related to combat stress reaction due to the large amount of caffeine ingested in war settings (Iancu, Dolberg, & Zohar, 1996). We had postulated that in addition to increasing anxiety, high caffeine intake would potentiate the anxiety-provoking effects of an exposure to a stressful situation, serving as a catalyst that causes the switch from an acute anxiety reaction to a more severe and debilitating reaction (acute stress disorder or posttraumatic stress disorder).

Individuals with anxiety disorders who avoid caffeinated products may be more sensitive to the psychostimulant effects of caffeine (Boulenger, Uhde, Wolff, & Post, 1984; Lee, Cameron, & Graden, 1985). More specifically, generalized anxiety disorder patients and, to some extent panic disorder patients, display anxiogenic effects of caffeine ingestion (higher anxiety scores, sweating, increased skin conductance and blood pressure; Bruce, Scott, Shine, & Lader, 1992).This increased caffeine sensitivity leads to decreased consumption (Lee et al., 1985). Caffeine is therefore believed to induce anxiety in anxiety disorder patients, as well as in individuals without underlying psychiatric illness (Mathew & Wilson, 1990).

CAFFEINISM AND DEPRESSIVE DISORDERS

Greden, Fontaine, Lubetsky, and Chamberlin (1978) reported that the depression scores among psychiatric patients increased proportionally with their caffeine intake. A study of psychiatric outpatients determined that those with retarded depression often self-medicated with high doses of caffeine, resulting in a state of agitated depression (Neil, Himmelhoch, Mallinger, Mallinger, & Hanin, 1978). Based on these limited studies, it cannot be determined whether patients become depressed and then self-medicate with caffeine or whether excessive caffeine ingestion plays a causal role in the depression (Clementz & Dailey, 1988).

CAFFEINISM AND EATING DISORDERS

Many patients with anorexia nervosa drink large quantities of beverages containing caffeine (e.g., coffee and diet cola), which have few calories and suppress the appetite while increasing energy and heightening vigilance (Sours, 1983). Diet cola contains more than 40 ml of caffeine per 12-oz can and is especially popular with anorectics because it provides a sweet-tasting, low-calorie drink in a potentially unlimited quantity for the self-starving individual. Sours (1983) described two patients with anorexia who used coffee and diet cola in excessive amounts and developed symptoms of caffeinism with reinforcing characteristics. In both cases, the patients unwillingly reduced caffeine intake, following the reinforcing properties the caffeine had for them. Bulimic patients may also use caffeine-containing products in a similar way (Kruger & Braunig, 1995).

CAFFEINISM AND RESTLESS LEGS SYNDROME

Restless legs syndrome, first described by the neurologist Thomas Willis (see Lutz, 1978), is characterized by tension, insomnia, inability to keep still, leg movements while going to sleep, and myoclonus. These symptoms are rather similar to those of excessive caffeine intake and Lutz postulated that the syndrome may result from caffeinism. He reported 62 patients over an 11-year period who were believed to suffer from the restless legs syndrome; the occurrence of the symptoms coincided with the initial consumption of caffeine-containing beverages or foods.

In others, this syndrome appears to have followed an increase in caffeine consumption. Some fluctuations in intensity were observed with varying degrees of caffeine intake. Cessation of caffeine intake (sometimes together with a benzodiazepine to improve sleep, sedation, and muscular symptoms) led to quick ablation of symptoms and general recovery. It is of interest that the first description of this entity (see Lutz, 1978) occurred in the time period when coffee and tea found their way to England, during the 17th century.

CAFFEINE USE IN PSYCHIATRIC INSTITUTIONS

High caffeine consumption has been noted in patients with bipolar I disorder, schizophrenia, and personality disorders; however, as discussed earlier, it is found less in patients with anxiety disorders who tend to refrain from caffeine use due to its anxiogenic properties. Studies of patients in psychiatric units have shown that chronic caffeine use may lead to clinically significant levels of anxiety and tension that could be reduced by decreasing caffeine consumption (Zaslove, Russell, & Ross, 1991). In a study of 83 psychiatric inpatients, Greden et al. (1978) reported that 22% were consumers of high amounts of caffeine (750 mg or more per day), similar to the report by Winstead (1976). These patients scored significantly higher on scores of anxiety and depression scales. They also reported more clinical symptoms; worse health; and greater use of cigarettes, alcohol, sedative–hypnotics, and minor tranquilizers.

Among psychiatric inpatients, the phenothiazine requirement was increased in patients who used caffeine compared with matched controls that did not use the drug (Shisslak et al., 1985). In a double-blind crossover study, decreased psychotic features, less irritability, and reduced anxiety were noted when psychiatric inpatients did not drink caffeinated beverages (DeFreitas & Schwartz, 1979). These findings have not been replicated, however (Mayo, Falkowski, & Jones, 1993). Inpatients may drink large quantities of tea and coffee to relieve thirst/dry mouth caused by tricyclic and antipsychotic medications side effects. Furthermore, inpatient settings, especially in the evening, may lead to increased potential of caffeine consumption. Thus, inpatients may be at a higher risk of caffeine intoxication.

OTHER DISORDERS

An additional *DSM-IV* diagnosis of note is the caffeine-induced sleep disorder, which may also manifest with caffeine intoxication. Caffeine is associated with a delay in falling asleep, an inability to remain asleep, and early morning awakening. Rarely, it may also lead to hypersomnia and parasomnia. Caffeine-induced sleep disorder should be diagnosed in patients with caffeine intoxication only if the sleep disturbance is in excess of that which would be expected from the intoxication (*DSM-IV*, 2000). It is important to remember that caffeine-related disorders are more likely to present with additional substance-related disorders. For example, about two thirds of persons who consume large quantities of caffeine every day also use or abuse sedative and hypnotic medications. Finally, the prevalence of premenstrual syndrome, especially moderate to severe cases, has been shown to increase with increased intake of caffeinated beverages (Rossignol, 1985).

CAFFEINE AND SUICIDE

Aside from the fact that caffeine ingestion is sometimes used for attempting or committing suicide, it has been suggested that coffee drinking is alternatively a possible risk factor for and protective factor against suicide, depending on the amount consumed. Klatsky et al. (1993) found that the use of coffee was related to a lower risk of suicide, progressively lower at a higher coffee intake. The relative risks (RR) for suicide in this study were 0.7 for drinkers of one to three cups/day, 0.6 for drinkers of four to six cups/day, and 0.2 for drinkers of six or more cups/day (although p values were significant only for the drinkers of six or more cups/day and no confidence intervals were reported).

In a 10-year follow-up study in an ongoing cohort study of 86,626 U.S. female registered nurses, Kawachi, Willet, Colditz, Stampfer, and Speizer (1996) reported age-adjusted RR of suicide of 0.34 for drinkers of two to three cups/day and 0.42 for drinkers of four or more cups/day. In terms of caffeine intake (coffee and noncoffee sources), the multivariate RR of suicide in the highest quintile (690 mg/day or more) was 0.33 (95% CI 0.13 to 0.87, p for trend = 0.002) compared with women in the lowest quintile (140 mg/day or less). Although the latter two studies demonstrated a significant inverse association between coffee drinking and the risk for suicide, studies examining heavy levels of coffee drinking (seven cups or more/day) demonstrated RR for suicide of up to 58% higher than for moderate drinkers.

In a survey of 43,166 subjects that were followed up for a mean of 14.6 years, Tanskanen et al. (2000b) demonstrated a J-shaped association between daily coffee intake and the risk of suicide. The age-adjusted risks (with 95% confidence limits) of suicide in this survey were 0.67 to 0.82 for moderate drinkers (two to seven cups/day), 1.32 for drinkers of eight or nine cups/day, and 1.69 for drinkers of ten or more cups/day. The protective effect has been attributed to caffeine's being a CNS stimulant. This speculation is supported by the experimental administration of small doses of caffeine (100 mg/day) that increases subjective feelings of well-being, self-confidence, and energy compared with placebo.

The higher relative risk for suicide in "heavy" coffee drinkers can be explained by the stress–diathesis model of the neurobiology of suicide suggested by Mann (1998). According to this model, reduced serotonergic and increased noradrenergic activity in the brain contributes to increased risk of suicide. It has been shown previously that caffeine can activate the noradrenaline neurons. These neurotransmitter mechanisms could influence the relationship between heavy coffee drinking and the risk of suicide, making it biologically plausible. However, solid evidence concerning the mechanism by which excessive coffee drinking influences the risk of suicide remains to be revealed.

LABORATORY ANALYSIS OF CAFFEINE

Caffeine levels are usually evaluated by gas–liquid chromatography or high-pressure liquid chromatography. Some reports indicate that analysis by the latter method is preferable because the lower quantities that would be sought in human toxicity are better measured by high-pressure liquid chromatography (Haddad & Winchester, 1983). Some correlations of caffeine blood levels and clinical effect appear to exist. Seizures occur with caffeine levels ranging from 79 to 199 µg/ml. Arrhythmias other than sinus tachycardia may be seen with levels greater than 180 µg/ml. Deaths have occurred with caffeine levels from 106 to 180 µg/ml (Ellenhorn, 1997), although patients with levels ranging from 190 to 200 µg/ml have been known to survive (Ellenhorn, 1997). A case of a patient that survived with serum caffeine of 405 µg/ml was reported; this is the highest serum caffeine level described with survival (Dunwiddie & Worth, 1982).

DIFFERENTIAL DIAGNOSIS

High intake of caffeine can produce symptoms that are indistinguishable from those of anxiety disorders (Greden, 1974). Caffeine withdrawal syndrome with its associated characteristic headache may also mimic anxiety. Thus, patients with caffeinism will generally be identified only by routine inquiry into their caffeine intake. However, this inquiry is rarely done in clinical settings. Although clinicians do ask about alcohol and drug usage, they rarely inquire about the habit of coffee drinking because caffeine is so commonly used.

According to the *DSM-IV* classification, the diagnosis of an anxiety disorder (i.e., panic disorder or generalized anxiety disorder) should be set only after excluding organic causes, such as medical disorders and medication and substance use. The psychiatrist should suspect caffeinism in cases in which people drink large quantities of coffee, do not respond to psychopharmacological agents, or have psychophysiological complaints, as well as hyperkinetic children (Greden, 1974).

It remains rare that caffeine intoxication is brought to clinical attention of medical personnel; other disorders should be considered for patients who present with features suggesting caffeine intoxication. The differential diagnosis should include withdrawal from sedative–hypnotics or alcohol, as well as abuse of substances such as anabolic steroids and other stimulants (i.e., amphetamines and cocaine). A urine sample may be needed to screen for these substances. The differential diagnosis should also include hyperthyroidism and pheochromocytoma, as well as anticholinergic intoxication, cardiomyopathy, myocardial infraction, hypoglycemia, sepsis, and migraine or tension headache.

Caffeine-induced anxiety disorder, which can occur during caffeine intoxication, is a *DSM-IV* diagnosis. The clinical picture may be similar to generalized anxiety disorder and the patient is irritable, wired, anxious, and insomniac. The diagnosis of caffeine-induced anxiety disorder depends upon linking the use of caffeine to the anxiety symptoms of concern. A trial of caffeine abstinence may aid in clarifying the diagnosis (Bruce & Lader, 1989). Patients with caffeine-induced intoxication may also be hard to differentiate from patients with exacerbations of schizophrenia, manic–depressive disorder, other anxiety disorders, and especially organic psychoses. The differential diagnosis also is important in restless children who have been exposed to caffeine (vs. attention deficit disorder) (Haddad & Winchester, 1983).

TREATMENT OF CAFFEINE TOXICITY AND OF EXCESSIVE USE

In 2001, 5,562 caffeine overdoses were reported to poison centers in the United States; half required treatment in a health care facility (Litovitz et al., 2002). Approximately two thirds of these cases occurred in young children and adolescents and more than half were intentional overdoses. The outcome was usually good and only one death was reported.

In adult and pediatric caffeine toxicity, symptomatic and supportive therapy is required. Due to its short half-life (3 to 6 hours), caffeine intoxication typically resolves quickly and without significant complications. The occurrence of seizures is dangerous and requires administration of antiseizure medication such as diazepam or phenobarbital. When resuscitation is needed, the prognosis is guarded and caffeine toxicity may become fatal. Beta blockers may be useful in caffeine-induced arrhythmias (Ellenhorn, 1997). Removal of any caffeine still in the gastrointestinal tract is beneficial. Charcoal hemoperfusion may be useful in patients with a potentially lethal ingestion who are exhibiting life-threatening complications (arrhythmias, severe central nervous system toxicity) (Ellenhorn). Because it is known to antagonize the excitatory effect of caffeine in the nervous system, IV glucose may lead to quick recovery in children with acute caffeine poisoning (Ellenhorn, 1997).

Complete recovery after acute toxicity in the adult usually occurs within 6 hours (Haddad & Winchester, 1983). Once the source of the symptoms is brought to the patient's attention, about half of the individuals will follow advice to use decaffeinated beverages. The other half appear reluctant to do so.

Methods of caffeine reduction include psychoeducation and behavior modification techniques (Bazire, 2000; Clementz & Dailey, 1988). First, recognition of problems of excessive caffeine intake (>750 mg/d) and likely benefits of reduction are needed. Second, identification of all current caffeine sources and the pattern of consumption should be examined. Then, through behavior-modification techniques, the patient and therapist should attempt gradual reduction of caffeine use (i.e., making weaker drinks, taken less often; increasing use of caffeine-free equivalent drinks, particularly at usual drinking times of the day). The use of analgesia (caffeine free, of course) for withdrawal headaches and muscle aches is allowed as symptomatic treatment. Benzodiazepines are rarely needed for relief of with-drawal symptoms and then for a few days only. Finally, setting a target for con-sumption that does not require complete abstinence (e.g., caffeine only on rising) is a possible objective.

CONCLUSIONS

Most regular caffeine users experience only subtle effects in mood and behavior that are often indistinguishable from changes in mood and behavior associated with normal behavior. On the other hand, caffeine may arguably be the most robust form of drug self-administration known to man (Griffiths & Mumford, 1995). A number of clinical reports document a high association of excessive caffeine intake with symptoms of anxiety, depression, mania, delirium, and psychosis (Victor, Lubetsky, & Greden, 1981).

Furthermore, many patients present for clinical evaluation complaining of diffuse somatic symptoms, such as sleep disturbances, headaches, tremulousness, tachycar-dia, and diarrhea. These symptoms may be due to caffeinism, but are often missed (Victor et al., 1981). Without accurate diagnosis, symptoms will tend to be treated in isolation, and additional iatrogenic problems develop because of use of analgesics or anticholinergics, often with frequent subsequent recurrence.

No certain diagnostic clues differentiate caffeinism from anxiety disorders and the two conditions can—and undoubtedly do—exist simultaneously (Greden, 1974). Affected subjects will be identified only by routine collection of historical data and rigorous clinical interview. Inquiry about caffeine intake during initial interviews with all anxiety patients is important; this will include use of coffee, tea, and over-the-counter medications, as well as alternative "medicines," in structured and oper-ationalized mental status forms. Such an approach would assist the identification of affected individuals and generate accurate prevalence data.

Many individuals complaining of anxiety will continue to receive substantial benefit from standard psychopharmacological agents. However, for an undetermined number of others, subtracting one drug—namely, caffeine—may be of benefit (Greden, 1974). In addition, researchers should probably consider caffeine use as a contaminating variable when evaluating psychopharmacological or hypnotic agents (Greden, 1974).

In conclusion, caffeine-induced symptoms are of clinical significance; caffeinism might complicate clinical symptomatology of other psychiatric disorders, produce additional reversible symptoms in patients with primary psychiatric disorders, or form part of a constellation of multiple-substance use (Bradley & Petree, 1990). Caffeinism remains an important clinical entity that is frequently underdiagnosed and may lead to significant morbidity. A greater sensitivity to the phenomenon is recommended for members of the medical profession.

REFERENCES

American Psychiatric Association (2000). *Diagnostic and statistical manual of mental disor-ders*, 4th ed. text rev. Washington, D.C.: American Psychiatric Association.

Bazire, S. (2000). *Psychotropic drug directory. The professionals' pocket handbook & aide memoire*. Wiltshire, England: Mark Allen Publishing.

Benjamin, L. T., Rogers, A. M., & Rosenbaum, A. (1991). Coca Cola, caffeine, and mental deficiency: Harry Hollingworth and the Chattanooga trial of 1911. *Journal of the History of the Behavioral Sciences, 27*, 42–55.

Boulenger, J. P., Uhde, T. W., Wolff, E. A., III, & Post, R. M. (1984). Increased sensitivity to caffeine in patients with panic disorder: Preliminary evidence. *Archives of General Psychiatry, 41*, 1067–1071.

Bradley, J. R., & Petree, A. (1990). Caffeine consumption, expectancies of caffeine-enhanced performance, and caffeinism symptoms among university students. *Journal of Drug Education, 20*, 319–328

Bruce, M. S., & Lader, M. (1989). Caffeine abstention in the management of anxiety disorders. *Psychological Medicine, 19*, 211–214.

Bruce, M., Scott, N., Shine, P., & Lader, M. (1992). Anxiogenic effects of caffeine in patients with anxiety disorders. *Archives of General Psychiatry, 49*, 867–869.

Carillo, J. A., & Benitez, J. (2000). Clinically significant interactions between dietary caffeine and medications. *Clinical Pharmacokinetics, 39*, 127–153.

Carillo, J. A., Herraiz, A. G., Ramos, S. I., & Benitez, J. (1998). Effects of caffeine withdrawal from the diet on the metabolism of clozapine in schizophrenic patients. *Journal of Clinical Psychopharmacology, 18*, 311–316.

Clementz, G. L., & Dailey, J. W. (1988). Psychotropic effects of caffeine. *American Family Physician, 37*, 167–172.

Cobb, S. (1974). Physiological changes in men whose jobs were abolished. *Journal of Psychosomatic Research, 18*, 245–258.

DeFreitas, B., & Schwartz, G. (1979). Effects of caffeine in chronic psychiatric patients. *American Journal of Psychiatry, 136*, 1337–1338.

Dunwiddie, T. V., & Worth, T. (1982). Sedative and anticonvulsant effects of adenosine analogs in mouse and rat. *The Journal of Pharmacology and Experimental Therapeutics, 220*, 70–76.

Ellenhorn, M. J. (1997). *Medical toxicology: Diagnosis and treatment of human poisoning.* Baltimore: Williams & Wilkins.

El Yacoubi, M., Ledent, C., Parmentier, M., Costentin, J., & Vaugeois, J. M. (2003). Caffeine reduces hypnotic effects of alcohol through adenosine A2A receptor blockade. *Neuropharmacology, 45*, 977–985.

Ferre, S., Fuxe, K., Von Euler, G., Johansson, B., & Fredholm, B. B. (1992). Adenosine–dopamine interactions in the brain. *Neuroscience, 51*, 501–512.

Ford, M. D., Delaney, K., Ling, L., Rose, R., & Erickson, T. (2001). *Clinical toxicology.* Philadelphia: W. B. Saunders Company.

Greden, J. F. (1974). Anxiety or caffeinism: A diagnostic dilemma. *American Journal of Psychiatry, 131*, 1089–1092.

Greden, J. F. (1976). The tea controversy in colonial America. *JAMA, 236*, 63–66.

Greden, J. F., Fontaine, P., Lubetsky, M., & Chamberlin, K. (1978). Anxiety and depression associated with caffeinism among psychiatric inpatients. *American Journal of Psychiatry, 135*, 963–966.

Griffiths, R. R. & Mumford, G. K. (1995). Caffeine—A drug of abuse? In F. E. Bloom & D. J. Kupfer (Eds.), *Psychopharmacology: The fourth generation of progress.* New York: Raven Press.

Haddad, L. M., & Winchester, J. F. (1983). *Clinical management of poisoning and drug overdose.* Philadelphia: W. B. Saunders Company.

Hagg, S., Spigset, O., Mjorndal, T., & Dahlquist, R. (2000). Effect of caffeine on clozapine pharmacokinetics in healthy volunteers. *British Journal of Pharmacology, 49*, 59–63.

Iancu, I., Dolberg, O. T., & Zohar, J. (1996). Is caffeine involved in the pathogenesis of combat stress reaction? *Military Medicine, 161*, 230–232.

Jacobson, K. A., van Gallen, P. J. M., & Williams, M. (1992). Adenosine receptors: Pharmacology, structure–activity relationships and therapeutic potential. *Journal of Medicinal Chemistry, 35*, 407–422.

Jeppensen, U., Loft, S., Poulsen, H. E., & Brosen, K. (1996). A fluvoxamine–caffeine interaction study. *Pharmacogenetics, 6*, 213–222.

Jokela, S., & Vartiainen, A. (1959). Caffeine poisoning. *Acta Pharmacologica, 15*, 331–334.

Kawachi, I., Willett, W. C., Colditz, G. A., Stampfer, M. J., & Speizer, F. E. (1996). A prospective study of coffee drinking and suicide in women. *Archives of Internal Medicine, 156*, 521–525.

Kendler, K. S., & Prescott, C. A. (1999). Caffeine intake, tolerance and withdrawal in women: A population-based twin study. *American Journal of Psychiatry, 156*, 223–228.

Klatsky, A. L., Armstrong, M. A., & Friedman, G. D. (1993). Coffee, tea, and mortality. *Annals of Epidemiology, 3*, 375–381.

Kruger, S., & Braunig, P. (1995). Abuse of body weight reducing agents in bulimia nervosa. *Nervenarzt, 66*, 66–69.

Lane, J. D., Adcock, R. A., Williams, R. B., & Kuhn, C. M. (1990). Caffeine effects on cardiovascular and neuroendocrine responses to acute psychosocial stress and their relationship to level of habitual caffeine consumption. *Psychosomatic Medicine, 52*, 320–336.

Lee, M. A., Cameron, O. G., & Greden, J. F. (1985). Anxiety and caffeine consumption in people with anxiety disorders. *Psychiatry Research, 15*, 211–217.

Litovitz, T. L., Klein–Schwartz, W., Rodgers, G. C., Cobaugh, D. J., Youniss, J., Omslaer, J. C., et al. (2002). 2001 Annual report of the American Association of Poison Control Centers toxic exposure surveillance system. *American Journal of Emergency Medicine, 20*, 391–452.

Lutz, E. G. (1978). Restless legs, anxiety and caffeinism. *Journal of Clinical Psychiatry, 39*, 693–698.

Mann, J. J. (1998). The neurobiology of suicide. *Nature Medicine, 4*, 25–30.

Mathew, R. J., & Wilson, W. H. (1990). Behavioral and cerebrovascular effects of caffeine in patients with anxiety disorders. *Acta Psychiatrica Scandinavica, 82*, 17–22.

Mayo, K. M., Falkowski, W., & Jones, C. A. (1993). Caffeine: Use and effects in long-stay psychiatric patients. *British Journal of Psychiatry, 162*, 543–545.

McCusker, R. R., Goldberger, B. A., & Cone, E. J. (2003). Caffeine content of specialty coffees. *Journal of Analytical Toxicology, 27*, 520–522.

Moffatt, A. C., Osselton, M. D. Widdop, B, & Galichet, L. Y. (Eds.). *Clarke's analysis of drugs and poisons in pharmaceuticals, body fluids and postmortem material*, 3rd ed. (Vol. II, pp. 736–738) London: Pharmaceutical Press.

Mueller, W. L. (1967), Coffee. In *Encyclopedia Americana*, international ed. (Vol. VII, pp. 209–211). New York: Americana Corporation.

Neil, J. F., Himmelhoch, J. M., Mallinger, A. G., Mallinger, J., & Hanin, I. (1978). Caffeinism complicating hypersomnic depressive episodes. *Comprehensive Psychiatry, 19*, 377–385.

O'Connell, S. E., & Zurzola, F.J. (1984). Rapid quantitative liquid chromatographic determination of caffeine levels in plasma after oral dosing. *Journal of Pharmaceutical Sciences, 73*, 1009–1011.

Porkka–Heiskanen, T., Strecker, R. E., Thakkar, M., Bjorkum, A. A., Greene, R. W., & McCarley, R. W. (1997). Adenosine: A mediator of the sleep-inducing effects of prolonged wakefulness. *Science, 276*, 1265–1268.

Radulovacki, M., Virus, R. M., Djuricic–Nedelson, M., & Green, R. D. (1984). Adenosine analogs and sleep in rats. *The Journal of Pharmacology and Experimental Therapeutics, 228*, 268–274.

Rasmussen, B. B., Nielsen, T. L., & Brosen, K. (1998). Fluvoxamine is a potent inhibitor of the metabolism of caffeine *in vitro. Pharmacology and Toxicology, 83,* 240–598.

Ross, G. W., Abbott, R. D., Petrovitch, H., Morens, D. M., Grandinetti, A., Tung, K. H., et al. (2000). Association of coffee and caffeine intake with the risk of Parkinson's disease. *JAMA, 283,* 2674–2679.

Rossignol, A. M. (1985). Caffeine-containing beverages and premenstrual syndrome in young women. *American Journal of Public Health, 75,* 1335–1337.

Satoh, S., Matsumura, H., Suzuki, F., & Hayaishi, O. (1996). Promotion of sleep mediated by the A2a-adenosine receptor and possible involvement of this receptor in the sleep induced by prostaglandin D2 in rats. *Proceedings of the National Academy of Sciences of the United States of America, 93,* 5980–5984.

Shanahan, M. P., & Hughes, R. N. (1986). Potentiation of performance-induced anxiety by caffeine in coffee. *Psychological Reports, 59,* 83–86.

Shils, M. E., Olson, J. A., Shike, M., & Ross, A. C., (Eds.) (1999). *Modern nutrition in health and disease,* 9th ed. Baltimore: Lipincott Williams & Wilkins

Shisslak, C. M., Buetler, L. E., Schreiber, S., Gaines, J. A., LaWall, J., & Crago, M. (1985). Patterns of caffeine use and prescribed medications in psychiatric inpatients. *Psychological Reports, 57,* 39–42.

Siegerist, H. E. (1943). Literary controversy over tea in 18th century in England. *Bulletin of the History of Medicine, 13,* 185.

Sours, J. A. (1983). Case reports of anorexia nervosa and caffeinism. *American Journal of Psychiatry, 140,* 235–236.

Strain, E. C., & Griffiths, R. R. (2000). Caffeine-related disorders. In B. J. Sadock & V. A. Sadock (Eds.), *Comprehensive textbook of psychiatry,* 7th ed. Philadelphia: Lippincott Williams & Wilkins.

Tanskanen, A., Tuomilehto, J., Viinamaki, H., Vartianien, E., Lehtonen, J., & Puska, P. (2000a). Joint heavy use of alcohol, cigarettes and coffee and the risk of suicide. *Addiction, 95,* 1699–1704.

Tanskanen, A., Tuomilehto, J., Viinamaki, H., Vartiainen, E., Lehtonen, J., & Puska, P. (2000b). Heavy coffee drinking and the risk of suicide. *European Journal of Epidemiology, 16,* 789–791.

Victor, B. S., Lubetsky, M., & Greden, J. F. (1981). Somatic manifestations of caffeinism. *Journal of Clinical Psychiatry, 42,* 185–188.

Williams, S. M. (1995). Purinoreceptors in central nervous system function. Targets for therapeutic intervention. In F. E. Bloom & D. J. Kupfer (Eds). *Psychopharmacology: The fourth generation of progress.* New York: Raven Press.

Winstead, D. K. (1976). Coffee consumption among psychiatric patients. *American Journal of Psychiatry, 133,* 1447–1450.

World Health Organization. (1992). *The ICD-10 classification of mental and behavioral disorders. Clinical description and diagnostic guidelines.* Geneva: World Health Organization.

Zaslove, M. O., Russell, R. L., & Ross, E. (1991). Effect of caffeine intake on psychotic inpatients. *British Journal of Psychiatry, 159,* 565–567.

Section V

Green and Black Teas

14 Catechins and Caffeine in Tea: A Review of Health Risks and Benefits

Raymond Cooper, Talash A. Likimani, D. James Morré, and Dorothy M. Morré

CONTENTS

INTRODUCTION

Teas from leaves of *Camellia sinensis*, a small plant growing mainly in China and southeast Asia, are generally consumed in forms referred to as black, oolong, or green teas. Although tea is consumed globally, it is cultivated in only about 30 countries worldwide. Successful tea cultivation requires moist humid climates provided most ideally by the slopes of northern India, Sri Lanka, Tibet, and southern China (Stella, 1992). The level of tea consumption varies around the world, but it is believed to be second only to that of water (Ahmad, Katiyar, & Mukhtar, 1998). Green tea is consumed predominantly in China, Japan, India, and a number of countries in North

Africa and the Middle East; black tea is consumed predominantly in Western and some Asian countries (Ahmad et al., 1998).

Health benefits have long been attributed to teas from *Camellia sinensis*; they were originally used as medicines for various illnesses (Chen & Yu, 1994). Their origins trace back 5,000 years to southwest China. Chinese medicine has traditionally stressed prevention. There is documentation that drinking tea was recommended to healthy people between 1100 and 200 B.C. (Yao & Chen, 1995). During the T'ang dynasty (618–907 A.D.), tea became the basis for a flourishing trade inside China. Subsequently, as the tea trade expanded, drinking tea has emerged worldwide as a pleasant and healthful practice.

Green tea is sold as fresh or dried leaves. In fresh leaves, total polyphenols comprise 20 to 35% by weight and catechins are 60 to 80% of total polyphenols (Lin, Tsai, Tsay, & Lin, 2003; Wang, Kim, & Lee, 2000). Green tea processing reduces total polyphenols by approximately 15%. Key ingredients, including the catechins and caffeine, are extracted by steeping the leaves in water (Blumenthal, Brickmann, Dinda, Goldberg, & Wollschlaeger, 2001) and are taken orally.

CATECHINS

Many of the natural substances in green tea that contribute to the majority of its health benefits have been identified (McKenna, Jones, & Hughes, 2002; Yang, Maliaka, & Meng, 2002). The major polyphenol belonging to the family of catechins found in green tea is (–)-epigallocatechin gallate (EGCg). Other catechins also present are catechin (C), epicatechin (EC), gallocatechin (GC), gallocatechin gallate (GCG), epigallocatechin (EGC), and epicatechin gallate (ECG) (Figure 14.1). Noncatechin polyphenols include caffeine, theanine, theaflavins, theobromine, theophylline, and phenolic acids such as gallic acid (Ahmad et al., 1998; Manning & Roberts, 2003). Sensitive and definitive analytical methods, mostly using HPLC and LC-MS techniques (Manning & Roberts, 2003), are now widely available for detection of these green tea constituents.

Quality control is improving and standardization (of the ratio and variation) of the catechins in commercially available green tea extracts is leading to availability of consistently prepared material. Because these preparations will in turn be used in clinical studies, confidence in the results of any future clinical evaluations will increase. Extracts of *Camellia sinensis* are frequently standardized to the specification of 98% catechins and <1% caffeine.

The major phenolic constituent, EGCg, has been implicated from many studies as responsible for the antioxidant and anticarcinogenic effects of green tea (Ahmad & Mukhtar, 1999; Yang et al., 2002). In addition to a high potential degree of efficacy from oral administration, the EGCg contained in tea is generally recognized as safe over a wide therapeutic range (equivalent to 5 to 20 cups of green tea). Green tea is consumed internationally as a food and is listed as GRAS (generally recognized as safe) (Duke, 1992).

THEAFLAVINS

The preparation of black tea requires that the fresh leaves be allowed to wither; then, they are crushed. A natural oxidative process, often erroneously referred to as fermentation, then takes place, resulting in the formation of higher molecular weight

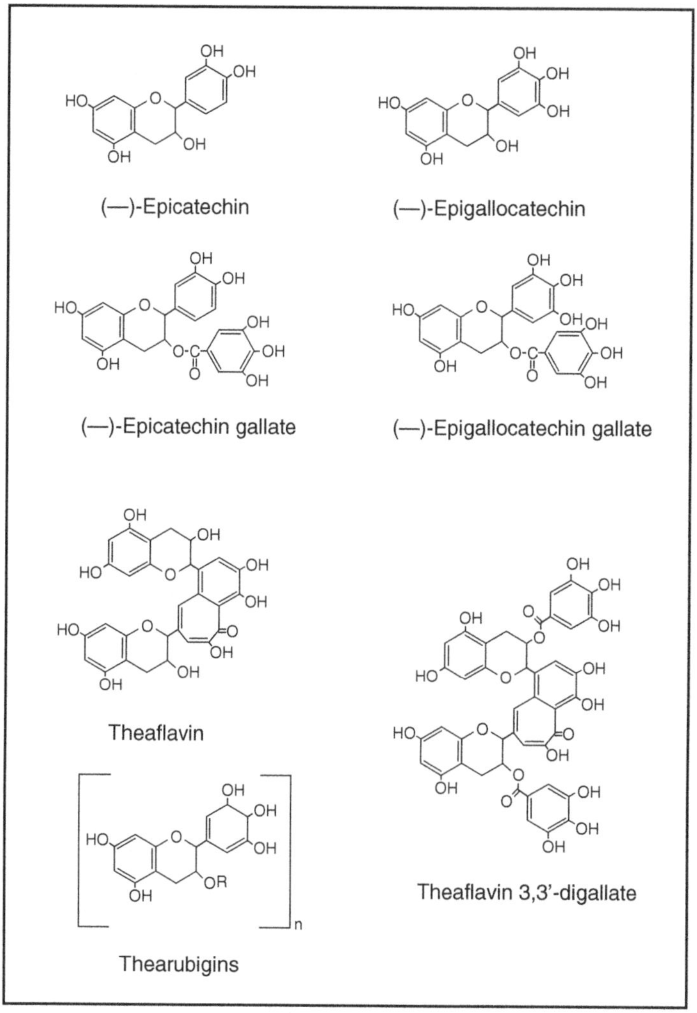

FIGURE 14.1 Molecular structures of tea constituents.

condensed polyphenolic constituents. As a result, black tea has a stronger, more tannic flavor. A less extensive and "incomplete" oxidative step leads to the preparation of a lighter flavored tea, popular in certain parts of Asia, known as oolong. During the process of oxidation, the catechins in the green tea are converted partially into the theaflavins. Black tea contains about 2% theaflavin and 6 to 30% thearubigins. Green tea does not generally contain these compounds (Table 14.1).

The oxidation process used to prepare black tea converts many of the lower molecular weight catechin (flavonoids) constituents in green tea leaves to more complex phenolics (Wang et al., 2000). Of the catechins originally present in green tea, 15% remain and the rest convert into theaflavins and thearubigins. The components of prepared black tea infusion (weight percent) include 3 to 6% theaflavin and

TABLE 14.1
Polyphenolic Constituents of Black and Green Teas

Compound	Green tea (mg/cup)	Black tea (mg/cup)
Catechin	60–125	30–60
Theaflavins	<0.25	3–6
Caffeine	20–50	30–60
L-theanine	20–40	20–40

12 to 18% thearubigin. The theaflavins and thearubigins are sources of bioactive flavonoids (Leung et al., 2001) and have health benefits similar to those of the catechins and less extensively polymerized flavonoids.

HEALTH BENEFITS OF TEA

Many publications, including clinical and epidemiological studies, have suggested the health benefits of green tea (Yang et al., 2002). Green tea is taken orally and contains catechins that are believed to prolong the life of norepinephrine in the synaptic cleft. The catechins activate thermogenesis and promote fat oxidation through inhibition of the enzyme that degrades norepinephrine, catechol-*o*-methyltransferase (Durand, Giacobino, & Giratdier, 1978).

The polyphenols found in green tea are among the dietary factors that may play a role in cancer protection and have recently been shown to have potent antioxidant and antitumor effects (Chow et al., 2001). One study determined the phenolic content of various teas and correlated those values to radical scavenging activity using a modified oxygen radical absorbance capacity (ORAC) assay at pH 5.5. Total flavonol content varied from 21.2 to 103.2 mg/g for regular tea and from 4.6 to 39.0 mg/g for decaffeinated teas. The ORAC value varied from 728 to 1686 Trolox equivalents/g tea for regular tea and from 507 to 845 Trolox equivalents/g for decaffeinated teas. There was a significant correlation of flavonol content to ORAC value ($r = 0.79$, $p = 0.0001$) for green tea extract. This large variation in flavonol content and ORAC value among various brands and types of tea might provide useful information in studies of nutrition and cancer prevention (Henning et al., 2003). It appears that caffeine contributes little to the ORAC values.

Green tea polyphenols have been reported to protect in varying degrees against certain cancers, including colon, rectal, bladder (Kemberling, Hampton, Keck, Gomez, & Salman, 2003), breast (Wu, Yu, Tseng, Hankin, & Pike, 2003), stomach, pancreatic, lung, esophageal, and prostate (Adhami, Ahmed, & Mukhtar, 2003; Bushman, 1998; Gao et al., 2002; Jian, Xie, Lee, & Binns, 2004). Mechanisms supporting anticarcinogenic and antitumor activity and several postulated mechanisms of action have been extensively reviewed (Cooper, Morré, & Morré, 2005a, b). Although there is a clear implication of a mechanism of action for EGCg and other catechins, the role of caffeine has not been linked to anticancer benefits. However, some health benefits are attributed to the combination of green tea and caffeine and these are reviewed here.

CAFFEINE

Classified as a stimulant of the central nervous system, caffeine is listed as GRAS when consumed in amounts found typically in foods (FDA, 2004). As reviewed by Eskenazi (1999), pregnant women have been advised by the FDA to "avoid caffeine-containing foods and drugs or consume them only sparingly." In a nested case-control study that used serum paraxanthine as a biologic marker for caffeine, Klebanoff, Levine, DerSimonian, Clemens, and Wilkins (1999) noted that moderate consumption of caffeine was unlikely to increase the risk of spontaneous abortion, although there may be risks associated with relatively high caffeine intake. The meta-analysis by Fernandes et al. (1998) revealed a small but statistically significant increase in the risks for spontaneous abortion and low birth weight babies in pregnant women consuming more than 150 mg caffeine per day. Bracken, Triche, Belanger, Hellenbrand, and Leaderer (2003) also observed a similar small reduction in birth weight with coffee consumption, that may become clinically important in women consuming 600 mg or more of caffeine daily.

More usual side effects of caffeine are insomnia, nervousness, restlessness, agitation, gastric irritation, nausea, vomiting, diuresis, fast heartbeat, arrhythmias, increased respiratory rate, muscle spasms, ringing in the ears, headache, delirium, and convulsions (McKevoy, 1998; Schulz, Hansel, & Taylor, 1998). If it is abruptly discontinued, physical withdrawal symptoms can sometimes result (McKevoy, 1998). Sleep disturbances in patients with acquired immunodeficiency syndrome (AIDS) may be exacerbated by caffeine (Dreher, 2003).

Conversely, with normal calcium intake, moderate caffeine intake (less than 300 mg per day) does not seem to increase osteoporosis risk significantly in most postmeno-pausal women (Lloyd et al., 2000; Massey, 2001; Massey & Whiting, 1993; Rapuri, Gallagher, Kinyama, & Ryschon, 2001). In people with high blood pressure, caffeine may result in further increase in blood pressure. Because of high excessive intake of caffeine, there is a possibility that products such as green tea, unless first decaf-feinated, or Yerba mate are unsafe when consumed in large amounts or for prolonged periods of time.

CAFFEINES AND TEAS

Low to moderate doses of caffeine are widely considered to enhance mental alertness and physical performance positively in some individuals (Heishman & Henningfield, 1994). Doses most often associated with increased alertness, energy, and concentration are generally in the 100- to 600-mg range (which varies according to gender). In a double-blind parallel group study designed to observe the response of 250 mg caffeine in two different age groups, Rees, Allen, and Lader (1999) concluded that caffeine induced a small but significant improvement in vigilance and psychomotor performance irrespective of age. In another double-blind randomized study, Kamimori et al. (2000) administered caffeine at three doses (2.2 [low], 4.3 [medium], and 8.6 [high] mg/kg body weight). Again, all these results indicate that high doses of caffeine have a significant and beneficial effect on alertness during prolonged wakefulness.

When tea alkaloids such as caffeine are present they inhibit phosphodiesterases. These enzymes prolong the life of cAMP in the cell, resulting in an increased and more sustained effect of norepinephrine on thermogenesis (Dreher, 2003). Tea catechins prolong the life of norepinephrine in the synaptic cleft.

TEA AND WEIGHT LOSS

A role for catechins in promoting weight loss is supported by animal studies (Kao, Hiipakka, & Liao, 2000; Sayama, Lin, Zheng, & Oguni, 2000). In one such study, the antiobesity effect of green tea was evaluated by feeding different levels of green tea (1 to 4% in the diet) to female mice for 4 months. The mice fed green tea showed significant suppression of food intake, body weight gain, and accumulation of fat tissue. Levels of cholesterol and triglycerides were lower. A direct beneficial effect leading to weight loss was indicated from decreased serum levels of leptin.

The mild increase in thermogenesis (increased caloric expenditure) associated with green tea intake is generally attributed to its caffeine content (Dulloo et al., 1999; Dulloo, Seydoux, Garardier, Chantre, & Vandermander, 2000). However, because green tea extract may stimulate thermogenesis to an extent much greater than can be attributed to its caffeine content, the thermogenic properties of green tea may be due to an interaction between caffeine and its high content of catechin–polyphenols. As already noted, a probable mechanism to explain the thermogenic effect of green tea is through an increase in levels of norepinephrine. Catechin–polyphenols are known to inhibit catechol-o-methyl-transferase, the enzyme that degrades norepinephrine.

A randomized, placebo-controlled study of 10 individuals was conducted to investigate whether a green tea extract could increase 24-h energy expenditure and fat oxidation in humans (Dulloo et al., 1999). Compared to the placebo, the green tea extract resulted in a significant increase in 24-h energy expenditure (4%; $P < 0.01$) and a significant decrease in 24-h respiratory quotient without a change in urinary nitrogen. During treatment with the green tea extract, 24-h urinary excretion of norepinephrine was higher than it was with the placebo. Treatment with caffeine in amounts equivalent to those found in the green tea extract (50 mg) had no effect on energy expenditure or fat oxidation, again suggesting that the thermogenic properties of green tea are due to compounds other than caffeine content alone.

One synergistic interaction between caffeine and catechin polyphenols appears to prolong sympathetic stimulation of thermogenesis (Dulloo et al., 1999, 2000)— a response not elicited by caffeine alone in amounts equivalent to those found in the green tea extract. It has been postulated that green tea extract may stimulate brown adipose tissue thermogenesis to an extent much greater than can be attributed to caffeine content; and when the thermogenic properties reside primarily in an interaction between the high content in catechin–polyphenols plus caffeine to sympathetically increase noradrenaline release (Dulloo et al., 2000).

In a double-blind human study (Jubel et al., 2000), a group of 10 males underwent a series of three separate 24-h tests of their energy expenditures and metabolism. Group 1 received 1500 mg green tea extract containing 8.4% caffeine (Arko Pharma) calculated as 150 mg caffeine, 270 mg EGCg taken in three equal doses with meals; group 2 received 150 mg caffeine; group 3 received placebo. No side effects or differences in heart rate were reported. Average energy expenditure was higher with the tea group over caffeine alone and the placebo group. The effect was reported as a 35 to 40% increase in thermogenesis in a normal human male (Cronin, 2000).

GREEN TEA BENEFITS IN BLOOD SUGAR CONTROL AND WEIGHT LOSS

A green tea preparation (Tegreen 97®, Pharmanex) helps to provide blood sugar control, body fat-burning properties, and weight-loss benefits in an experimental setting of Metabolic Syndrome × Subjects—a precursor to type-2 diabetes (Yu, Zhu, & Yin, 2003)—and builds on a greater body of knowledge related to two significant health issues today: weight gain and lack of blood sugar control. The study examined the effects of Tegreen 97 in enhancing insulin sensitivity and improving glucose–lipid metabolism.

In addition, the research examined the effects of the proprietary green tea supplement in lowering body weight and weight of abdominal fat and inhibiting angiogenesis, which is the formation and differentiation of blood vessels, a key pathological process in the development of abnormal cells. Angiogenesis is hypothesized to play an important role in development of obesity. The results of the study showed enhanced insulin sensitivity, improved glucose–lipid metabolism, increased fat burning and decreased body fat percentage, and lowered body weight associated with inhibited angiogenesis.

GREEN TEA AND EXERCISE ENDURANCE

Balb/c mice given green tea extract at a dose of 0.5% of their weight regularly over 10 weeks increased their endurance in exercise (swimming in an adjustable-current water pool) by up to 24% (Murase, Haramizu, Shimotoyodome, Nagasawa, & Tokimitsu, 2004). The green tea extract appeared to stimulate the use of fatty acids by the muscle, reducing carbohydrate use and allowing for longer exercise times. Green tea's effect on fatty acid uptake—speeding up fat breakdown—may help in weight loss.

Effects of EGCg alone, when fed to mice, appear weak by comparison, so there appear to be contributions from other components of the green tea. No marked effects in improvement in endurance capacity were seen after a single dose, suggesting that the response required habitual green tea extract intake—for example, upregulation of muscular beta-oxidation. Muscular beta-oxidation was demonstrated to be higher in green tea extract-fed mice than controls, suggesting that the green tea enhanced the capacity of muscle to catabolize lipids and use fatty acids as an energy source.

COMBINED EFFECTS OF CAFFEINE AND
POLYPHENOLS ON THERMOGENESIS AND OBESITY

Obesity can be treated only by reducing energy intake or by increasing energy expenditure. Thermogenesis and fat oxidation are to a large extent under control of the sympathetic nervous system (SNS). Therefore, any approach that interferes with the SNS and its neurotransmitter norepinephrine may be used in obesity management. In this context, there has been a lot of interest in potential thermogenic effects of many compounds extracted from plants, such as caffeine from coffee, which has been shown to potentiate thermogenesis induced by sympathetic stimuli (Dulloo, 1993; 1998).

Dulloo et al. (1999) investigated the effects of caffeine and polyphenols on energy expenditure and fat oxidation. Ten healthy men were subjected to a respiratory chamber for 24 h and randomly assigned among three treatments comprising green tea extract (50 mg caffeine and 90 mg epigallocatechin gallate), caffeine (50 mg), and placebo, three times a day. The outcomes measured were 24-h energy expenditure, respiratory quotient, and urinary excretion of nitrogen and catecholamines. Treatment with the green tea extract resulted in a significant increase in 24-h energy expenditure and a significant decrease in 24-h respiratory quotient without any change in urinary nitrogen. However, treatment with 50 mg caffeine alone—the amount equivalent to that found in the green tea extract— had no effect on energy expenditure or respiratory quotient. The implication is that green tea has thermogenic properties and promotes fat oxidation as a result of a combined effect of caffeine and polyphenols beyond that explained by caffeine alone.

The research of Dulloo and colleagues (Dulloo, Fathi, Mensi, & Girardier, 1996; Dulloo et al., 1999, 2000) establishes that green tea catechins in combination with caffeine may modestly increase metabolism. Caffeine increases sympathetic tone by binding to adenosine receptors inhibiting phospodiesterase and increasing catechol levels. In the past 10 years, green tea has a history of investigation for thermogenesis in promoting weight loss through stimulating thermogenesis (Dulloo et al., 1996, 1999, 2000).

In vitro research in rats (Durand et al., 1978) looked at adipose tissue comparing enhancement of thermogenesis by tea, ephedra, and caffeine (Dulloo et al., 1996, 1999). The tea used in the study contained 8% caffeine. Dulloo et al. (1999) studied the effects of green tea on 10 healthy young men (age 25) who ranged in body type from lean to mildly overweight. They were given a Western diet of 13% protein, 40% fat, and 47% carbohydrates. The study was conducted over 6 weeks and they were given two capsules of green tea + 50 mg caffeine, 50 mg caffeine alone, or a placebo with each meal. The researchers measured energy expenditure in a respiratory chamber and respiration quotient. A lower respiratory quotient means more fats are metabolized by the body for energy. The results showed that those taking the green tea experienced a significant increase in 24-h energy expenditure and a significant decrease in 24-h respiratory quotient over those taking caffeine alone or placebo.

CAFFEINE AND THIAMINE

Using a mixture of thiamine, arginine, caffeine, and citric acid (TACC), Muroyama and colleagues (Muroyama, Murosaki, Yamamoto, Odaka, et al., 2003; Muroyama, Murosaki, Yamamoto, Ishijima, & Toh, 2003) investigated the antiobesity effects in non-insulin-dependent diabetic KK mice and on lipid metabolism in healthy subjects. Results from the animal studies suggested that TACC is effective in reducing adipose tissue mass as well as improving disorders in lipid metabolism. Furthermore, results from the clinical studies suggest that TACC may be effective in reducing body fat in obese subjects.

OTHER THERMOGENIC AGENTS

Yerba maté (*Ilex paraquariensis*) is often taken orally as a tea and is used as a stimulant to relieve mental and physical fatigue (Blumenthal, Goldberg, & Brinckmann, 2000). The thermogenic effect arises from a combined effect of caffeine, green tea, cacao, and Yerba maté, which also contains theobromine. A study that evaluated the thermogenic effects of commercially available plant preparations found Yerba maté to be the best preparation for increasing the proportion of oxidized fat, resulting in a favorable decrease in body fat (Martinet, Hostettmann, & Schultz, 2000).

Cocoa contains methylxanthines, flavonoids, tyramine, phenylethylamine (PEA), magnesium, and possibly N-acylethanolamines. Cocoa has CNS stimulant, cardiac stimulant, coronary dilatory, and diuretic actions (Wolters Kluwer Co., 1999). Theobromine is the major methylxanthine found in cocoa and has only 10% of the cardiac activity of caffeine. In one study, consumption of 1.5 g/kg body weight of chocolate had no acute hemodynamic or physiologic effects on the hearts of healthy, young adults. Effects of cacao are similar to green tea for thermogenesis due to the presence of the methylxanthines.

CAFFEINE, CATECHINS, AND CANCER

According to Conney (2003), many observers have observed a broad spectrum of cancer chemopreventive activity in tea and some of its constituents in several organ systems in experimental animals. Caffeine, (–)-epigallocatechin gallate, and tea were found to have inhibitory effects in animal models of carcinogenesis. These substances appear to work, at least in part, by enhancing apoptosis in DNA-damaged cells or in tumors. Research to date provides a rationale for clinical trials on the potential chemopreventive effects of caffeine, EGCg, and tea on the formation of cancer of the skin, mouth, esophagus, stomach, and colon in people with precancerous lesions and a high risk of developing these cancers.

In a key study, Yoshizawa et al. (1987) showed an inhibitory effect of topical applications of EGCg on tumor promotion by teleocidin on mouse skin initiated previously with DMBA. Fujita et al. (1989) showed an inhibitory effect of oral administration of EGCg on N-ethyl-N'-nitro-N-nitrosoguanidine-induced duodenal carcinogenesis. Oral administration to rodents of green tea, black tea, EGCg, or a green tea polyphenol fraction has been reported to inhibit chemically induced carcinogenesis in many organs, including esophagus, stomach, duodenum, colon, lung, liver, and pancreas (Higdon & Frei, 2003; Katiyar & Mukhtar, 1996; Yang & Wang, 1993, Yang et al., 2002).

Although many studies showed inhibitory effects of caffeine administration on carcinogenesis in animal models, some showed a stimulatory effect of caffeine administration on carcinogenesis. Accordingly, the effects of caffeine on carcinogenesis are complex, and whether caffeine inhibits or stimulates carcinogenesis depends on the experimental model used. More detailed mechanistic studies are needed to determine why caffeine inhibits carcinogenesis in some animal models and stimulates it in others (Conney, 2003).

CONCLUSIONS

Catechins are polyphenols comprising epigallocatechin gallate (EGCg), epigallocatechin (EGC), epicatechin gallate (ECG), and epicatechin (EC). Oxidation results in the formation of higher molecular weight condensed polyphenolic constituents known as theaflavins. Catechins and theaflavins seem to be responsible for many of the proposed benefits of tea. EGCg is the major phenolic constituent and has been implicated from many studies as responsible for the antioxidant and anticarcinogenic health benefits of green tea. Noncatechin polyphenols include caffeine, theanine, theaflavins, theobromine, theophylline, and phenolic acids such as gallic acid (Ahmad et al., 1998; Manning & Roberts, 2003).

Caffeine is a methylxanthine compound and a known stimulant of the central nervous system. Low to moderate doses of caffeine are widely considered to enhance mental alertness and physical performance positively in some individuals. Doses most often associated with increased alertness, energy, and concentration are generally in the 100- to 600-mg range (Heishman & Henningfield, 1994).

The research of Dulloo et al. (1996, 1999, 2000) establishes that green tea catechins in combination with caffeine may modestly increase metabolism. Several studies have shown the role of catechins in promoting weight loss in animal studies (Kao et al., 2000; Sayama et al., 2000). In one study, different levels of green tea were administered to female mice. Mice fed green tea resulted in significant suppression of food intake, body weight gain, and accumulation of fat tissue. In human trials, treatment with 50 mg caffeine alone (the amount equivalent to that found in the green tea extract) had no effect on energy expenditure or respiratory quotient. In contrast, treatment with green tea extract resulted in significant increase in energy expenditure and significant decrease in respiratory quotient over caffeine alone or placebo.

Because the green tea extract may stimulate thermogenesis to an extent greater than can be attributed to its caffeine content, the thermogenic properties of green tea may be due to an interaction between caffeine and its high content of catechin–polyphenols. The probable mechanism explaining the thermogenic effect of green tea is through an increase in levels of norephinephrine. Catechin–polyphenols are known to inhibit catechol-*o*-methyltrasferase, the enzyme that degrades norephinephirine.

The tea alkaloids inhibit phosphodiesterases, which prolong the life of cAMP in the cell, resulting in an increased and more sustained effect of norepinephrine on thermogenesis (Dulloo et al., 1999).

Other thermogenic agents include Yerba maté (*Ilex paraquariensis*), cocoa, and proprietary products such as Total Control® (Herbalife Internation). These products also contain a combination of caffeine, green tea, cacao, and polyphenols (Martinet, et al., 2000; Wolters Kluwer Co., 1999; Yu et al., 2003).

Tea and some of its constituents are known to have a broad spectrum of cancer chemopreventive activity in skin, mouth, esophagus, stomach, and colon cancers. These substances appear to work, at least in part, by enhancing apoptosis in DNA-damaged cells or in tumors. However, caffeine administration on carcinogenesis in animal models showed inhibitory and stimulatory effects, leading to the conclusion that the effects of caffeine on carcinogenesis are complex. More detailed mechanistic studies are needed to determine why caffeine inhibits carcinogenesis in some animal models and stimulates it in others (Conney, 2003).

REFERENCES

Adhami, V. M., Ahmad, N., & Mukhtar, H. (2003). Molecular targets for green tea in prostate cancer prevention. *Journal of Nutrition, 133,* 2417S–2424S.

Ahmad, N., Katiyar, S. K., & Mukhtar, H. (1998). Cancer chemoprevention by tea polyphenols. In C. Ioannide (Ed.), *Nutrition and chemical toxicity* (pp. 301–343). Sussex, England: John Wiley & Sons.

Ahmad, N., & Mukhtar, H. (1999). Green tea polyphenols and cancer biologic mechanisms and practical implications. *Nutrition Reviews, 57,* 78–83.

Blumenthal, M., Brinckmann, J., Dinda, K., Goldberg, A., & Wollschlaeger, B. (2001). *The ABC clinical guide to herbs* (pp. 335–349). Austin, TX: American Botanical Council.

Blumenthal, M., Goldberg, A., & Brinckmann, J. (2000). Maté. *Herbal Medicine: Expanded Commission E Monographs* (pp. 249–252). Boston, MA: Intergrative Medicine Communications.

Bracken, M. B., Triche, E. W., Belanger, K., Hellenbrand, K., & Leaderer, B. P. (2003). Association of maternal caffeine consumption with decrements in fetal growth. *American Journal of Epidemiology, 157,* 456–466.

Bushman, J. L. (1998). Green tea and cancer in humans: A review of the literature. *Nutrition & Cancer, 31,* 151–159.

Chen, Z. M., & Yu, Y. M. (1994). Tea. In C. J. Arntzen and E. M. Ritter (Eds.), *Encyclopedia of agriculture* (pp. 281–288). San Diego, CA: Science Academic Press.

Chow, H. H., Cai, Y., Alberts, D. S., Hakim, I., Dorr, R., Shahi, F., et al. (2001). Phase I pharmacokinetic study of tea polyphenols following single-dose administration of epigallocatechin gallate and polyphenon E. *Cancer Epidemiological Biomarkers Previews, 10,* 53–58.

Conney, A. H. (2003). Enzyme induction and dietary chemicals as approaches to cancer chemoprevention: The seventh DeWitt S. Goodman Lecture. *Cancer Research, 63,* 7005–7031.

Cooper, R., Morre, D. J., & Morré, D. M. (2005a). Medicinal benefits of green tea. Part I. Review of non-cancer health benefits. *Journal of Alternative & Complementary Medicine, 11,* 521–528.

Cooper, R., Morré, D. J., & Morré, D. M. (2005b). Medicinal benefits of green tea. Part II: Review of anticancer properties. *Journal of Alternative & Complementary Medicine, 11,* 639–652.

Cronin, J. R. (2000). Green tea extract stokes thermogenesis: Will it replace ephedra? *Alternative & Complementary Therapies, 6,* 296–300.

Dreher, H. M. (2003). Measuring health status in HIV disease: Challenges from a sleep study. *Holistic Nursing Practitioner, 17,* 81–90.

Duke, J. (1992). *Handbook of phytochemical constituents of GRAS herbs.* Boca Raton, FL: CRC Press.

Dulloo, A. G. (1993). Epinephrine, xanthines and prostaglandin-inhibitors: Actions and interaction in the stimulation of thermogenesis. *International Journal of Obesity Related to Metabolism Disorders, 17,* S35–S40.

Dulloo, A. G. (1998). Spicing fat for combustion. *British Journal of Nutrition, 80,* 493–494.

Dulloo, A. G., Duret, C., Rohrer, D., Girardier, L., Mensi, N., Fathi, M., et al. (1999). Efficacy of a green tea extract rich in catechin polyphenols and caffeine in increasing 24-h energy expenditure and fat oxidation in humans. *American Journal of Clininical Nutrition, 70,* 1040–1045.

Dulloo, A. G., Fathi, M., Mensi, N., & Girardier, L. (1996). Twenty-four hour energy expenditure and urinary catecholamines of humans consuming low to moderate amounts of medium-chain-triglycerides: A dose–response study in a respiratory chamber. *European Journal of Clinical Nutrition, 50,* 152–158.

Dulloo, A. G., Seydoux, J., Girardier, L, Chantre, P., & Vandermander, J. (2000). Green tea and thermogenesis: Interactions between catechins–polyphenols, caffeine and sympathetic activity. *International Journal of Obesity Related to Metabolism Disorders, 24,* 252–258.

Durand, J., Giacobino, J. P., & Girardier, L. (1978). Catechol-O-methyl-transferase activity in whole brown adipose tissue of rats *in vitro. Experientia Suppl., 32,* 45–53.

Eskenazi, B. (1999). Caffeine—Filtering the facts. *New England Journal of Medicine, 341,* 1688–1689.

FDA. Center for Food Safety and Applied Nutrition, Office of Premarket Approval. (2004). EAFUS: A food additive database. Available at: vm.cfsan.fda.gov/~dms/eafus.html.

Fernandes, O., Sabharwal, M., Smiley, T., Pastuszak, A., Koren, G., & Einarson, T. (1998). Moderate to heavy caffeine consumption during pregnancy and relationship to spontaneous abortion and abnormal fetal growth: A meta-analysis. *Reproductive Toxicology, 12,* 435–444.

Fujita Y., Yamane Y., Tanaka T., Kuwata K., Okuzumi J., Takahashi T., et al. (1989). Inhibitory effect of (–)-epigallocatechin gallate on carcinogenesis with N-ethyl-N'-nitro-N-nitrosoguanidine in mouse duodenum. *Japan Journal of Cancer Research, 80,* 503–505.

Gao, C. M., Takezaki, T., Wu, J. Z., Li, Z. Y., Liu, Y. T., Li, S. P., et al. (2002). Glutathione-S-transferases M1 (GSTM1) and GSTT1 genotype, smoking, consumption of alcohol and tea and risk of esophageal and stomach cancers: A case-control study of a high-incidence area in Jiangsu Province, China. *Cancer Letters, 188,* 95–102.

Heishman, S. J., & Henningfield, J. E. (1994). Is caffeine a drug of dependence? Criteria and comparisons. *Pharmacopsychoecologia, 7,* 127–136.

Henning, S. M., Fajardo–Lira, C., Lee, H. W., Youssefian, A. A., Go, V. L., & Heber, D. (2003). Catechin content of 18 teas and a green tea extract supplement correlates with the antioxidant capacity. *Nutrition & Cancer, 45,* 226–235.

Higdon, J. V., & Frei, B. (2003). Tea catechins and polyphenols: Health effects, metabolism, and antioxidant functions. *Critical Reviews in Food Science & Nutrition, 43,* 89–143.

Jian, L., Xie, L. P., Lee, A. H., & Binns, C. W. (2004). Protective effect of green tea against prostate cancer: A case-controlled study in southeast China. *International Journal of Cancer, 108*, 130–135.

Jubel, C., Armand, M., Pafumi, Y., Rosier, C., Vandermander, J., & Lairon, D. (2000). Green tea extract (AR25) inhibits lipoysis of triglycerides in gastric and duodenal medium *in vitro. Journal of Nutritional Biochemistry, 11*, 45–51.

Kamimori, G. H., Penetar, D. M, Headley, D. B, Thorne, D. R., Otterstetter, R., & Belenky, G. (2000). Effect of three caffeine doses on plasma catecholamines and alertness during prolonged wakefulness. *European Journal of Clinical Pharmacology, 56*, 537–544.

Kao, Y. H., Hiipakka, R. A., & Liao, S. (2000). Modulation of endocrine systems and food intake by green tea epigallocatechin gallate. *Endocrinology, 141*, 980–987.

Katiyar, S. K., & Mukhtar, H. (1996). Tea in chemoprevention of cancer: Epidemiologic and experimental studies (review). *International Journal of Oncology, 8*, 221–238.

Kemberling, J. L., Hampton, J. A., Keck, R. W., Gomez, M. A., & Selman, S. H. (2003). Inhibition of bladder tumor growth by the green tea derivative epigallocatechin-3-gallate. *Journal of Urology, 170*, 773–776.

Klebanoff, M. A., Levine, R. J, DerSimonian, R., Clemens, J. D., & Wilkins, D. G. (1999). Maternal serum paraxanthine, a caffeine metabolite, and the risk of spontaneous abortion. *New England Journal of Medicine, 341*, 1639–1644.

Leung, L. K., Su, Y., Chen, R., Zhang, Z., Huang, Y., & Chen, Z. -Y. (2001). Theaflavins in black tea and catechins in green tea are equally effective antioxidants. *Journal of Nutrition, 131,* 2248–2251.

Lin, Y. S., Tsai, Y. J., Tsay, J. S., & Lin, J.K. (2003). Factors affecting the levels of tea polyphenols and caffeine in tea leaves. *Journal of Agriculture & Food Chemistry, 51*, 1864–1873.

Lloyd, T., Johnson–Rollings, N., Eggli, D. F., Kieselhorst, K., Mauger, E. A., & Cusatis, D. C. (2000). Bone status among postmenopausal women with different habitual caffeine intakes: a longitudinal investigation. *Journal of American College of Nutrition, 19*, 256–261.

Manning, J., & Roberts, J. C. (2003). Analysis of catechin content of commercial green tea products. *Journal of Herbal Pharmacotherapy, 3*, 19–32.

Martinet, A., Hostettmann, K., & Schultz, Y. (2000). Thermogenic effects of commercially available plant preparations aimed at treating human obesity. *Phytomedicine, 6*, 231–238.

Massey, L. K. (2001). Is caffeine a risk factor for bone loss in the elderly? *American Journal of Clinical Nutrition, 2001, 74*, 569–570.

Massey, L. K., & Whiting, S. J. (1993). Caffeine, urinary calcium, calcium metabolism and bone. *Journal of Nutrition, 123*, 1611–1614.

McKenna, D. J, Jones K., & Hughes, K. (2002). *Botanical medicines: The desk reference for major herbal supplements* (pp. 597–639). New York: The Haworth Herbal Press.

McKevoy, G. K., Ed. (1998). *AHFS drug information,* Bethesda, MD: American Society of Health-System Pharmacists.

Murase, T., Haramizu, S., Shimotoyodome, A., Nagasawa, A., & Tokimitsu, I. (2004). Green tea extract improves endurance capacity and increases muscle lipid oxidation in mice. *American Journal of Physiology, Regulatory, Integrative and Comparative Physiology, 288*, R708–R715.

Muroyama, K., Murosaki, S., Yamamoto, Y., Ishijima, A., & Toh, Y. (2003). Effects of intake of a mixture of thiamin, arginine, caffeine, and citric acid on adiposity in healthy subjects with high percent body fat. *Bioscience Biotechnology Biochemistry, 67*, 2325–2333.

Muroyama, K., Murosaki, S., Yamamoto, Y., Odaka, H., Chung, H. C., & Miyoshi, M. (2003). Anti-obesity effects of a mixture of thiamin, arginine, caffeine, and citric acid in non-insulin dependent diabetic KK mice. *Journal Nutrition Science Vitaminology, 49,* 56–63.

Rapuri, P. B., Gallagher, J. C., Kinyamu, H. K., & Ryschon, K. L. (2001). Caffeine intake increases the rate of bone loss in elderly women and interacts with vitamin D receptor genotypes. *American Journal of Clinical Nutrition, 74,* 694–700.

Rees, K., Allen, D., & Lader, M. (1999). The influences of age and caffeine on psychomotor and cognitive function. *Psychopharmacology* (Berl), *145,* 181–188.

Wolters Kluwer Co. (2003). Review of natural products by facts and comparisons.

Sayama, K., Lin, S., Zheng, G., & Oguni, I. (2000). Effects of green tea on growth, food utilization and lipid metabolism in mice. *In Vivo, 14,* 481–4.

Schulz, V., Hansel, R., & Tyler, V. E. (1998). *Rational phytotherapy: A physician's guide to herbal medicine.* New York: Springer.

Stella, A. (1992). *The book of tea.* Italy: Mondadori Publishing.

Wang, L. F., Kim, D. M., & Lee, C. Y. (2000). Effects of heat processing and storage on flavanols and sensory qualities of green tea beverages. *Journal of Agricultural Food Chemistry, 48,* 4227–4232.

Wu, A. H., Yu, M. C., Tseng, C. C., Hankin, J., & Pike M. C. (2003). Green tea and risk of breast cancer in Asian Americans. *International Journal of Cancer, 106,* 574–579.

Yang, C. S., Maliaka, P., & Meng, X. (2002). Inhibition of carcinogenesis by tea. *Annual Reviews of Pharmacology Toxicology, 42,* 25–54.

Yang, C. S., & Wang, Z. Y. (1993). Tea and cancer. *Journal of the National Cancer Institute, 85,* 1038–1049.

Yao, G. K., & Chen, P. F. (1995). *Tea drinking and health* (pp. 6–7). Shanghai: Shanghai Culture Publishers.

Yoshizawa, S., Horiuchi, T., Fujiki, H., Yoshida, T., Okuda, T., & Sugimura, T. (1987). Antitumor promoting activity of (–)-epigallocatechin gallate, the main constituent of "tannin" in green tea. *Phytotherapy Research, 1,* 44–47.

Yu, H., Zhu, Z., & Yin, W. (2003). Tegreen improves glucose and lipid metabolism in obese rats that have features similar to metabolic syndrome X. *FASEB Journal, 17,* A318.

Section VI

Integration and Conclusion

15 Caffeine, Physiology, Pathology, and Behavior

Barry D. Smith, Uma Gupta, and B. S. Gupta

CONTENTS

Arousal theory has long held that neural arousal and its downstream consequences are basic to behavior and health. Mediated, at least in part, by complex interactions among the brainstem reticular formation, limbic system, hypothalamus, and cortex, arousal impacts heart rate, blood pressure, muscle tension, and other psychophysiological parameters that reflect autonomic and somatic innervation.

Acute and chronic optimal arousal level is seen as falling near the middle of a theoretical arousal continuum. When arousal is extremely high or extremely low on a chronic basis, physical health problems and abnormal patterns of behavior may result. Anxiety disorders, for example, are marked by abnormally high levels of neurally mediated arousal, and very low arousal is often seen in depressive disorders. The chapters in this volume addressing the effects of caffeine on health and behavior provide considerable information relevant to arousal theory.

The widespread consumption of caffeine, its arousal-inducing properties, and its potential as a factor in physical and psychological health have virtually mandated the scientific study of the drug. Research in psychopharmacology, psychology, psychiatry, biochemistry, neuroscience, and related fields has for decades been directed toward the achievement of a better understanding of the processing and effects of caffeine. Researchers have accordingly studied the pharmacokinetics and pharmacodynamics of the drug and addressed its impact on health and behavior. The consistent aim of the plethora of investigations has been to develop and refine a series of improving causal models to explain the impact of caffeine, arousal, and their consequences.

Basic to these causal models is an understanding of the physiological mechanisms that underlie the effects of the drug, and Astrid Nehlig has provided a detailed review of the relevant human and animal studies. As she points out, the primary brain mechanisms for caffeine differ substantially from those of other stimulants such as cocaine and amphetamine. Unlike these latter drugs, which act primarily in the dopamine system, low doses of caffeine act principally to inhibit adenosine A2a receptors. Higher doses also act on other adenosine receptors and on the dopamine system, but in a different way than is the case for cocaine and amphetamine. Caffeine activates brain circuitry dealing with locomotor activity, sleep, and mood state, but not addiction and reward. Thus, the overall neurophysiological impact of caffeine is primarily on arousal.

The largest and most controversial literature on coffee and caffeine is that concerned with the effects of its consumption on the cardiovascular system. Despite decades of study and numerous investigations, firm and final conclusions remain elusive. However, the four chapters in this volume thoroughly review the relevant literature and attempt to understand, if not entirely resolve, the complex findings. In all cases, the reviewers note that not all investigations covered by their chapters are consistent, thus necessitating development of integrative conclusions that attempt to take discrepancies into account.

James reasons that because caffeine elevates blood pressure and blood pressure is a major factor in CHD, chronic caffeine consumption contributes to the disorder. Wei and Schwertner conclude that there is a likely relationship between coffee consumption and LDL cholesterol elevation due primarily to the diterpenes in coffee rather than the caffeine. Smith and colleagues, in two chapters dealing with the acute and chronic cardiovascular effects of coffee and caffeine, conclude that the overall relationship between consumption and CHD is J-shaped or U-shaped, such that low consumption may reduce and high consumption increase the probability of developing heart disease.

At least three refinements of these overall conclusions are possible. First, it is clear that substances other than caffeine found in coffee and tea can also have potential cardiovascular effects. There is certainly evidence that the diterpenes in coffee—cafestol and kahweol—are likely responsible for LDL cholesterol elevations, and coffee contains other substances that may likewise affect health. Similarly, the antioxidant effects of catechins in tea may have a CHD protective effect (Cheng, 2005; Hernandez, Rodriguez–Rodriguez, & Sanchez–Muniz, 2004). Second, coffee preparation method appears to be important. In particular, coffee prepared using boiling methods is more strongly associated with cholesterol elevation and CHD than is coffee prepared with filtering methods. Finally, genetic factors may play a larger role in the tendency to consume caffeine and the cardiovascular consequences of its consumption than has thus far been realized (Carrillo & Benitez, 1994; Luciano, Kirk, Heath, & Martin, 2005). Overall, however, it is clear that considerably more research is needed before we will have a full understanding of the contributions of coffee and caffeine to cardiovascular disease.

Issues related to the menstrual cycle, including menstrual physiology, related disorders, and fertility, have long been studied. Among studies found in this literature are numerous investigations devoted to understanding the impact of interactions between caffeine and the variable physiology of the cycle. It is clear from our two chapters on these topics that caffeine very likely does affect aspects of menstrual function and that its metabolism is differentially affected by phases of the cycle.

As Vo and her colleagues point out, caffeine appears to increase levels of reproductive hormones during the follicular phase. In addition, the drug increases the duration of menses and shortens the menstrual cycle. At the same time, the physiology of the luteal phase delays caffeine elimination. As to fertility, Northstone and Golding review all major studies carried out to date and conclude that any association between caffeine and fertility impairment is weak and inconsistent. Finally, Vo concludes that caffeine consumption is unrelated or weakly related to premenstrual syndrome, though more research on this topic is clearly needed.

Four additional chapters address the impact of caffeine on behavior and related psychological functioning. In particular, the authors review relevant literature concerned with mood, performance, and psychopathology. Smit and Rogers point to several caffeine effects related to mood. In particular, the drug increases energetic arousal in a dose–response fashion, and low doses work to improve hedonic tone and reduce anxiety; high doses increase tense arousal. Stafford, Rusted, and Yeomans note that caffeine increases alertness, especially when the subject is fatigued, and improves psychomotor performance, particularly when sustained attention is required; there is no consistent effect on memory. They also note that performance effects vary with dose, task characteristics, baseline arousal, and fatigue.

In their studies of letter transformation performance, Gupta and Gupta found that a low dose of caffeine facilitates performance, while a high dose inhibits it. Most adversely affected are storage, rehearsal, and updating operations. They conclude that the fundamental effect of arousal agents is to change the individual's state and alter the tendency to action within a task. This may suggest that caffeine modifies a central selection process that governs cognitive operations.

Finally in this section, Iancu addresses the role of caffeine in psychopathology. He concludes that excessive consumption of the drug can cause or contribute to anxiety, depression, delirium, mania, and even psychosis. Physical consequences of chronically high doses include headaches, sleep disturbance, tremulousness, diarrhea, and tachycardia—all symptoms of caffeinism. Short of this formal diagnosis, caffeine may exacerbate the symptoms of anxiety disorders that arise primarily from other causes. Iancu suggests that, in many cases, it may be possible to treat the patient's symptoms by reducing or eliminating caffeine consumption, rather than prescribing psychiatric drugs to treat the disorder.

Our final chapter, by Cooper, Morré, Likimani, and Morré, addresses the effects of green and black teas on health. They point to the important potential for the catechins in tea to have beneficial effects in weight control and reduction and note that the interaction of catechins with caffeine may induce thermogenesis. In addition, there is evidence for chemoprotective effects of catechins in some forms of cancer, though they may also stimulate carcinogenesis in other cases. It is important to note that relatively few studies of the catechins have been conducted thus far, so the evidence is preliminary (Graf, Milbury, & Blumberg, 2005). Moreover, some have concluded that thus far no definitive support for the cancer chemoprevention hypothesis exists (Scalbert, Manash, Morand, Remesy, & Jimenez, 2005; Arts & Hollman, 2005). Thus, again, much additional research is needed.

Two themes that run through virtually every chapter are that more research is needed and that we must improve our research designs to include as many relevant control variables as possible. Thus far, the nature and extent of the variables examined and the control conditions imposed and assessed have varied substantially from one laboratory and one investigation to another. This fact alone makes it difficult to compare results across studies and limits the generalizability of the findings in any given study.

It should be possible to correct the problems seen in many previous studies without great difficulty. More laboratory studies involving randomized designs are clearly needed. In these investigations, double-blind procedures should be followed whenever possible, and measurement of the caffeine doses administered needs to be precise. In addition, it is important to consider that some investigators administer absolute doses of caffeine, whereas others weight-titrate the dose in milligrams per kilogram.

It would obviously be best if one of these methods were chosen for all studies. Because that is unlikely, it is important that researchers using weight titration report the mean number of milligrams actually consumed in each dosing condition and preferably the mean weight of participants in each as well. The use of multiple doses (and placebo) in each study is also desirable because this permits an assessment of the dose–response relationship as it applies to the particular area of investigation.

Laboratory investigators should also assess and take into account the conditions under which their participants are tested. Are the subjects fully alert or fatigued? What time of day are they tested? Is this uniform across groups or conditions? How aroused is each participant before caffeine or placebo is administered? Assessment of baseline arousal can provide a more accurate assessment of drug effects by examining not only the absolute effect of the drug, but also the change from baseline.

An even more important issue is the effect of caffeine deprivation. As several chapter authors note, most laboratory studies involve depriving participants of caffeine for a period of time prior to their entering the experiment. In some studies, subjects are asked to abstain from caffeine for anywhere from a few hours to overnight before reporting to the laboratory. This procedure, while arguably necessary in many studies, greatly complicates interpretation of data. When subjects are deprived, they are subject to withdrawal effects, which are then reversed by the caffeine dose given in the laboratory.

Under these conditions, we must ask whether the observed effects on results are due to a direct effect of caffeine or whether the reversal of withdrawal is responsible for outcomes. In other words, is there a net beneficial or detrimental effect of caffeine over and above that of withdrawal reversal? One possible (though only partial) solution to this problem is to apply the experimental and control conditions of the study to groups of participants who do not regularly consume caffeine. Obviously, because the drug is found in so many consumables, we are unlikely to find subjects who perfectly fit this ideal. However, we can select those who say they do not drink coffee, tea, or other caffeinated beverages and do not consume chocolate or medications containing caffeine. By comparing results of users and nonusers, we can at least partially avert the deprivation-reversal interpretation problem.

In nonlaboratory investigations such as prospective and retrospective studies, it is important to assess a number of variables often not taken into account. For one thing, studies focusing on coffee or tea consumption and calculating overall caffeine intake on that basis are obviously ignoring all other sources of the drug, including such major ones as caffeinated soft drinks and energy drinks. Not only does this omission greatly underestimate total caffeine consumption, but it also makes estimates inconsistent. For example, one participant may consume 500 mg of caffeine in coffee per day, while another may drink the same amount of coffee, but also consume 300 mg in soft drinks and chocolate. If the study assesses only coffee intake, both subjects would be listed as consuming a total of 500 mg. In another case, a participant who reports no coffee consumption at all will be listed as 0 mg, even though he or she may be consuming several hundred milligrams in tea and soft drinks. The effect of not assessing other sources of caffeine is thus to introduce considerable extraneous variance.

Under such circumstances, how can we then arrive at a reasonable estimate of the contribution of caffeine to heart disease, menstrual function, mood, performance, psychopathology, or any other variable that might be a focus of the study? The bottom line is that we should ideally attempt to determine each participant's overall level of caffeine consumption, not his or her consumption based on only one source. Beyond the need to assess all major sources of caffeine in each study is the fact that very few studies have been conducted on the effects of the drug when it appears in soft drinks, chocolate, energy drinks, or medications, and relatively few of tea. All these sources of caffeine need to be subjected to considerable additional investigation, in part because each source of the drug contains other substances that may also be important, just as the diterpenes in coffee may independently contribute to heart disease.

Nonlaboratory studies should ideally also assess some or all of several variables, depending on the focus of the study. Of particular importance here is the method by which each participant typically prepares coffee. Does the method used basically involve boiling or filtering? Other variables included here would be the type of coffee—caffeinated or decaffeinated—use of milk products, sugar or other sweeteners in coffee or tea, smoking status, alcohol consumption, and relevant dietary factors.

Another issue is that when coffee consumption is studied, one factor almost never addressed is the type of coffee and its corresponding caffeine content. Tanzania Peaberry, for example, is 1.42% caffeine, whereas Mocha Matari is only 1.01%. Thus, a cup of one coffee may contain markedly more caffeine than does the same size cup of another. Finally, because the (assumed) standard cup size varies from one study to another, some investigators do calculations based on 5-oz cups and others on 6- or 7-oz cups. This should ideally be standardized across studies or, at the very least, carefully taken into account in comparing studies.

Although we still have considerable distance to cover in the quest to understand the effects of caffeine and coffee on health and behavior, the chapters in this book make it clear that great progress has already been made. They also address the broader issues raised by arousal theory and contribute to our understanding of the origins and impact of arousal on physical and psychological health, as well as behavior. If future studies act on some of the methodological recommendations here, we may make more rapid progress toward the goal of fully understanding the effects of the most widely consumed drug in the world.

REFERENCES

Arts, I. C., & Hollman, P. C. (2005). Polyphenols and disease risk in epidemiologic studies. *American Journal of Clinical Nutrition, 81*, 317S–325S.

Carrillo, J. A., & Benitez, J. (1994). Caffeine metabolism in a healthy Spanish population: N-acetylator phenotype and oxidation pathways. *Clinical Pharmacology Therapy, 55*, 293–304.

Cheng, T. O. (2005). Will green tea be even better than black tea to increase coronary flow velocity reserve? *American Journal of Cardiology, 94*, 1223.

Graf, B. A., Milbury, P. E., & Blumberg, J. B. (2005). Flavonols, favones, flavanones, and human health: Epidemiological evidence. *Journal of Medicine & Food, 8*, 281–290.

Hernandez, T. T., Rodriguez–Rodriguez, E., & Sanchez–Muniz, F. J. (2004). The green tea, a good choice for cardiovascular disease prevention? *Archives of Latinoamerican Nutrition, 54*, 380–394.

Luciano, M., Kirk, K. M., Health A. C., & Martin, N. G. (2005). The genetics of tea and coffee drinking and references for source of caffeine in a large community sample of Australian twins. *Addiction, 1000*, 1510–1517.

Scalbert, A., Manach, C., Morand, C., Remesy, C. & Jimenez, L. (2005). Dietary polyphenols and the prevention of diseases. *Critical Reviews Food Science Nutrition, 45*, 287–306.

Index

For Product Safety Concerns and Information please contact our EU
representative GPSR@taylorandfrancis.com Taylor & Francis Verlag GmbH,
Kaufingerstraße 24, 80331 München, Germany

Printed and bound by CPI Group (UK) Ltd, Croydon, CR0 4YY
01/05/2025
01858534-0001